Sepsis Management

Jordi Rello • Jeffrey Lipman • Thiago Lisboa

Editors

Sepsis Management

PIRO and MODS

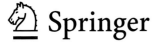 Springer

Editors
Dr. Jordi Rello
Critical Care Department
Vall d'Hebron University Hospital
Ps. Vall d'Hebron 119-129
Anexe AG-5a planta
08035 Barcelona
Spain

Prof. Jeffrey Lipman
Critical Care and Anaesthesiology
The University of Queensland, Brisbane
Queensland
Australia

Department of Intensive Care Medicine
Royal Brisbane and Women's Hospital
Herston Road
4029 Herston, Brisbane
Queensland
Australia

Thiago Lisboa, MD
Critical Care Department and Infection
Control Committee
Hospital de Clinicas de Porto Alegre
Porto Alegre
Brazil

Intensive Care Unit, Hospital Santa Rita
Rede Institucional
de Pesquisa e Inovação em Medicina
Intensiva (RIPIMI)
Complexo Hospitalar Santa Casa
Porto Alegre
Brazil

ISBN 978-3-642-03518-0   e-ISBN 978-3-642-03519-7
DOI 10.1007/978-3-642-03519-7
Springer Heidelberg Dordrecht London New York

Library of Congress Control Number: 2011937715

Springer is part of Springer Science+Business Media (www.springer.com)

Contents

Multiorgan Dysfunction Syndrome (MODS): What is New?

1

Jean-Louis Vincent, Marjorie Beumier, Antoine Herpain, and Katia Donadello

1.1   Introduction

Multiorgan dysfunction syndrome (MODS) was defined by the ACCP/SCCM conference almost 20 years ago as the situation in an acutely ill patient whereby organ function is disrupted such that it is unable to maintain homeostasis (Bone et al. 1992). Importantly, MODS is a dynamic process, changing over time according to various host-related factors and as the patient responds (or not) to therapeutic interventions. In this chapter, we will discuss some of the current concepts surrounding MODS, and highlight recent advances in our understanding of the pathophysiology and treatment for this condition.

1.2   Current Concepts

1.2.1   Intensive Care Unit (ICU) Patients Seldom Die from a Single Acute Organ Failure

Particularly with today's advanced organ support systems, ICU patients rarely die from a single organ failure. With rare exceptions, e.g., extended cerebral hemorrhage, large cerebral tumor with herniation, or acute liver injury, most ICU non-survivors will develop and die with dysfunction of multiple organs. There are

J.-L. Vincent (✉)
Department of Intensive Care, Erasme Hospital,
Université Libre de Bruxelles, Brussels, Belgium
e-mail: jlvincen@ulb.ac.be

M. Beumier • A. Herpain • K. Donadello
Department of Intensive Care, Erasme Hospital,
Université Libre de Bruxelles, Brussels, Belgium

J. Rello (eds.), *Sepsis Management*,
DOI 10.1007/978-3-642-03519-7_1, © Springer-Verlag Berlin Heidelberg 2012

relatively few data documenting causes of death in ICU patients, but in a study of 3,700 critically ill patients over a 7-year period, Mayr et al. reported that the cause of death in the ICU was acute, refractory multiple organ failure in 47% of cases, and chronic refractory multiple organ failure accounted for another 12% of deaths (Mayr et al. 2006). In a study of non-cardiac surgical ICU patients in 21 Brazilian ICUs, Lobo et al. reported that multiple organ failure was the leading cause of death, occurring in 53% of patients (Lobo et al. 2011).

1.2.2   Organ Failure Is Often a Marker of the Severity of Illness

Although individual organ failures rarely lead to death, they are associated with increased mortality. For example, acute renal failure is associated with mortality rates of 30–50%, and these have not really decreased over time (Ympa et al. 2005). Likewise, acute respiratory failure is associated with mortality rates of about 30–40%, although the death rate from acute respiratory distress syndrome has probably decreased over the years (Zambon and Vincent 2008), and mortality rates as low as 20% have recently been reported in patients with acute lung injury (ALI) (Rice 2009).

1.2.3   MOF Is a Package

Ultimately, the death rate of patients with any given organ failure is between 20% and 40%. Not surprisingly, patients with multiple organ failures have higher mortality rates than those with single organ failure. In a study of patients admitted to 1 of 35 French ICUs between 1997 and 2004, 69% of patients with severe sepsis had more than one organ dysfunction at some point during their ICU stay (Guidet et al. 2005). These patients had hospital mortality rates of 49%, compared to 11.3% for patients with just one organ dysfunction. Moreover, there is a relationship between the number of failing organs and death. In the Sepsis Occurrence in Acutely Ill Patients (SOAP) study, which studied 3,147 patients in 198 ICUs across Europe, ICU mortality rates increased with increasing numbers of failing organs from 6% in patients with no organ dysfunction on admission to 65% in those with four or more organ failures (Vincent et al. 2006) (Fig. 1.1). In emergency department patients with suspected sepsis, each additional organ dysfunction increased the adjusted 1-year mortality hazard by 82% (Shapiro et al. 2006). Hence, just counting the number of organs failing provides a fair estimate of the chances of survival.

   Patterns of organ failure differ among ICU patients, but there are no clear associations of specific patterns with mortality. For example, there do not seem to be any prognostic differences between respiratory followed by renal failure compared to a reverse pattern where renal failure is followed by respiratory failure. There are several reasons for this, including the fact that the functions of many organ systems are intertwined. Identification of organ failure is also easier for certain organs than for others. For example, respiratory failure is often identified early, but this is probably

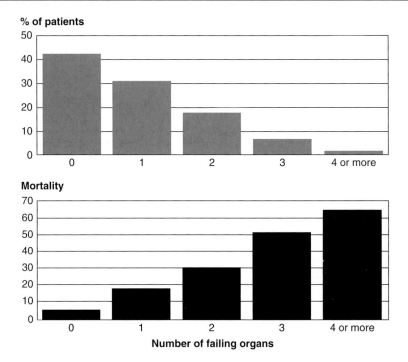

Fig. 1.1 Frequency of organ failure on admission and corresponding ICU mortality in patients enrolled in the SOAP study. Patients with no organ dysfunction on admission had ICU mortality rates of 6%, while those with four or more organ failures had mortality rates of 65% (From Vincent et al. (2006) with permission)

because it is rapidly manifest by hypoxemia and easily recognized by an infiltrate on chest X ray; in contrast, liver dysfunction may occur relatively early, but we have no good diagnostic test as the commonly used bilirubin levels increase relatively late in patients with liver failure.

1.3   Pathophysiology of MODS

The pathophysiology of MODS is not fully understood, and various mechanisms have been proposed, including microcirculatory dysfunction, mitochondrial dysfunction, metabolic alterations, hormonal alterations, and immune dysregulation (Abraham and Singer 2007). As MODS is a whole body disease, microcirculatory dysfunction resulting in tissue hypoperfusion and hypoxia is likely a key global mechanism. Persistent microcirculatory alterations have been fairly widely reported to be associated with multiple organ dysfunction and with increased mortality in patients with septic shock (Sakr et al. 2004). The inflammatory response may also play a role, with cytokines and other mediators having direct toxic effects, but also being associated with increased oxygen demand, altered oxygen extraction, and impaired cardiac function, this indirectly affecting tissue oxygenation (Abraham and Singer 2007). Markers of the inflammatory response have been associated with organ dysfunction and death. In 313 consecutive ICU patients, high C-reactive protein (CRP) levels on admission were associated with more severe organ dysfunction than normal CRP levels (Lobo et al. 2003). Moreover, CRP levels correlated with the number of failing organs. Levels of another widely studied marker of sepsis, procalcitonin, were reported to be correlated with severity of sepsis (Ugarte et al. 1999) and of organ dysfunction as assessed by the sequential organ failure assessment (SOFA) score (Endo et al. 2008). Blood lactate levels, a surrogate marker of inadequate tissue oxygenation, have also been shown to be correlated with SOFA scores in ICU patients, particularly in the early part of the ICU stay (Jansen et al. 2009). Increasingly, the role of cross-talk within and between injured organs and cells is being appreciated as vital in the development and propagation of multiple organ failure (Clark and Coopersmith 2007; Li et al. 2009).

1.4   Prevention and Treatment of MODS

With the lack of specific therapeutic interventions for MODS, prevention or limitation of organ dysfunction is the principal factor in the management of patients with or at risk of MODS.

Adequate resuscitative measures must be instituted early in patients with shock, as highlighted in the study on early goal-directed therapy by Rivers et al. (Rivers et al. 2001). The implications of different aspects of the Rivers protocol are still debated, e.g., use of central venous oxygenation ($ScvO_2$), and several studies are evaluating these facets prospectively at a multicenter level. Nevertheless, the emphasis on early intervention remains valid. Hence, fluids, including blood products when indicated, should be administered in sufficient quantities as soon as possible. Dobutamine may be needed to increase cardiac output and may also improve the microcirculation (De Backer et al. 2006a). The endpoints of resuscitation are important, but, as there are no specific markers of MODS that can be targeted, they are difficult to define. Clearly, a blood pressure level alone is not adequate. Patients may be normotensive but still have marked microcirculatory disturbances (Sakr et al. 2004). The Surviving Sepsis Campaign guidelines recommend that the mean arterial pressure (MAP) be maintained at 65 mmHg (Dellinger et al. 2008), but this must be adapted to the individual patient as some patients may need a higher MAP. Clinical surrogates for adequate tissue oxygenation may be used as endpoints and include hemodynamic stability without vasopressors, adequate urine output, adequate skin perfusion, and unaltered mental status. In the early stages of severe sepsis, resuscitation can be guided by maintaining a $ScvO_2 > 70\%$ (Rivers et al. 2001). All these measures should be combined and complemented by lactate levels – normal around 1 mEq/L, shock >2 mEq/L – which, although not ideal, are still the best marker we have of altered tissue perfusion, particularly when repeated measurements are used.

In terms of specific treatments, these are very limited. Anti-inflammatory therapies have not been shown to be effective, except for activated protein C (Bernard et al.

2001), and even these results have been queried. However, other options continue to be developed, and several are undergoing clinical trials, including toll-like receptor (TLR)-4 and thrombomodulin. Extracorporeal removal of mediators may also help, although further study is needed to optimize this approach (Vincent 2009).

Resuscitation of the microcirculation is a relatively new treatment option and still considered experimental as there are no data that demonstrate improved outcomes with therapies directed at improving microcirculatory parameters. Various established therapies, e.g., fluids (Ospina-Tascon et al. 2010), blood transfusions (Sakr et al. 2007), dobutamine (De Backer et al. 2006a), and activated protein C (De Backer et al. 2006b), have been shown to improve the microcirculation, and the next step is to demonstrate that this can be associated with reduced organ failure and improved survival.

1.5 Conclusion

Much has been learned about the condition of MODS since it was first described in association with sepsis in the 1970s, but much remains unclear. Important aspects of the pathophysiology and pathogenesis have been revealed, but precise mechanisms need further study. The importance of early and adequate resuscitation has been clearly established, but specific therapies remain elusive. Current focus on targeting the microcirculation and development of techniques to aid cellular repair may help limit the development of multiorgan failure and improve outcomes in the future.

References

Abraham E, Singer M (2007) Mechanisms of sepsis-induced organ dysfunction. Crit Care Med 35:2408–2416

Bernard GR, Vincent JL, Laterre PF, LaRosa SP, Dhainaut JF, Lopez-Rodriguez A, Steingrub JS, Garber GE, Helterbrand JD, Ely EW, Fisher CJ Jr (2001) Efficacy and safety of recombinant human activated protein C for severe sepsis. N Engl J Med 344:699–709

Bone RC, Balk RA, Cerra FB, Dellinger RP, Fein AM, Knaus WA, Schein RM, Sibbald WJ (1992) Definitions for sepsis and organ failure and guidelines for the use of innovative therapies in sepsis. The ACCP/SCCM Consensus Conference Committee. American College of Chest Physicians/Society of Critical Care Medicine. Chest 101:1644–1655

Clark JA, Coopersmith CM (2007) Intestinal crosstalk: a new paradigm for understanding the gut as the "motor" of critical illness. Shock 28:384–393

De Backer D, Creteur J, Dubois MJ, Sakr Y, Koch M, Verdant C, Vincent JL (2006a) The effects of dobutamine on microcirculatory alterations in patients with septic shock are independent of its systemic effects. Crit Care Med 34:403–408

De Backer D, Verdant C, Chierego M, Koch M, Gullo A, Vincent JL (2006b) Effects of drotrecogin alfa activated on microcirculatory alterations in patients with severe sepsis. Crit Care Med 34:1918–1924

Dellinger RP, Levy MM, Carlet JM, Bion J, Parker MM, Jaeschke R, Reinhart K, Angus DC, Brun-Buisson C, Beale R, Calandra T, Dhainaut JF, Gerlach H, Harvey M, Marini JJ, Marshall J, Ranieri M, Ramsay G, Sevransky J, Thompson BT, Townsend S, Vender JS, Zimmerman JL, Vincent JL (2008) Surviving Sepsis Campaign: international guidelines for management of severe sepsis and septic shock: 2008. Crit Care Med 36:296–327

Endo S, Aikawa N, Fujishima S, Sekine I, Kogawa K, Yamamoto Y, Kushimoto S, Yukioka H, Kato N, Totsuka K, Kikuchi K, Ikeda T, Ikeda K, Yamada H, Harada K, Satomura S (2008) Usefulness of procalcitonin serum level for the discrimination of severe sepsis from sepsis: a multicenter prospective study. J Infect Chemother 14:244–249

Guidet B, Aegerter P, Gauzit R, Meshaka P, Dreyfuss D (2005) Incidence and impact of organ dysfunctions associated with sepsis. Chest 127:942–951

Jansen TC, van Bommel J, Woodward R, Mulder PG, Bakker J (2009) Association between blood lactate levels, Sequential Organ Failure Assessment subscores, and 28-day mortality during early and late intensive care unit stay: a retrospective observational study. Crit Care Med 37:2369–2374

Li X, Hassoun HT, Santora R, Rabb H (2009) Organ crosstalk: the role of the kidney. Curr Opin Crit Care 15:481–487

Lobo SM, Lobo FR, Bota DP, Lopes-Ferreira F, Soliman HM, Melot C, Vincent JL (2003) C-reactive protein levels correlate with mortality and organ failure in critically ill patients. Chest 123:2043–2049

Lobo SM, Rezende E, Knibel MF, Silva NB, Paramo JA, Nacul FE, Mendes CL, Assuncao M, Costa RC, Grion CC, Pinto SF, Mello PM, Maia MO, Duarte PA, Gutierrez F, Silva JJ, Lopes MR, Mellot C (2011) Early determinants of death due to multiple organ failure after noncardiac surgery in high-risk patients. Anesth Analg 112(4):877–883

Mayr VD, Dunser MW, Greil V, Jochberger S, Luckner G, Ulmer H, Friesenecker BE, Takala J, Hasibeder WR (2006) Causes of death and determinants of outcome in critically ill patients. Crit Care 10:R154

Ospina-Tascon G, Neves AP, Occhipinti G, Donadello K, Buchele G, Simion D, Chierego ML, Silva TO, Fonseca A, Vincent JL, De Backer D (2010) Effects of fluids on microvascular perfusion in patients with severe sepsis. Intensive Care Med 36:949–955

Rice TW (2009) Omega-3 (n-3) fatty acid, gamma-linolenic acid (GLA) and anti-oxidant supplementation in acute lung injury (OMEGA trial) (abstract). Crit Care Med 37:A408

Rivers E, Nguyen B, Havstad S, Ressler J, Muzzin A, Knoblich B, Peterson E, Tomlanovich M (2001) Early goal-directed therapy in the treatment of severe sepsis and septic shock. N Engl J Med 345:1368–1377

Sakr Y, Dubois MJ, De Backer D, Creteur J, Vincent JL (2004) Persistent microcirculatory alterations are associated with organ failure and death in patients with septic shock. Crit Care Med 32:1825–1831

Sakr Y, Chierego M, Piagnerelli M, Verdant C, Dubois MJ, Koch M, Creteur J, Gullo A, Vincent JL, De Backer D (2007) Microvascular response to red blood cell transfusion in patients with severe sepsis. Crit Care Med 35:1639–1644

Shapiro N, Howell MD, Bates DW, Angus DC, Ngo L, Talmor D (2006) The association of sepsis syndrome and organ dysfunction with mortality in emergency department patients with suspected infection. Ann Emerg Med 48:583–590, 590

Ugarte H, Silva E, Mercan D, De Mendonca A, Vincent JL (1999) Procalcitonin used as a marker of infection in the intensive care unit. Crit Care Med 27:498–504

Vincent JL (2009) Sepsis: clearing the blood in sepsis. Nat Rev Nephrol 5:559–560

Vincent JL, Sakr Y, Sprung CL, Ranieri VM, Reinhart K, Gerlach H, Moreno R, Carlet J, Le Gall JR, Payen D (2006) Sepsis in European intensive care units: results of the SOAP study. Crit Care Med 34:344–353

Ympa YP, Sakr Y, Reinhart K, Vincent JL (2005) Has mortality from acute renal failure decreased? A systematic review of the literature. Am J Med 118:827–832

Zambon M, Vincent JL (2008) Mortality rates for patients with acute lung injury/ARDS have decreased over time. Chest 133:1120–1127

MODS Scores: Which One Should I Use?

2

Rui Moreno and Andrew Rhodes

The symptoms usually set in within twenty-four hours, and rarely later than the third or fourth day. There is a chill or chilliness, with moderate fever at first, which gradually rises and is marked by daily remissions and even intermissions. The pulse is small and compressible, and may reach 120 or higher. Gastro-intestinal disturbances are common, the tongue is red at the margin, and the dorsum is dry and dark. There may be early delirium or marked mental prostration and apathy. At the disease progresses there may be pallor of the face or a yellowish tint. Capillary haemorrhages are not uncommon. Death may occur within twenty-four hours, and in fatal cases life is rarely prolonged for more than seven or eight days.

William Osler
The Principles and Practice of Medicine, 1898

2.1 Introduction

The Multiple Organ Dysfunction/Failure syndrome (MODS) nowadays represents the leading cause of death in the Intensive Care Unit (ICU) (Vincent et al. 2003, 2009; Azoulay et al. 2009; Tibby 2010; Knaus et al. 1985; Deitch 1992; Tran 1994). Described initially by Tilney et al. after severe haemorrhage and shock following abdominal aortic surgery (Tilney et al. 1973), MODS has been subsequently described in association with infection (Fry et al. 1980; Bell et al. 1983), severe acute pancreatitis (Tran and Cuesta 1992), burns (Marshall and Dimick 1983), shock (Henao et al. 1991) and trauma (Faist et al. 1983).

R. Moreno (✉)
Unidade de Cuidados Intensivos Polivalente,
Hospital de St. António dos Capuchos,
Centro Hospitalar de Lisboa Central,
E.P.E, Lisbon, Portugal
e-mail: r.moreno@mail.telepac.pt

A. Rhodes
Department of Intensive Care Medicine,
St George's Healthcare NHS Trust, London, UK

J. Rello (eds.), *Sepsis Management*,
DOI 10.1007/978-3-642-03519-7_2, © Springer-Verlag Berlin Heidelberg 2012

Since the publication in 1985 by Knaus of a practical scale to access and quantify MODS (Knaus et al. 1985), several systems have been proposed, evaluated and published. The last published systems are the Multiple Organ Dysfunction score (MODS) by John Marshall et al. (1995), the Logistic Organ Dysfunction score (LODS) by Jean-Roger Le Gall et al. (1996) and the Sequential Organ Failure Assessment (SOFA) score developed by a working group of the European Society of Intensive Care Medicine (ESICM) (Vincent et al. 1996).

In MODS, time is an extremely important dimension. The deterioration in the function of several organs and systems, which prevents them functioning in a normal fashion without medical support, takes time to develop. This time-dependence produces a practical incapacity to predict or to describe MODS in a rigorous way, using static models, performed only once at ICU admission or after 24 hours in the ICU.

As stressed by the American College of Chest Physicians/Society of Critical Care Medicine Consensus Conference, there is a need to build databases to test and validate optimal criteria for the description of MODS and in which several variables can be tested against outcome (1992). As a consequence of this appeal several attempts to develop such kinds of models have appeared in the literature (Marshall et al. 1995; Le Gall et al. 1996; Vincent et al. 1996; Bernard 1997).

All the modern systems have been developed based on common assumptions and methodologies (Vincent et al. 1996):
- Able to describe the increasing dysfunction of individual organs and to evaluate MODS as a continuum of dysfunction/failure instead of a binary outcome (present/absent);
- Developed to be used repeatedly, since MODS is not a static condition and the degree of dysfunction/failure changes with time during the course of the evolution of the pathological process;
- Based on simple and objective measures to evaluate each organ/system. They need to be available routinely in all ICUs, being specific for the evaluated organ and independent from baseline characteristics of the patients;
- All the variables chosen should ideally be independent from therapy, although this condition is very hard to meet in real life (Marshall et al. 1995).

All the existing MODS scores present some limitations that will be discussed later on. It should be mentioned that these kind of systems should be viewed as complementary to general severity scores (APACHE, SAPS, MPM) and not as an alternative to them. They have been designed to describe a patient's evolution and not to forecast their prognosis, they use a very small set of simple variables, and they can be used in the large majority of intensive care patients (Vincent et al. 1996; Bertleff and Bruining 1997).

This process of repeated, sequential estimation of the MODS is relatively new in Intensive Care Medicine, and therefore there is little unanimity or agreement about which organs should be assessed or the variables that should be used. Many of these systems have been proposed in the past (Knaus et al. 1985; Fry et al. 1980; Marshall et al. 1995; Le Gall et al. 1996; Vincent et al. 1996; Elebute and Stoner 1983; Stevens 1983; Goris et al. 1985; Chang et al. 1988; Meek et al. 1991; Baumgartner et al. 1992; Bernard et al. 1995), with small differences mainly in the type of variables

Table 2.1 Types of variables used in the MODS systems

Organ/system	Physiological variable	Therapeutic variable
Respiratory	PaO_2/FiO_2	Mechanical ventilation PEEP level
Cardiovascular	Arterial pressure	Use of vasoactive drugs
Renal	Urinary output Serum urea Serum creatinine	Use of dialysis
Haematological	Platelets Leukocytes Haematocrit	Use of blood and blood products
Neurological	Glasgow Coma Scale	Use of sedation

Adapted from Marshal et al. (1997b)
PEEP positive end-expiratory pressure

used (Table 2.1) (Bertleff and Bruining 1997; Marshall et al. 1997a). In almost all cases, all the recent systems evaluate six organs/systems: respiratory, cardiovascular, renal, haematological, neurological and hepatic.

The objective of this review is to present the main systems in use today as well as their potential applications.

2.2   Organ System Failure (OSF) Score

The OSF score, described by William Knaus et al. in 1985 (Knaus et al. 1985), is the oldest of the systems currently in use. This system describes MODS as a binary phenomenon (absence/present); it does not allow the quantification of intermediate degrees of MODS. It should ideally be evaluated daily, for the entire ICU stay. An extensive review of its use has been published by Zimmerman et al. (1996a, b). It is rarely used today, having been progressively replaced by subsequent systems.

It evaluates five organs/systems: respiratory, cardiovascular, renal, haematological and neurological (Table 2.2). Some modifications have been published, such as the one by Garden et al., where hepatic failure was added to the list (Garden et al. 1985).

2.3   Multiple Organ Dysfunction Score (MODS)

The MODS score was described in 1995 by John Marshall et al. (1995). Developed based on an extensive revision of the literature, it has been subsequently tested and validated in a sample of surgical patients. This system was also submitted to some external validations, such as the one from Jacobs et al. on a sample of patients with septic shock, demonstrating a good behaviour, both in non-operative and in post-operative patients (Jacobs et al. 1999).

It assesses six organs/systems, with a score for each variable of between 0 (normality) and 4 (failure) points: respiratory, cardiovascular, renal, haematological,

Table 2.2 Organ System Failure (OSF) score

Respiratory (1 or more of the following):
- Respiratory rate ≤5 or ≥49 cycles/min
- $PaCO_2 \geq 50$ mmHg
- $DAaO_2 \geq 350$ mmHg[a]
- Ventilatory dependence (should only be scored after the 3rd day of organ failure)

Cardiovascular (1 or more of the following):
- Pulse ≤54 beats/min
- Mean arterial pressure ≤49 mmHg
- Ventricular tachycardia, ventricular fibrillation or both
- Seum pH ≤7.24 with $PaCO_2 \leq 49$ mmHg

Renal (1 or more of the following)[b]:
- Urinary output ≤479 mL/24 h or ≤159 mL in 8 h
- Urea ≥100 mg/dL
- Creatinine ≥3.5 mg/dL

Haematological (1 or more of the following):
- Leukocytes ≤1,000/mm³
- Platelets ≤20,000/mm³
- Haematocrit ≤20%

Neurological (1 or more of the following)[c]:
- Glasgow Coma Scale ≤6 in the absence of sedation at any time during the day

Adapted from Knaus et al. (1985)

[a]$DAaO_2 = [(713 \times FiO_2) - PaCO_2/0.8] - PaO_2$

[b]Excluded patients on chronic dialysis before hospital admission

[c]If the patient is entubated, score the verbal component as follows:
 Seems able to speak: 5 points
 Questionable ability to speak: 3 points
 Does not seems able to speak: 2 points

neurological and hepatic, for a maximum of 24 points in a given day (Table 2.3). The worst values on each day for each organ system are later summated to compute the value of the MODS score for that day. The baseline and serial component scores have been described by the same authors based on data from 16 Canadian ICUs (Cook et al. 2001) where the six organ systems comprising MODS were measured at ICU admission (baseline scores) and daily thereafter. The change in organ dysfunction each day (serial scores) was calculated as daily component scores minus the corresponding baseline component scores. Using multivariable analysis (Cox regression), the authors were able to demonstrate that when each organ system was analyzed individually, both the baseline and serial MODS for the cardiovascular, respiratory, renal, central nervous system and haematologic components were significantly associated with ICU mortality, but the baseline hepatic score was not. The relative risk of mortality related to organ dysfunction varied significantly over time and between organ systems, with only four organs/systems being both associated at baseline and serially with mortality: cardiovascular (baseline relative risk [RR], 1.5; serial RR, 1.4), respiratory (baseline RR, 1.4; serial RR, 1.4), renal (baseline RR,

Table 2.3 Multiple Organ Dysfunction Score (MODS)

	0	1	2	3	4
Respiratory[a]					
PaO$_2$/FiO$_2$, mm^3	>300	226–300	151–225	76–150	≤75
Renal[b]					
Serum creatinine, µmol/L	≤100	101–200	201–350	351–500	>500
Hepatic[c]					
Serum Bilirubin, µmol/L	≤20	21–60	61–120	121–240	>240
Cardiovascular[c]					
PAR	≤10.0	10.1–15.0	15.1–20.0	20.1–30.0	>30.0
Haematological Platelets (× 1,000/mm^3)	>120	81–120	51–80	21–50	≤20
Neurological[d]					
Glasgow Coma Scale	15	13–14	10–12	7–9	≤6

Adapted from Marshall et al. (1995)
[a]Independently from mechanical ventilation, with or without PEEP
[b]Independently from dialysis being used
[c]The pressure-adjusted heart rate, PAR, is computed as:

$$PAR = \frac{Heart\ rate\ (beats/minute)}{Mean\ arterial\ pressure\ (mmHg)} \times Central\ venous\ pressure\ (mmHg)$$

[d]The Glasgow Coma Scale should be evaluated in a conservative way. If the patient is sedated it should be scored as normal unless intrinsic lesions of the central nervous system exist

1.3; serial RR, 1.5) and central nervous system (baseline RR, 1.6; serial RR, 1.7). The results of this study support very well the theoretical concept that MODS scores must be evaluated serially, at least daily, because although patterns vary by system, daily MODS component scores provide additional prognostic value over the baseline MODS.

The MODS system presents a significant difference when compared to all other modern methods: the method chosen to assess and quantify cardiovascular function. While in the other systems cardiovascular dysfunction/failure is assessed though a combination of physiological parameter and/or therapeutic variables, in the MODS score the evaluation of cardiovascular dysfunction/failure is made using a composite variable, the pressure-adjusted heart rate (PAR). This fact makes its computation more complex, requiring the measure of a central venous pressure, despite the fact that it presents a very good discriminative capability when compared with the other systems (Moreno et al. 1997).

It has been demonstrated that this system presents a better discriminative capability than the daily APACHE II or OSF (Jacobs et al. 1999). It has been used in an increasing number of studies (Gonçalves et al. 1998; Maziak et al. 1998; Pinilla et al. 1998; Staubach et al. 1998). However, Zygun et al. demonstrated that its capability to predict outcome was limited (Zygun et al. 2005). Also, when formally compared with the SOFA score, the MODS seems to evaluate cardiovascular dysfunction less well than the SOFA score (Bota et al. 2002), and presents a lower discriminative capability and lower association with outcome compared with the

SOFA score for the determination of non-neurological organ dysfunction in patients with severe traumatic brain injury (Zygun et al. 2006). In a similar study, Khwannimit in 2008 performed a serial assessment and comparison of the MODS, SOFA and LODS scores in their ability to predict ICU mortality in 2,054 patients. The aROC curves were all very high (0.892 for the MODS, 0.907 for the SOFA, and 0.920 for the LODS), but no statistical difference existed between all maximum scores and the APACHE II score (Khwannimit 2008).

2.4   Logistic Organ Dysfunction Score (LODS)

Proposed by Jean-Roger Le Gall et al. (1997), this system was developed using more sophisticated statistical techniques to choose and weight the variables in a large multicenter multinational database, comprising data from 13,152 consecutive admissions to 137 ICUs in 12 countries. However, the database utilized (the same that was used to develop the SAPS II and MPM II models) data from just the first 24 h after ICU admission, and so the LODS was developed without any data after the first ICU day.

To compute the LODS, each organ/system receives a score between 0 and 5 points, the latter being possible to assign to the most severe forms of cardiovascular, neurological and renal system dysfunction (for the respiratory and haematological systems the maximum is 3 points and for liver 1). The maximum score is 22 points. All the variables must be measured at least once. The value chosen is the most deranged during the first 24 h after ICU admission, with missing values being considered as normal in the computation of the score.

It comprises the evaluation of six organs/systems: respiratory, cardiovascular, renal, haematological, neurological and hepatic, and is the only one of the published systems that allows the computation of the predicted mortality at hospital discharge based on the amount of organ dysfunction/failure assessed 24 h after ICU admission (Table 2.4).

The computation of the probability of mortality at hospital discharge is made using the equation:

$$\text{Probability of death} = \frac{e^{-3.4043 + 0.4173 \times \text{LOD score}}}{1 + e^{-3.4043 + 0.4173 \times \text{LOD score}}}$$

Despite the fact that the LODS was not initially validated for repeated use during the ICU stay, in a study of 1,685 patients in French ICUs, the LODS was shown to be accurate in characterising the progression of organ dysfunction during the first week of ICU stay (Timsit et al. 2002). The predicted value varies between 3.2% in patients without any organ dysfunction/failure up to 99.7% in patients with 22 points (failure of all the six analysed systems). In a preliminary analysis it seems to present a deficient calibration and a lower discriminative capability than the other systems (Moreno et al. 1997). It was utilised for the first time in 1999 (Soufir et al. 1999).

Table 2.4 Logistic Organ Dysfunction Score (LODS)

	Increase in severity/decreasing value			Normal	Increase in severity/increasing value		
	5	3	1	0	1	3	5
Neurological							
Glasgow Coma Scale	3–5	6–8	9–13	14–15	–	–	–
Cardiovascular							
Heart rate (beats/min)	<30 or	–	–	30–139 e	≥140 or	–	–
Systolic blood pressure (mmHg)	<40			90–239	240–269	≥270	–
Renal							
Serum urea, mmol/L (g/L) or				<6 (<0.36)	6–9.9 (0.36–0.59)	10–19.9 (0.6–1.19)	
blood urea nitrogen, mmol/L (md/dL)				<6 (<17) e	6–9.9 (17–27.9) or	10–19.9 (28–55.9)	
Serum creatinine, µmol/L (mg/dL)				<106 (<1.2) e	106–140 (1.2–1.59)	or≥141 (≥ 1.60)	
Urinary output (L/dia)	< 0.5	0.5–0.74		0.75–9.99		or≥10.0	
Respiratory							
PaO_2 (mmHg)/FiO_2 [a]		< 150	≥ 150	Without mechanical ventilation or CPAP			
Haematological							
Leukocytes (× 1,000/mm³)		<1.0	1.0–2.4 or	2.5–49.9 e	≥ 50.0		
Platelets (× 1,000/mm³)			<50	≥50			
Hepatic							
Serum Bilirubin, µmol/L (mg/dL)				< 34.2 (< 2.0) e	≥ 34.2 (≥ 2.0) or		
Prothrombin time [b]			(< 25%)	<3 (≥ 25%)	≥3		

Adapted from Le Gall et al. (1997)
[a] Only if mechanical ventilation or CPAP
[b] Seconds above control (% of the control)

2.5   Sequential Organ Failure Assessment (SOFA) Score

Developed in 1994 by a panel of experts from the ESICM, based on a review of the literature, the Sequential Organ Failure Assessment (SOFA) score was originally named the Sepsis-related Organ Failure Assessment score. The fact that it functions well even in patients without sepsis is responsible for the change in the name, and according to the recommendation of the authors, it is applicable to all types of critically ill patients (Vincent et al. 1996).

It quantifies the dysfunction/failure of six organs/systems: respiratory, cardiovascular, renal, haematological, neurological and hepatic (Table 2.5), scored from 0 (normal function) up to 4 points (severe failure). It presents a maximum score of 24 points.

It has been validated in quite different contexts, such as unselected critically ill patients (Vincent et al. 1998) and even trauma (Antonelli et al. 1999). Subsequent to the original publication, several derived measures have been proposed, allowing a more detailed evaluation of the evolutive patterns of the critically ill patient (Moreno et al. 1999). It has been used in several clinical studies (Di Filippo et al. 1998; Fiore et al. 1998; Briegel et al. 1999; Hynninen et al. 1999). Because it was developed based on expert opinion, it needed a very careful validation to evaluate the chosen variables and their limits. In a retrospective evaluation during the first 24 h of ICU stay in 1,643 patients with early severe sepsis, the SOFA score demonstrated a good relationship with mortality and an acceptable distribution of the patients into the several groups (Vincent et al. 1996). Later, the Working Group of the European Society of Intensive Care Medicine conducted a prospective validation in 1,449 patients (11,417 patient days) in 40 ICUs in Europe, North America, South America and Australia during a 1-month period (Vincent et al. 1998). Based on this study, several derived measures were proposed, destined to become a more rigorous quantification of MODS, allowing the separated evaluation of the amount of organ dysfunction/failure present at admission (admission SOFA), the amount of organ dysfunction/failure that appears during the ICU stay (delta SOFA) and the cumulative dysfunction/failure suffered by the patient during the ICU stay (total maximum SOFA) (Moreno et al. 1999).

It should be noted that the best discriminative power was obtained by the total maximum SOFA (area under the curve ROC 0.847 ± 0.012) followed by the admission SOFA (area under the ROC curve 0.772 ± 0.015) and for the delta SOFA (area under the ROC curve 0.742 ± 0.017). Among the six analysed organs/systems, the best discriminative power was obtained by the cardiovascular (area under the ROC curve 0.802 ± 0.015), renal (0.739 ± 0.016) and respiratory (0.736 ± 0.016). In multivariable analysis the most significant contribution for the prognosis was presented by the cardiovascular system (odds ratio 1.68, 95% confidence interval 1.49–1.91), followed by the renal (odds-ratio 1.46, 1.29–1.64), neurological (odds ratio 1.40, 1.28–1.55), coagulation (odds ratio 1.22, 1.06–1.40) and respiratory systems (odds ratio 1.18, 1.01–1.38). An independent contribution to prognosis from the hepatic dysfunction/failure could not be demonstrated (odds ratio 0.82, 0.60–1.11).

Table 2.5 Sequential Organ Failure Assessment (SOFA) score

	0	1	2	3	4
Respiratory[a]					
PaO₂/FiO₂, mm³	>400	≤400	≤300ᵃ	≤200ᵃ	≤100ᵃ
Haematological					
Platelets (×1,000/mm³)	>150	≤150	≤100	≤50	≤20
Liver					
Serum Bilirubin, mg/dL (μmol/L)	<1.2 (<20)	1.2–1.9 (20–32)	2.0–5.9 (33–101)	6.0–11.9 (102–204)	>12.0 (>204)
Cardiovascular					
Hypotension	MAPᵇ ≥70	MAP<70	Dopamine ≤5 or Dobutamine (any dose)	Dopamine>5 or adrenaline ≤0.1 or noradrenaline ≤0.1	Dopamine>15 or adrenaline>0.1 or noradrenaline>0.1
Neurological					
Glasgow Coma Scale	15	13–14	10–12	6–9	<6
Renal					
Serum creatinine, mg/dL (μmol/L) or	<1.2 (<110)	1.2–1.9 (110–170)	2.0–3.4 (171–299)	3.5–4.9 (300–440)	>5.0 (>440)
Urinary output (L/day)				<0.5	<0.2

Adapted from Vincent et al. (1996)

Vasoactive drugs should be given by continuous I.V. infusion for at least 1 h. Doses are presented in micrograms/kg/min

ᵃWith ventilatory support

ᵇMAP mean arterial pressure, mmHg

Fig. 2.1 Mean time (days) to reach maximum SOFA score in patients with organ failure. Values are presented as mean +/-Ł 95% confidence intervals for the mean. Adapted from Moreno et al. (1999)

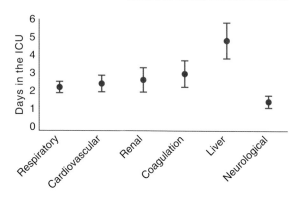

The relative contribution for prognosis of the organ dysfunction/failure present at admission was 1.36 (95% confidence interval 1.30–1.42) for a point increase in the admission SOFA and of 1.37 (1.30–1.43) for a point increase in the delta SOFA. It should be noted that the capacity of the delta SOFA to distinguish the survivors from those who died was smaller than that of the total maximum SOFA and than the admission SOFA. This fact enhances the importance of the degree of physiological dysfunction present at ICU admission to the prognosis (Knaus et al. 1991; Lemeshow et al. 1993; Wagner et al. 1994) as well as the cumulative organ failure (Knaus et al. 1985; Marshall et al. 1995). It is worth noting that, unlike what is frequently described, the maximum organ dysfunction/failure was reached quickly after admission to the ICU, with medium values varying between 0.8 days (95% confidence interval 0.6–0.9 days) for the central nervous system and 1.4 days (95% confidence interval 1.2–1.5 days) for the respiratory system. If the analysis is limited to organ failure (SOFA≥3 points), the time needed to reach the maximum values was larger (average 2.9±1.1 days). The central nervous system was the first to fail; the respiratory, cardiovascular, renal and coagulation organs/systems occupied an intermediate position; and the hepatic was the last (Fig. 2.1).

Why should we use the total maximum SOFA score instead of a simpler measure? Daily evaluation could not capture the total degree of suffered insult for the patient during the course of their disease. Different organs are affected in this complex process at different points in time (Deitch 1992) and a daily evaluation, although attractive, can miss the cumulative suffered insult. It was demonstrated that mortality of MODS depends on the number of organs in failure (Knaus et al. 1985; Marshall et al. 1995; Zimmerman et al. 1996a), on the gravity of the dysfunction/failure (Marshall et al. 1995; Le Gall et al. 1996), on the peculiar combination of organs in failure (Zimmerman et al. 1996a; Hébert et al. 1993; Fagon et al. 1993) and on the duration of the failure (Knaus et al. 1985; Zimmerman et al. 1996a). The SOFA system, following the path of previous works by Marshall et al. (1995), allows the quantification of all these conditions. Alternative approaches were proposed, based on the daily application of severity scores (Chang et al. 1988; Wagner et al. 1994; Chang 1989; Lemeshow et al. 1994; Rogers and Fuller 1994; Yzerman et al. 1996; Pittet et al. 1996), but they are usually limited to the first days in the ICU (Wagner et al. 1994; Lemeshow et al. 1994) or were not validated later (Jacobs et al. 1992). Moreover, the authors (Moreno et al. 1999) described the relationship between the maximum SOFA score and ICU mortality though the equation:

$$\text{Probability of death} = \frac{e^{4.0473+0.2790 \text{ (total maximum SOFA score)}}}{1 + e^{4.0473+0.2790 \text{ (total maximum SOFA score)}}}$$

2.6 Which System to Use?

The main difference in modern MODS scores is the way they access and quantify the cardiovascular system: the SOFA score uses mean arterial pressure and level of adrenergic support, LODS uses systolic blood pressure and heart rate, and the MODS a composite variable, the pressure-adjusted heart rate (PAR). The first formal comparison among them was presented in 1997 at the ESICM Congress, and it seems to indicate a better discrimination from MODS and SOFA scores than the others (Moreno et al. 1997). However, the low number of analysed patients requires further confirmation.

At the moment, and missing better information, each ICU should use the system that:

- Has been tested and validated in their population;
- Can minimise the number of missing values;
- Is easier to compute and register.

When we compare these systems with general severity scores, they give us a very important complementary piece of information in our evaluation of the critically ill patient, since they describe the evolution of the individual patient better and are more sensitive to change in the clinical status caused by the evolution of the disease, the response to therapy or the development of complications.

When used alone, MODS scores seem to have a limited capability to forecast prognosis, as demonstrated clearly by Zygun et al., when studying SOFA and MODS in a database of 1,436 patients admitted to a multisystem ICU in the Calgary Health Region over a 1-year period (Zygun et al. 2005). They concluded that for ICU and hospital mortality, there was very little practical difference between the SOFA and MODS scores in their ability to discriminate outcomes as determined by the area under the ROC. However, compared to previous literature, the discriminatory ability of both scores in this population was weak. As well, the calibration of the models was poor for both scores. The SOFA cardiovascular component score performed better than the MOD cardiovascular component score in the discrimination of both ICU and hospital mortality. These results are important because they question the appropriateness of using organ dysfunction scores as a "surrogate" for mortality in clinical trials as proposed by several authors and suggest further work is necessary to better understand the temporal relationship and course of organ failure with mortality (Vincent and Moreno 2010).

Some attempts have been made to transform MODS in order to replace general severity scores. However, even in the largest of these studies (Kajdacsy-Balla

Amaral et al. 2005), using data from 748 patients admitted to ICUs in six countries, the authors had to adjust the SOFA score for patient age and the presence of infection in order to better predict mortality, and calibration was unbalanced among different countries. These results are almost certainly explained by the absence in these mixed models of an adequate evaluation of the most important prognostic determinants in the critically ill patient: predisposition (age, chronic health status, co-morbid diseases, etc.).

Other similar attempts using combinations of general severity scores (e.g., SAPS II) and MODS (e.g., LODS) were not able to demonstrate the validity or the potential benefits of this approach clearly (Timsit et al. 2001). The same has been demonstrated by Minne et al. (combining the APACHE II/III plus SOFA), but the results are not completely conclusive, despite slightly better behaviour of the combined score with any of the individual scores (Minne et al. 2008). Similar results were found by Ho et al. combining the SOFA score with APACHE II (Ho 2007).

2.7   The Application of MODS in the Daily Life of an ICU

All MODS aim at describing the critically ill patient. Several aggregated measures have been proposed to help in that description (Moreno et al. 1999; Bernard 1998; Marshall 1999). The most important are:

- *Admission score*: reflects the condition of the patient at ICU admission. It depends mainly on ICU admission policies and pre-ICU factors, and allows the user to have a baseline assessment of the condition of the patient at admission. It can be used as entry (or exclusion) criteria for clinical trials or to evaluate the comparability of groups before the assignment to a certain therapy or management strategy;
- *Daily score*: this is the sum of the individual scores for the different organs/systems evaluated by the score on a given day. It is especially useful when analysed in a serial way in order to monitor the evolution of a given patient;
- *Delta score*: this is the difference between the maximum score and the admission score, and reflects the degree of organ dysfunction/failure that develops after ICU admission, being especially useful for monitoring the impact on the patients of events that happen after ICU admission;
- *Total maximum score*: this is the sum of the maximum score for each organ/system during the entire ICU stay. It reflects the cumulative insult suffered by the patient, taking into account that the timing for maximum dysfunction/failure differs among different organs/systems;
- *Organ failure free days*: for a certain organ during a certain period of time (usually 28 days), this is the number of days presented by the patient alive and without failure of the specific organ/system. It is especially useful as an aggregated measure of morbidity in survivors and of mortality in non-survivors.

2.8   Conclusion

The best treatment for sepsis and MODS is, without any doubt, prevention. Unfortunately, this is not possible in many cases. While we wait for the development of new diagnostic and therapeutic instruments, the use of objective scores for the evaluation and quantification of the gravity of our patients' situations should be advocated. This use should not be restricted to experimental or almost-experimental contexts, but should be implemented in daily clinical practice.

It is still too early for these instruments to provide us with decisive help in the complex decision-making process of deciding who to treat, when to treat and how to treat a patient, or when deciding that we should concentrate our efforts in providing a death with dignity to those who are beyond the scope of our intervention. In other words, in fulfilling our duties to our patients and to society, accomplishing what Hippocrates called in general terms "the duty of Medicine," as stated below. But it is our strong belief that these measures constitute a step in the right direction.

> In general terms [the duty of medicine] is to do away with the sufferings of the sick, to lessen the violence of their diseases, and to refuse to treat those who are over-mastered by their diseases, realizing that in such cases medicine is powerless
>
> Hippocrates, 400 BC

References

Antonelli M, Moreno M, Vincent JL, Spung CL, Mendonça A, Passariello M, Riccioni L, Osborn J, SOFA Group (1999) Application of SOFA score to trauma patients. Intensive Care Med 25:389–394

Azoulay E, Metnitz B, Sprung CL, Timsit JF, Lemaire F, Bauer P, Schlemmer B, Moreno R, Metnitz P (2009) End-of-life practices in 282 intensive care units: data from the SAPS 3 database. Intensive Care Med 35:623–630

Baumgartner JD, Bula C, Vaney C et al (1992) A novel score for predicting the mortality of septic shock patients. Crit Care Med 20:953

Bell RC, Coalson JJ, Smith JD, Johanson WG (1983) Multiple organ failure and infection in adult respiratory distress syndrome. Ann Intern Med 99:293–298

Bernard G (1997) The Brussels score. Sepsis 1:43–44

Bernard GR (1998) Quantification of organ dysfunction: seeking standardization. Crit Care Med 26:1767–1768

Bernard GR, Doig BG, Hudson G et al (1995) Quantification of organ failure for clinical trials and clinical practice (abstract). Am J Respir Crit Care Med 151:A323

Bertleff MJ, Bruining HA (1997) How should multiple organ dysfunction syndrome be assessed? A review of the variations in current scoring systems. Eur J Surg 163:405–409

Bota DP, Melot C, Ferreira FL, Ba VN, Vincent JL (2002) The Multiple Organ Dysfunction Score (MODS) versus the Sequential Organ Failure Assessment (SOFA) score in outcome prediction. Intensive Care Med 28:1619–1624

Briegel J, Forst H, Haller M, Schelling G, Kilger E, Kuprat G, Hemmer B, Lenhart A, Heyduck M, Stoll C, Peter K (1999) Stress doses of hydrocortisone reverse hyperdynamic septic shock: a prospective, randomized, double-blind, single-center study. Crit Care Med 27:723–732

Chang RW (1989) Individual outcome prediction models for intensive care units. Lancet i:143–146

Chang RW, Jacobs S, Lee B (1988) Predicting outcome among intensive care unit patients using computerised trend analysis of daily Apache II scores corrected for organ system failure. Intensive Care Med 14:558–566

Cook R, Cook D, Tilley J, Lee KA, Marshall J, Canadian Critical Care Trials Group (2001) Multiple organ dysfunction: baseline and serial component scores. Crit Care Med 29: 2046–2050

Deitch EA (1992) Multiple organ failure: pathophysiology and potential future therapy. Ann Surg 216:117–134

Di Filippo A, De Gaudio AR, Novelli A et al (1998) Continuous infusion of vancomycin in methicillin-resistant *staphylococcus* infection. Chemotherapy 44:63–68

Elebute EA, Stoner HB (1983) The grading of sepsis. Br J Surg 70:29–31

Fagon JY, Chastre J, Novara A, Medioni P, Gilbert C (1993) Characterization of intensive care unit patients using a model based on the presence or absence of organ dysfunctions and/or infection: the ODIN model. Intensive Care Med 19:137–144

Faist E, Baue AE, Dittmer H, Heberer G (1983) Multiple organ failure in polytrauma patients. J Trauma 23:775–787

Fiore G, Donadio PP, Gianferrari P et al (1998) CVVH in postoperative care of liver transplantation. Minerva Anestesiol 64:83–87

Fry DE, Pearlstein L, Fulton RL, Polk HC (1980) Multiple system organ failure. The role of uncontrolled infection. Arch Surg 115:136–140

Garden OJ, Motyl H, Gilmour WH, Utley RJ, Carter DC (1985) Prediction of outcome following acute variceal haemorrhage. Br J Surg 72:91–95

Gonçalves JA, Hydo LJ, Barie PS (1998) Factors influencing outcome of prolonged norepinephrine therapy for shock in critical surgical illness. Shock 10:231–236

Goris RJA, Te Boekhorst tP, Nuytinck JKS, Gimbrère JSF (1985) Multiple-organ failure. Generalized autodestructive inflammation? Arch Surg 120:1109–1115

Hébert PC, Drummond AJ, Singer J, Bernard GR, Russell JA (1993) A simple multiple system organ failure scoring system predicts mortality of patients who have sepsis syndrome. Chest 104:230–235

Henao FJ, Daes JE, Dennis RJ (1991) Risk factors for multiorgan failure: a case-control study. J Trauma 31:74–80

Ho K (2007) Combining sequential organ failure assessment (SOFA) score with acute physiology and chronic health evaluation (APACHE) II score to predict hospital mortality of critically ill patients. Anaesth Intensive Care 35:515–521

Hynninen M, Valtonen M, Markkanen H et al (1999) Interleukin 1 receptor antagonist and E-selectin concentrations: a comparison in patients with severe acute pancreatitis and severe sepsis. J Crit Care 14:63–68

Jacobs S, Arnold A, Clyburn PA, Willis BA (1992) The Riyadh intensive care program applied to a mortality analysis of a teaching hospital intensive care unit. Anaesthesia 47:775–780

Jacobs S, Zuleika M, Mphansa T (1999) The multiple organ dysfunction score as a descriptor of patient outcome in septic shock compared with two other scoring systems. Crit Care Med 27:741–744

Kajdacsy-Balla Amaral AC, Andrade FM, Moreno R, Artigas A, Cantraine F, Vincent JF (2005) Use of the Sequential Organ Failure Assessment score as a severity score. Intensive Care Med 31:243–249

Khwannimit B (2008) Serial evaluation of the MODS, SOFA and LOD scores to predict ICU mortality in mixed critically ill patients. J Med Assoc Thai 91:1336–1342

Knaus WA, Draper EA, Wagner DP, Zimmerman JE (1985) Prognosis in acute organ-system failure. Ann Surg 202:685–693

Knaus WA, Wagner DP, Draper EA, Zimmerman JE, Bergner M, Bastos PG, Sirio CA, Murphy DJ, Lotring T, Damiano A, Harrell FE Jr (1991) The APACHE III prognostic system. Risk prediction of hospital mortality for critically ill hospitalized adults. Chest 100:1619–1636

Le Gall JR, Klar J, Lemeshow S, Saulnier F, Alberti C, Artigas A, Teres D, The ICU scoring group (1996) The logistic organ dysfunction system. A new way to assess organ dysfunction in the intensive care unit. JAMA 276:802–810

Le Gall JR, Klar J, Lemeshow S (1997) How to assess organ dysfunction in the intensive care unit? The logistic organ dysfunction (LOD) system. Sepsis 1:45–47

Lemeshow S, Teres D, Klar J, Avrunin JS, Gehlbach SH, Rapoport J (1993) Mortality Probability Models (MPM II) based on an international cohort of intensive care unit patients. JAMA 270:2478–2486

Lemeshow S, Klar J, Teres D, Avrunin JS, Gehlbach SH, Rapoport J, Rué M (1994) Mortality probability models for patients in the intensive care unit for 48 or 72 hours: a prospective, multicenter study. Crit Care Med 22:1351–1358

Marshall J (1999) Charting the course of critical illness: prognostication and outcome description in the intensive care unit. Crit Care Med 27:676–678

Marshall WG, Dimick AR (1983) Natural history of major burns with multiple subsystem failure. J Trauma 23:102–105

Marshall JC, Cook DA, Christou NV, Bernard GR, Sprung CL, Sibbald WJ (1995) Multiple organ dysfunction score: a reliable descriptor of a complex clinical outcome. Crit Care Med 23:1638–1652

Marshall JD, Bernard G, Le Gall JR, Vincent JL (1997a) The measurement of organ dysfunction/failure as an ICU outcome. Sepsis 1:41

Marshall JD, Bernard G, Le Gall JR, Vincent JL (1997b) Conclusions. Sepsis 1:55–57

Maziak DE, Lindsay TF, Marshall JC et al (1998) The impact of multiple organ dysfunction on mortality following ruptured abdominal aortic aneurysm repair. Ann Vasc Surg 12:93–100

Meek M, Munster AM, Winchurch RA et al (1991) The Baltimore sepsis scale: measurement of sepsis in patients with burns using a new scoring system. J Burn Care Rehabil 12:564

Members of the American College of Chest Physicians and the Society of Critical Care Medicine Consensus Conference Committee (1992) American College of Chest Physicians / Society of Critical Care Medicine Consensus Conference: definitions of sepsis and multiple organ failure and guidelines for the use of innovative therapies in sepsis. Crit Care Med 20:864–874

Minne L, Abu-Hanna A, de Jonge E (2008) Evaluation of SOFA-based models for predicting mortality in the ICU: a systematic review. Crit Care 12:R61

Moreno R, Pereira E, Matos R, Fevereiro T (1997) The evaluation of cardiovascular dysfunction/failure in multiple organ failure (abstract). Intensive Care Med 23:S153

Moreno R, Vincent JL, Matos R, Mendonça A, Cantraine F, Thijs L, Takala J, Sprung C, Antonelli M, Bruining H, Willatts S, on behalf of the Working Group on "Sepsis-related problems" of the European Society of Intensive Care Medicine (1999) The use of maximum SOFA score to quantify organ dysfunction/failure in intensive care. Results of a prospective, multicentre study. Intensive Care Med 25:686–696

Pinilla JC, Hayes P, Laverty W et al (1998) The C-reactive protein to prealbumin ratio correlates with the severity of multiple organ dysfunction. Surgery 124:799–805

Pittet D, Thiévent B, Wenzel RP, Li N, Auckenthaler R, Suter PM (1996) Bedside prediction of mortality from bacteriemic sepsis. A dynamic analysis of ICU patients. Am J Respir Crit Care Med 153:684–693

Rogers J, Fuller HD (1994) Use of daily acute physiology and chronic health evaluation (APACHE) II scores to predict individual patient survival rate. Crit Care Med 22:1402–1405

Soufir L, Timsits JF, Mahe C et al (1999) Attributable morbidity and mortality of catheter-related septicemia in critically ill patients: a matched, risk-adjusted, cohort study. Infect Control Hosp Epidemiol 20:396–401

Staubach KH, Schroder J, Stuber F et al (1998) Effect of pentoxifylline in severe sepsis: results of a randomized, double-blind, placebo-controlled study. Arch Surg 133:94–100

Stevens LE (1983) Gauging the severity of surgical sepsis. Arch Surg 118:1190–1192

Tibby SM (2010) Does PELOD measure organ dysfunction...and is organ function a valid surrogate for death? Intensive Care Med 46:4–7

Tilney NL, Baily GL, Morgan AP (1973) Sequential system failure after rupture of abdominal aortic aneurisms: an unsolved problem in postoperative care. Ann Surg 178:117–122

Timsit JF, Fosse JP, Troche G, De Lassence A, Alberti C, Garrouste-Orgeas M, Azoulay E, Chevret S, Moine P, Cohen Y (2001) Accuracy of a composite score using daily SAPS II and LOD scores for predicting hospital mortality in ICU patients hospitalized for more than 72 h. Intensive Care Med 27:1012–1021

Timsit JF, Fosse JP, Troché G, De Lassenc A, Alberti C, Garrouste-Orgeas M, Bornstain C, Adrie C, Cheval C, Chevret S, OUTCOMEREA Study Group (2002) Calibration and discrimination by daily Logistic Organ Dysfunction scoring comparatively with daily Sequential Organ Failure Assessment scoring for predicting hospital mortality in critically ill patients. Crit Care Med 30:2003–2013

Tran DD (1994) Age, chronic disease, sepsis, organ system failure and mortality in the elderly admitted to the intensive care medicine. Intensive Care Med 20:S110

Tran DD, Cuesta MA (1992) Evaluation of severity in patients with acute pancreatitis. Am J Gastroenterol 87:604–608

Vincent JL, Moreno R (2010) Clinical review: scoring systems in the critically ill. Crit Care 14:207 DOI: 10.1186/cc8204

Vincent JL, Moreno R, Takala J, Willats S, De Mendonça A, Bruining H, Reinhart CK, Suter PM, Thijs LG (1996) The SOFA (sepsis-related organ failure assessment) score to describe organ dysfunction/failure. Intensive Care Med 22:707–710

Vincent JL, de Mendonça A, Cantraine F, Moreno R, Takala J, Suter P, Sprung C, Colardyn F, Blecher S, on behalf of the working group on "sepsis-related problems" of the European Society of Intensive Care Medicine (1998) Use of the SOFA score to assess the incidence of organ dysfunction/failure in intensive care units: results of a multicentric, prospective study. Crit Care Med 26:1793–1800

Vincent JL, Sakr Y, Moreno R, Sprung C, Reinhart K, Payen D, Ranieri VM, Carlet J, Gerlach H, Le Gall JR, on behalf of the SOAP investigators (2003) Epidemiology of ICU acquired infection: results of the SOAP study (Abstract). Crit Care Med 31:A126

Vincent JL, Rello J, Marshall J, Silva E, Anzueto A, Martin CD, Moreno R, Lipman J, Gomersall C, Sakr Y, Reinhart K, EPIC II Group of Investigators (2009) International study of the prevalence and outcomes of infection in intensive care units. JAMA 302:2323–2329

Wagner DP, Knaus WA, Harrel FE Jr, Zimmerman JE, Watts C (1994) Daily prognostic estimates for critically ill adults in intensive care units: results from a prospective, multicenter, inception cohort analysis. Crit Care Med 22:1359–1372

Yzerman EP, Boelens HA, Tjhie JH, Kluytmans JA, Mouton JW, Verbrugh HA (1996) Delta APACHE II for predicting course and outcome of nosocomial Staphylococcus aureus bacteremia and its relation to host defense. J Infect Dis 173:914–919

Zimmerman JE, Knaus WA, Sun X, Wagner DP (1996a) Severity stratification and outcome prediction for multisystem organ failure and dysfunction. World J Surg 20:401–405

Zimmerman JE, Knaus WA, Wagner DP, Sun X, Hakim RB, Nystrom PO (1996b) A comparison of risks and outcomes for patients with organ failure: 1982–1990. Crit Care Med 24: 1633–1641

Zygun DA, Laupland KB, Fick GH, Sandham JD, Doig CJ (2005) Limited ability of SOFA and MOD scores to discriminate outcome: a prospective evaluation in 1,436 patients. Can J Anaesth 52:302–308

Zygun D, Berthiaume L, Laupland K, Kortbeek J, Doig C (2006) SOFA is superior to MOD score for the determination of non-neurologic organ dysfunction in patients with severe traumatic brain injury: a cohort study. Crit Care 10:R115

Why Guidelines Require Reform

3

Andrew Rhodes, Maurizio Cecconi, and Rui Moreno

3.1   Introduction

Clinical practice guidelines are nowadays seen as a necessity in order to summarize an ever-burgeoning amount of published evidence into a simple format that practicing clinicians can read, digest and implement in order to improve a patient's outcome. Their use has also been advocated to reduce the gap between bench and bedside, to standardize clinical practice with the avoidance of inappropriate variations, to reduce the risk of legal claims and as a tool for quality assurance. Indeed, even a cursory inspection of PubMed reveals just how vast the published evidence is. In 2009 alone, there were 7,082 papers published that are retrieved when searching on the term "critical care." If we also consider other databases, with the knowledge that a significant issue exists concerning language bias and publication bias (Grégoire et al. 1995), the volume is even greater.

This is obviously far in excess of what the average person can hope to read, so there needs to be a mechanism for summarizing these data in a format that provides clear, robust and evidence-based recommendations that can then be used at the bedside. More than 2,000 guidelines can now be found in a search in PubMed, covering all aspects of medical care. For the guidelines to be trusted, however, all the mechanisms that are behind the development and the dissemination of the recommendation must be well understood and trusted. This means that the guidelines have to be developed independent of vested interests, and they must be relevant and objective

A. Rhodes (✉) • M. Cecconi
Department of Intensive Care Medicine, St George's Healthcare NHS Trust,
London, UK
e-mail: andyr@sgul.ac.uk

R. Moreno
Unidade de Cuidados Intensivos Polivalente, Hospital de St. António dos Capuchos,
Centro Hospitalar de Lisboa Central, E.P.E, Lisbon, Portugal

J. Rello (eds.), *Sepsis Management*,
DOI 10.1007/978-3-642-03519-7_3, © Springer-Verlag Berlin Heidelberg 2012

in making recommendations that both support decision-making processes and impact on clinical care (Grol 2010). By necessity this requires input into the process from all stake-holding groups, including patients, administrators and politicians, but also must be developed in a multi-disciplinary and multi-specialty approach. There is little point having a strong recommendation from a clinical practice guideline that insists that a certain modality of treatment should be used in a group of patients if that modality is neither available nor affordable. The result will inevitably be seen as a politically motivated "wish list" rather than a sensible decision-making tool.

3.2   Generating Guidelines and the Controversies of Evidence-Based Medicine

George Browman described in 2010 in an editorial published in the Journal of Surgical Oncology that "the main challenge of the evidence-based movement in guideline development is to ensure that we do not simply replace the tyranny of authority (i.e., experts) with the tyranny of methodology" (Browman 2010). This statement sums up many of the controversies that pertain to guideline development in a simple but punchy statement. Many of the basic principles behind guideline development have been well established for many years (Shekelle et al. 1999; Grimshaw and Russell 1993), although the publication of many examples has been rightly criticized for falling short of this high standard (Grilli et al. 2000; Shaneyfelt et al. 1999).

Amerling has recently pointed out the distinction between guidelines and textbooks (Amerling et al. 2008). Guidelines can be educational, but are fundamentally distinct from textbooks because of a series of reasons.

Textbook chapters are usually single or double authored and are as authoritative as the individual authors. Different textbooks exist covering more or less the same subjects, giving a spectrum of opinion. Authors are free, indeed encouraged, to scan ahead and make predictions about where the field is going, based on as yet unpublished data. Financing usually comes from publishers who then market the product in the hope of making a profit, or at least recouping their expenses. On the other hand, guidelines result from the deliberations and contributions of a "panel of experts" formed into "working groups" or "panels." Frequently these experts have relationships with industry that may or may not influence their decision-making abilities. These panels review the literature and then make specific treatment-based recommendations. Guidelines are generally sponsored implicitly or explicitly by industry, sometimes through the funding of specialty societies. The industry expects to recover their investment through increased sales of their products, based on guideline recommendations (which are distributed for free). All these points need deep consideration before using them to change clinical practice, an even more difficult exercise (Landucci 2004; Poole et al. 2008), especially when different strategies and actions are combined into "bundles of care" (Machado and Freitas 2008).

In 2003, in response to these concerns with regards to guideline development, an international group of researchers from 13 countries—the Appraisal of Guidelines, Research and Evaluation (AGREE) collaboration—developed and validated a tool to specifically assess the quality of the guideline development process. Importantly this instrument assesses neither the clinical content nor the quality of the evidence of any given guideline; however it does assess the processes involved in the development of the guideline itself (The AGREE Collaboration 2003). The AGREE collaboration's appraisal instrument contains six main domains that assess the quality of any given guideline. These six domains describe: (1) the scope and purpose of the project (2) stakeholder development (3) the rigor of development (4) clarity and presentation of the document (5) applicability and (6) editorial independence. This tool was validated for appraisee acceptability and also for quality assessment of guidelines, finding that national policy-making guidelines (with greater resource backing) tended to be of higher quality in terms of rigor of development. These domains describe in depth exactly how a guideline development process should proceed. We will describe each of these domains in a little more detail, and it is recommended that the reader considers each of these domains in relation to a set of guidelines with which he/she is familiar.

3.2.1 Scope and Purpose

This domain describes the overall objectives of the project. It needs to address the questions to be answered and the patients upon whom the guidelines are to be focused. Specific details of these are absolutely necessary, as the evidence base sitting behind many of the recommendations within the guideline should have been extracted from studies focusing on these identical patients. When guidelines are extrapolated from one patient group to another, then the evidence base weakens and may become fundamentally flawed. In conscience, the reader needs to understand very clearly why any specific guideline was identified as a priority by the group proposing and presenting it, and why it was developed at that specific moment in time. Unfortunately, many times, the answer to this question is the pre-release of a new drug or device that is then recommended within the guideline in order to increase awareness and sales of the product.

3.2.2 Stakeholder Involvement

This domain pertains to the guideline development group's composition and also to the target audience. The target audience needs to be described as the recommendations are made specifically for them. The composition of the development group has a major influence on the final output of the project (Institute of Medicine 2009). This is not only pertinent to individuals with vested interests, but also and perhaps more importantly to ensuring that all appropriate professional groups are included. Often the interpretation of evidence from one specialty is different to the views as seen from another. All relevant parties must therefore be contributing to the process with methods of gaining consensus being agreed upon up front. In addition, it is important that the views of the patients (or their advocates) are also sought. What may be perfectly acceptable and intuitive to a clinician, even with the best of intentions, may be completely unacceptable to a patient. These views must be balanced somehow within the process. Prior to the guideline being released, there must be some testing of the reliability of the recommendations. This may mean having a pilot phase project or some wider peer review process to ensure that the recommendations are sensible and based on a sound rationale. This should be prior to wider dispersion, which has the potential for major detrimental effects if the recommendations are subsequently proved to be wrong.

3.2.3   Rigor of Development

In any evidence-based methodology, the processes involved in the acquisition, assessment and analysis of the data, and then the conversion to a recommendation, are of paramount importance. The methodology needs to be stated up front so that every reader can be confident of the methodology chosen.

Any data acquired must be found with the search strategies clearly described in a systematic fashion, similar to the methodology of the Cochrane group. The methods used for formulating the recommendations must be described together with the potential risks, benefits and side effects that are possible as a consequence. It is worth considering at this stage the likely difference between the efficacy of any given treatment from the published trials and its potential effectiveness in a real-life setting. There needs to be a clear link between the evidence base and the recommendation that fully explains the assumptions made to get from one to the other. It is vital, as said above, that these steps undergo a rigorous peer review and that a mechanism is put into place to update the recommendation when new data becomes available (GRADE Working Group 2004; Guyatt et al. 2006; Schünemann et al. 2006).

The question of whether we should provide a discrete "grade" for recommendations has recently been discussed (Browman 2010). Discriminating between a strong and weak recommendation is often difficult when the data are not as strong as would be hoped for, or even when data are completely lacking, but the treatment choice is obvious. An example of this is in the taking of blood cultures in the assessment of septicemia. There are no data from randomized controlled studies that tell us that taking blood cultures is beneficial for patients, and such studies are unlikely ever to be performed. A strong recommendation to use this technique, however, is obviously correct, although would be difficult to justify in objective evidence-based assessments. It is therefore perhaps more useful for the recommendation to simply describe in plain language what is being suggested, in order to convey the areas of strength, weakness or uncertainty.

One way of getting the areas of potential conflict over to the readers of a set of guidelines would be to publish a transcript of the arguments used during the process. This would be strengthened further if the peer review process, and subsequent changes to the document, were also to be available to the bedside clinicians. Where the recommendation has been contentious, then a description of how consensus was reached should be described, perhaps even with the results of any vote if that was how agreement was achieved.

The differing results between the various mechanisms of assessing and grading the evidence are worth considering, as demonstrated in some of the changing conclusions between the 2004 and 2008 recommendations from the Surviving Sepsis Campaign (Dellinger et al. 2004, 2008) and also the methods this group used to gain consensus when disparate views arose (Jaeschke et al. 2008). The important point to recognize is that differing methodologies may bring differing results. In the first set of Surviving Sepsis guidelines, each clinical trial used to support recommendations was assessed based on an evidence-based methodology that took into consideration the presence or absence of important elements such as concealed randomization, blinded outcome adjudication, intention to treat analysis and explicit definitions of primary outcomes. The goal was total consensus, which was reached in all recommendations except two. In those two circumstances the solution was achieved with sub-recommendations that expressed some of the differences in expert opinion. When there was difference of opinion about grading of a clinical trial, an outside epidemiologist was consulted. This occurred in one circumstance with resolution of differences. At the end, the system used for achieving consensus was a table grading the evidence from level A (supported by at least two level I investigations) to E (supported by level IV or V evidence only).

When the 2008 revision was implemented (Dellinger et al. 2008), the GRADE system (GRADE Working Group 2004) was used. This system did not use the A to E classification, but instead used two complementary parameters to classify each recommendation: the concept of strong (grade 1) versus weak (grade 2) recommendations, and the quality of evidence as high (grade A), moderate (grade B), low (grade C) or very low (grade D). This introduced a potential bias because the strong/weak classification is based on soft data: the opinion of the panel. As it is written in the original manuscript "The world is not dangerous because of those who do harm but because of those who look at it without doing anything" the committee assessed whether the desirable effects of adherence will outweigh the undesirable effects, and the strength of a recommendation reflects the group's degree of confidence in that assessment. A strong recommendation in favour of an intervention reflects that the desirable effects of adherence to a recommendation (beneficial health outcomes, less burden on staff and patients, and cost savings) will clearly outweigh the undesirable effects (harms, more burden, and greater costs). A weak recommendation in favor of an intervention indicates that the desirable effects of adherence to a recommendation probably will outweigh the undesirable effects, but the panel is not confident about these tradeoffs – either because some of the evidence is low quality (and thus there remains uncertainty regarding the benefits and risks) or the benefits and downsides are closely balanced. While the degree of confidence is a continuum and there is no precise threshold between a strong and a weak recommendation, the presence of important concerns about one or more of the preceding factors makes a weak recommendation more likely. A strong recommendation is worded as "we recommend" and a weak recommendation as "we suggest."

3.2.4   Clarity and Presentation

For any clinical practice guideline to be of use, it has to be in a format that is easy to read and understand and can then be implemented. This means that the presentation of the guideline must be clear and precise. Lengthy and turgid documents that hide the recommendations within reams of text are unlikely to be of much use to implement change in behavior and/or treatment strategies. The recommendations must be specific and unambiguous, with the differing options for treatment clearly described. The more successful documents are not simply a published text, but are supplemented with on line tools that aid the transition from traditional care to the new recommended ways of practicing. A recent example of this is the bundle methodology described by the Institute of Healthcare Improvement in the United States and used to change the behaviors of clinicians within the Surviving Sepsis Campaign (Berwick 2008; Levy et al. 2004). This unproven and relatively controversial methodology has been assessed by some as the new "holy grail" (Marwick and Davey 2009; Thomas 2007) and by others as almost useless (Wip and Napolitano 2009 #11061). This is certainly an area where we need more science and less emotion.

3.2.5   Applicability

It is nonsense to suggest that simply publishing a recommendation will result in significant change in clinician behavior. The barriers preventing such change need to be acknowledged and discussed in a guideline document. These barriers may be related to cost and finance, or may be organizational in nature. Whatever the cause, the impediment should be described and methods of overcoming the hurdle suggested. In parallel with this should be a methodology for auditing the uptake and implementation of the guideline into routine clinical practice. Without a change in behavior, the development of the guideline itself becomes of little worth.

3.2.6   Editorial Independence

In recent years there has been considerable interest and controversy concerning this domain. Many guidelines have been called into question with respect to their relationship to their funding bodies or the (potential) vested interests of the individual members. The potential conflicts of interest that can impact on guideline development are complex and do not simply relate to financial entanglements with interested parties. Academic interests can often be far more rigid and also a lot more difficult to either describe or disclose.

3.3   Implementing Guidelines into Clinical Practice

In recent years, despite many improvements in our methods for evaluating evidence generated from clinical research (GRADE Working Group 2004; Jaeschke et al. 2008), little has been published about how to integrate research data into clinical practice while maintaining the efficacy of the original intervention, or in other words about how to ensure that the same intervention has a high degree of effectiveness. In the rush to move from the bench to the bedside and in the desire to translate promising research into outcome improvements for many, researchers can be tempted to forget some of the fundamental principles of scientific endeavor: to validate their results and to insure the integrity of any given data.

Central to this whole discussion is the concept of bundles of care. These were introduced to "force" process change and to therefore alter clinicians' behavior in order to implement new and confirmed research data. They have been incorporated into the practice of many different aspects of care, often with little evidence to support their use. Areas where they have been used include the "ventilator bundle" or the "ventilator-associated pneumonia (VAP) bundle," a series of measures to prevent VAP (Wip and Napolitano 2009), and the "catheter-bundles," a series of measures to prevent catheter-related bloodstream infections (Pronovost et al. 2006).

Part of the problem with this process is the drift away from bundles simply being used to translate research into practice. They are now used for quality improvement (Marwick and Davey 2009), the measurement of clinical or organizational performance and in some spheres for justification of reimbursement (Marwick and Davey 2009). If all components of a bundle are uncontroversial, then there is no problem. When not all elements of a bundle are equally important (some maybe eventually even have antagonist effects), controversy arises (Gao et al. 2005; Ferrer et al. 2008). This raises the question as to whether similar standards that have been used to assess evidence have been applied to bundle generation. And here the answer is clearly no.

It is imperative that when assessing evidence for incorporation into a bundle, the grounding and rationale of that evidence must be robust. In order to do this we need to have reliable, open and transparent instruments that can weigh the evidence, taking into account both the internal and external validity of the underpinning studies. If the rationale for using any specific variable is not strong, then the bundle methodology may force its use in inappropriate patients with resulting harm (Bertolini et al. 2007; Kanji et al. 2007). We strongly believe that any bundle of care, once drafted, should then enter a validation phase in an independent cohort of patients before being used to mandate any change in practice. This is especially important before administrators or funders of health care take control of these tools to drive quality control, legal or benchmarking issues or for reimbursement purposes. This validation should test the effect of the different elements of the bundle in patients with different baseline characteristics being evaluated with the same rigor that we ask for other fields of science.

3.4   Conclusions

The development of a rigorous set of clinical practice guidelines is a complex and costly business. It has been estimated that a detailed set of guideline recommendations will cost more than $400,000 to produce and take a considerable period of time. It is vital, therefore, that appropriate systems are in place to ensure these projects are performed with the rigor that they deserve, and that then the recommendations from them are dispersed and implemented in an appropriate fashion. Many recent guidelines that have been produced fail to successfully fulfill all of the above-described domains . The only way that these processes will ever be fully trusted is if the process is open and transparent, and the methodology used is validated and reliable. We believe that the guidelines when published should not simply be a stand-alone textual document, but must include a methodology for ensuring dispersion and then monitoring uptake and implementation.

References

Amerling R, Winchester JF, Ronco C (2008) Guidelines have done more harm than good. Blood Purif 26:73–76

Bertolini G, Rossi C, Anghileri A, Livigni S, Addis A, Poole D (2007) Use of Drotrecogin alfa (activated) in Italian intensive care units: the results of a nationwide survey. Intensive Care Med 33:426–434

Berwick DM (2008) The science of improvement. JAMA 299:1182–1184

Browman GP (2010) Evidence-based clinical practice guideline development: principles, challenges, and accountability to evidence. J Surg Oncol 101:1–2

Dellinger RP, Carlet JM, Masur H, Gerlach H, Calandra T, Cohen J, Gea-Banacloche J, Keh D, Marshall JC, Parker MM, Ramsay G, Zimmerman JL, Vincent JL, Levy MM (2004) Surviving Sepsis Campaign guidelines for the management of severe sepsis and septic shock. Intensive Care Med 30:536–555

Dellinger RP, Levy MM, Carlet JM, Bion J, Parker MM, Jaeschke R, Reinhart K, Angus DC, Brun-Buisson C, Beale R, Calandra T, Dhainaut JF, Gerlach H, Harvey M, Marini JJ, Marshall J, Ranieri M, Ramsay G, Sevransky J, Thompson BT, Townsend S, Vender JS, Zimmerman JL, Vincent JL (2008) Surviving Sepsis Campaign: international guidelines for management of severe sepsis and septic shock: 2008. Intensive Care Med 34:17–60

Ferrer R, Artigas A, Levy MM, Blanco J, González-Días G, Garnacho-Montero J, Ibáñez J, Palencia E, Quintana M, de la Torre-Prados MV, Edusepsis Study Group (2008) Improvement in process of care and outcome after a multicenter severe sepsis educational program in Spain. JAMA 299:2294–2303

Gao F, Melody T, Daniels DF, Giles S, Fox S (2005) The impact of compliance with 6-hour and 24-hour sepsis bundles on hospital mortality in patients with severe sepsis: a prospective observational study. Crit Care 9:R764–R770

GRADE Working Group (2004) Grading quality of evidence and strength of recommendations. Br Med J 328:1–8

Grégoire G, Derderian F, Le Lorier J (1995) Selecting the language of the publications included in a meta-analysis: is there a tower of babel bias? J Clin Epidemiol 48:159–163

Grilli R, Magrini N, Penna A, Mura G, Liberati A (2000) Practice guidelines developed by specialty societies. The need for a critical appraisal. Lancet 355:103–106

Grimshaw JM, Russell IT (1993) Achieving health gain through clinical guidelines. I: developing scientifically valid guidelines. Qual Health Care 2:243–248

Grol R (2010) Has guideline development gone astray? Yes. Br Med J 340:c306. doi:10.1136/bmj.c306

Guyatt G, Gutterman D, Baumann MH, Addrizzo-Harris D, Hylek EM, Phillips B (2006) Grading strength of recommendations and quality of evidence in clinical guidelines: report from an American College of Chest Physicians task force. Chest 129:174–182

Institute of Medicine (2009) Conflict of interest in medical research, education and practice. National Academics Press, Washington

Jaeschke R, Guyatt GH, Dellinger P, Schünemann H, Levy MM, Kunz R, Norris S, Bion J, GRADE Working Group (2008) Use of GRADE grid to reach decisions on clinical practice guidelines when consensus is elusive. Br Med J 337:a744. doi:10.1136/bmj.a744

Kanji S, Perreault MM, Chant C, Williamson D, Burry L (2007) Evaluating the use of Drotrecogin alfa (activated) in adult severe sepsis: a Canadian multicenter observational study. Intensive Care Med 33:517–523

Landucci D (2004) The surviving sepsis guidelines: "lost in translation". Crit Care Med 32: 1598–1600

Levy MM, Pronovost PJ, Dellinger RP, Townsend S, Resar RK, Clemmer TP, Ramsay G (2004) Sepsis change bundles: converting guidelines into meaningful change in behavior and clinical outcome. Crit Care Med 320:S595–S597

Machado FR, Freitas FGR (2008) Controversies of surviving sepsis campaign bundles: should we use them? Shock 30:34–40

Marwick C, Davey P (2009) Care bundles: the holy grail of infectious risk management in hospital? Curr Opin Infect Dis 22:364–369

Poole D, Bertolini G, Garattini S (2008) Errors in the approval process and post-marketing evaluation of drotrecogin alfa (activated) for the treatment of severe sepsis. Lancet Infect Dis 9:67–72

Pronovost P, Needham D, Berenholtz S, Sinopoli D, Chu H, Cosgrove S, Sexton B, Hyzy R, Welsh R, Roth G, Bander J, Kepros J, Goeschel C (2006) An intervention to decrease catheter-related bloodstream infections in the ICU. N Engl J Med 355:2725–2732

Schünemann HJ, Jaeschke R, Cook DJ, Bria WF, El-Solh AA, Ernst A, Fahy BF, Gould MK, Horan KL, Krishnan JA, Manthous CA, Maurer JR, McNicholas WT, Oxman AD, Rubenfeld G, Turino GM, Guyatt G, ATS Documents Development and Implementation Committee (2006) An official ATS statement: grading the quality of evidence and strength of recommendations in ATS guidelines and recommendations. Am J Respir Crit Care Med 174:605–614

Shaneyfelt TM, Mayo-Smith MF, Rothwangl J (1999) Are guidelines following guidelines? The methodological quality of clinical practice guidelines in the peer-reviewed medical literature. JAMA 281:1900–1905

Shekelle PG, Woolf SH, Eccles M, Grimshaw J (1999) Clinical guidelines: developing guidelines. Br Med J 318:593–596

The AGREE Collaboration (2003) Development and validation of an international appraisal instrument for assessing the quality of clinical practice guidelines: the AGREE project. Qual Saf Health Care 12:18–23

Thomas KW (2007) Adoption of sepsis bundles in the emergency room and intensive care unit: a model for quality improvement. Crit Care Med 35:1210–1212

Wip C, Napolitano L (2009) Bundles to prevent ventilator-associated pneumonia: how valuable are they? Curr Opin Infect Dis 22:159–166

PIRO Concept and Clinical Failure

4

Thiago Lisboa and Jordi Rello

4.1 Introduction

In 2001, a consensus conference on sepsis definitions was convened, sponsored by several major medical societies (Levy et al. 2003). The participants at this meeting agreed that the SIRS concept was not helpful and should no longer be used per se, but rather that the systemic inflammatory response syndrome (SIRS) criteria should be incorporated into a longer list of signs of sepsis. This list includes biological signs of inflammation (e.g., increased concentrations of C-reactive protein [CRP] or procalcitonin), hemodynamic parameters [e.g., increased cardiac output, low systemic vascular resistance (SVR), low oxygen extraction ratio], signs of altered tissue perfusion (e.g., altered skin perfusion, reduced urine output), and signs of organ dysfunction (e.g., increased urea and creatinine, low platelet count or other coagulation abnormalities, and hyperbilirubinemia).

A system for the grading of sepsis uses clinical and laboratory parameters to aid diagnosis and patient classification, with each element being divided according to degree of involvement (e.g., infection can be classified as localized, extended, or generalized; immune response can be classified as limited, appropriate, or excessive; organ dysfunction can be classified as mild, moderate, severe) (Vincent 2009;

Thiago Lisboa (✉)
Critical Care Department and Infection Control Committee,
Hospital de Clinicas de Porto Alegre,
Porto Alegre, Brazil

Intensive Care Unit, Hospital Santa Rita, Rede Institucional
de Pesquisa e Inovação em Medicina Intensiva (RIPIMI),
Complexo Hospitalar Santa Casa, Porto Alegre, Brazil
e-mail: tlisboa@hotmail.com

J. Rello
Critical Care Department, Vall d'Hebron University Hospital,
Ps. Vall d'Hebron 119-129, Anexe AG-5a planta,
08035 Barcelona, Spain

J. Rello (eds.), *Sepsis Management*,
DOI 10.1007/978-3-642-03519-7_4, © Springer-Verlag Berlin Heidelberg 2012

Moreno et al. 2009). This approach may be useful for assessment of patients with higher risk for clinical failure and allow a follow-up and tailoring of the treatment in order to obtain optimal therapeutics.

4.2 Why the PIRO Concept?

A sepsis severity staging system focused on predisposition, insult, deleterious response, and organ failure (PIRO), and interaction among these different domains, could provide a useful basis for severity assessment and has potential for identifying specific subgroups for therapeutic interventions.

The complexity of sepsis might be better understood after assessment of these aspects of the disease. Predisposition factors such as the genetic profile of an individual are likely to be a major determinant of the lifetime predisposition to sepsis, and progress continues to be made in identifying relevant candidate genes. But the presence of comorbid conditions and age are also important predisposing factors that affect outcomes in pneumonia patients. The site of infection, and the nature and spread of the pathogen within the body are also important features, including the presence of bacteremia and radiological spread pattern. Although some elements of the variables that affect the host response to infection are easy to identify (age, nutritional status, sex, co-morbid conditions, and so on), others are more complex and arise from interactions among inflammation, coagulation, and sepsis. Development of shock and hypoxemia are important factors related with the host response to infection. Use of biomarkers might help to identify response patterns, helping to assess severity. Finally, development of organ dysfunction is a clear sign of poor evolution (Rosolem et al. 2010; Rello 2008).

Severe sepsis occurs as a result of a wide array of community-acquired and nosocomial infections including pneumonia, peritonitis, soft-tissue infection, meningitis, and viral diseases. Septic patients represent a heterogeneous group of severely ill patients. The severity of illness is certainly due to a combination of the type and intensity of the initial insult, impacting on a patient with comorbidities and individual genetic backgrounds that imply different patterns of immune response. The combination of the previously mentioned factors may result in organ dysfunction and death. Sepsis should not be seen as a disease, but as a syndrome encompassing a group of diseases. Oncologists learned this about evaluating cancer patients long ago. Cancer has many etiologies with significantly distinct clinical courses and therapeutic responses. The TNM model divides the patients with solid tumors according to "T," which refers to tumor characteristics such as size and histology; "N," which identifies the presence of metastasis to regional lymph nodes; and "M," which indicates the presence of distant metastases. Each area of the system is correlated with the probability of survival at 5 years and response to therapy (Marshall et al. 2003).

Due to these similarities, the PIRO concept was proposed with the aim to improve sepsis staging. In addition, organizing these patients into more homogeneous groups may help to improve patient management, determine the prognosis, and aid the inclusion of such patients in clinical studies (Rabello et al. 2009).

4.2.1   Predisposition

Premorbid factors such as age, gender, comorbidities, and the presence and degree of immunosuppression have an impact on the prognosis of patients with sepsis, influencing both the course of the disease and the management of patients. In addition, genetic variability has become increasingly important in determining the risk of death in septic patients.

Racial differences (Vincent 2009), and age and gender differences (Martin et al. 2006; Wichmann et al. 2000; Romo et al. 2004; Vincent et al. 2006) may have an impact on outcomes. Chronic predisposing conditions such as cirrhosis, diabetes, and chronic obstructive pulmonary disease (COPD) and immunosuppression may predispose patients to sepsis, specific pathogens, and worse outcomes. However, each factor may have a different impact on the other three PIRO components (Vincent 2009), affecting the magnitude of response (e.g., immunosuppression) or increasing the risk for development of acute organ dysfunction (e.g., chronic renal failure). These are complex relationships with multiple confounding factors, and further research is needed to clearly define which factors should be taken into account and to identify how knowledge of increased risks can be translated into improved clinical outcomes.

4.2.2   Infection

In the case of sepsis, the insult to the body is the infection, and the characteristics of the insult are its site, type, and extension, which have great impact on the prognosis (Rosolem et al. 2010). Just as the "T" in the TNM system describes the aspect of the surgically treatable cancer, the "I" describes that aspect of the septic process that responds to conventional anti-infective therapy. Four key aspects related to the underlying infection can influence management and prognosis in patients with sepsis: the source, degree, hospital-acquired versus community-acquired, and microorganism involved (Vincent et al. 2003a). Recently, studies have proposed new strategies to evaluate the infection and, consequently, to increase our ability to accurately stratify the severity of the disease. In this context, our group recently tested the hypothesis that bacterial load may be associated with outcomes in patients with pneumococcal pneumonia. Patients with $\geq 10^3$ copies/mL of *Streptococcus pneumoniae* DNA in their blood were associated with having a higher risk for septic shock ($OR = 8.0$), need for mechanical ventilation ($OR = 10.5$), and hospital mortality ($OR = 5.43$) (Rello et al. 2009). Whereas previous studies have suggested that severe sepsis is related to delay in therapy or an exaggerated host inflammatory response, this study suggests for the first time that insult, the bacterial burden, also plays a key role in the development multiple organ dysfunction syndrome (MODS). In addition, data on the virulence of microorganisms may provide valuable clues to the development of strategies directed at pathogen-specific targets (Veesenmeyer et al. 2009). Also, the emergence of a community-acquired methicillin-resistant *Staphylococcus aureus* (MRSA) strain has increased concerns about the role of exotoxins and other bacterial products in the pathogenesis of severe infections, such as Panton-Valentine leukocidin and hematoxin. In cases of pneumococcal pneumonia, the role of toxins such as pneumolysin in the pathophysiology and new therapeutic possibilities targeting these toxins should also be further assessed.

4.2.3 Response

Response represents the host response to infection, and it is the component of sepsis responsible for most adverse events. Modulation of the host response to infection has been proposed for decades with limited efficacy (Eichacker et al. 2002). It is proposed that selection of specific biological markers have to be tailored to the treatment strategy being employed. In the same way as hormone receptor status is used to stratify patients with breast carcinoma, an indicator of dysregulation of the coagulation system might be valuable for making a decision about whether to institute therapy with drotrecogin alfa (activated) (Vincent 2009), and the adrenal function may predict the response to corticosteroids (Oppert et al. 2005; Annane et al. 2002). However, due to controversial results, tailored-therapy strategies based on biomarkers are yet to be validated in patients with severe sepsis (Marshall et al. 2009).

Response modulation, with the use of macrolides for example, has been associated with improved survival in patients with severe community-acquired pneumonia. This effect is independent of their antimicrobial activity and seems to be associated with the immunomodulatory effects on the cytokine response to macrolides (Parnham 2005). This effect is the likely explanation for the improved survival found with macrolide combination therapy of bacteremic pneumococcal pneumonia. Biomarkers such as cytokines, CRP, procalcitonin, and cortisol identified as markers of host response to sepsis may improve traditional scoring factors in predicting outcomes and guiding response to therapy (Póvoa 2008), but this approach has yet to be validated.

4.2.4 Organ Dysfunction

By analogy with the TNM system, the presence of organ dysfunction in sepsis is similar to the presence of metastatic disease in cancer and is an important determinant of prognosis (Rodriguez et al. 2009). In a PIRO-based approach to a patient with severe sepsis, the presence, number, and severity of organ dysfunctions may be useful not only to predict prognosis, but also to predict the response to adjunctive therapies (Bernard et al. 2001). Organ dysfunction in severe sepsis is not a simple "present" or "absent" variable, but presents a continuous spectrum of varying severity in different organs over time (Vincent et al. 2003b). The degree of organ involvement can be assessed with various scoring systems, such as the sequential organ failure assessment (Vincent et al. 1998) (SOFA). Thus, with repeated scores, a dynamic picture of the effects of sepsis on individual or global organ dysfunction can be developed. Sequential assessment of the SOFA score during the first few days of ICU admission has been shown to be a good indicator of prognosis, with an increase in SOFA score during the first 48 h in the ICU predicting a mortality rate of at least 50% (Ferreira et al. 2001).

4.3 PIRO Concept and Clinical Failure

Early clinical recognition of therapeutic failure is of paramount importance if corrective measures are to be taken. While this will intuitively make sense to clinicians, data available on this issue are very limited. Several studies have suggested that clinical failure might be assessed through clinical resolution parameters to discriminate patients who are responding to antibiotic treatment from those who are not.

In VAP patients, the performance of a systematic approach to clinical variables with the Clinical Pulmonary Infection Score (CPIS) to identify which patients with VAP are responding to therapy has been described. Only hypoxemia, a clinical response aspect, was discovered to distinguish survivors from nonsurvivors as early as day 3 of therapy for VAP. Moreover, they reported that the PaO_2/FiO_2 ratio improves over 250 in survivors, and this improvement happens before the improvement of the other components of the score (white blood cell count, fever, secretions, and radiographic abnormalities). Thus, the PaO_2/FiO_2 ratio might represent a very accurate and rapid measure of the patient's response to therapy and can tailor the appropriate duration of therapy (Luna et al. 2003).

Our group described that changes in clinical resolution parameters, such as fever, hypoxemia, or WBC count, are associated with clinical response to infection and significant differences in the clinical course of VAP according the pathogen associated with the VAP episode (Vidaur et al. 2005, 2008). In addition, our group described the relevance of using C-reactive protein, a response biomarker, as a surrogate for an appropriate empirical antibiotic treatment, suggesting that in those patients whose CRP levels fail to decrease after 4 days of antibiotic treatment, recognizing clinical failure and reassessing the patient are necessary (Lisboa et al. 2008b). These studies, although specific for VAP, show how clinical variables included in a systematic PIRO approach might help to assess clinical evolution and clinical failure (Lisboa et al. 2008a).

Optimization of therapy based on this novel approach is a strategy that should be evaluated, as higher risk patients might benefit from more aggressive strategies or adjunctive therapy. As PIRO allows a more appropriate stratification of patients into different severity groups, clinical trials designed to evaluate therapeutic strategies for severe sepsis patients should use this tool in analysis of outcomes. It might help to identify specific subgroups of patients who would benefit more from specific therapeutic strategies. Knowledge of the severity of illness and risk stratification allowed by a PIRO system approach could be a crucial therapy optimization and minimize the risk of clinical failure.

References

Annane D, Sébille V, Charpentier C, Bollaert PE, François B, Korach JM et al (2002) Effect of treatment with low doses of hydrocortisone and fludrocortisone on mortality in patients with septic shock. JAMA 288(7):862–871, Erratum in: JAMA. 2008;300(14):1652. Chaumet-Riffaut, Philippe [corrected to Chaumet-Riffaud, Philippe]

Bernard GR, Vincent JL, Laterre PF, LaRosa SP, Dhainaut JF, Lopez-Rodriguez A, Steingrub JS, Garber GE, Helterbrand JD, Ely EW, Fisher CJ Jr, Recombinant human protein C Worldwide Evaluation in Severe Sepsis (PROWESS) study group (2001) Efficacy and safety of recombinant human activated protein C for severe sepsis. N Engl J Med 344(10):699–709

Eichacker PQ, Gerstenberger EP, Banks SM, Cui X, Natanson C (2002) Meta-analysis of acute lung injury and acute respiratory distress syndrome trials testing low tidal volumes. Am J Respir Crit Care Med 166(11):1510–1514

Ferreira FL, Bota DP, Bross A, Mélot C, Vincent JL (2001) Serial evaluation of the SOFA score to predict outcome in critically ill patients. JAMA 286(14):1754–1758

Levy MM, Fink MP, Marshall JC, Abraham E, Angus D, Cook D, Cohen J, Opal SM, Vincent JL, Ramsay G, SCCM/ESICM/ACCP/ATS/SIS (2003) 2001 SCCM/ESICM/ACCP/ATS/SIS International Sepsis Definitions Conference. Crit Care Med 31(4):1250–1256

Lisboa T, Diaz E, Sa-Borges M et al (2008a) The ventilator-associated pneumonia PIRO score: a tool for predicting ICU mortality and health-care resources use in ventilator-associated pneumonia. Chest 134(6):1208–1216

Lisboa T, Seligman R, Diaz E et al (2008b) C-reactive protein correlates with bacterial load and appropriate antibiotic therapy in suspected ventilator-associated pneumonia. Crit Care Med 36(1):166–171

Luna CM, Blancazo D, Niederman MS et al (2003) Resolution of ventilator-associated pneumonia: prospective evaluation of the clinical pulmonary infection score as an early clinical predictor of outcome. Crit Care Med 31(3):676–682

Marshall JC, Vincent JL, Fink MP, Cook DJ, Rubenfeld G, Foster D et al (2003) Measures, markers and mediators: toward a staging system for clinical sepsis. A report of the Fifth Toronto Sepsis Roundtable, Toronto, Ontario, Canada, October 25–26, 2000. Crit Care Med 31(5):1560–1567

Marshall JC, Reinhart K, International Sepsis Forum (2009) Biomarkers of sepsis. Crit Care Med 37(7):2290–2298

Martin GS, Mannino DM, Moss M (2006) The effect of age on the development and outcome of adult sepsis. Crit Care Med 34(1):15–21

Moreno RP, Diogo AC, Afonso S (2009) Risk stratification in severe sepsis: organ failure scores or PIRO? In: Rello J, Díaz E, Rodríguez A (eds) Management of sepsis: the PIRO approach. Springer, New York, pp 1–9

Oppert M, Schindler R, Husung C, Offermann K, Gräf KJ, Boenisch O et al (2005) Low-dose hydrocortisone improves shock reversal and reduces cytokine levels in early hyperdynamic septic shock. Crit Care Med 33(11):2457–2464

Parnham MJ (2005) Immunomodulatory effects of antimicrobials in the therapy of respiratory tract infections. Curr Opin Infect Dis 18(2):125–131

Póvoa P (2008) Serum markers in community-acquired pneumonia and ventilator-associated pneumonia. Curr Opin Infect Dis 21(2):157–162

Rabello L, Rosolem M, Leal J et al (2009) Understanding the PIRO concept: from theory to clinical practice. Rev Bras Ter Intensiva 22(1):64–68

Rello J (2008) Demographics, guidelines and clinical experience in severe community-acquired pneumonia. Crit Care 12(Suppl 6):S2

Rello J, Lisboa T, Lujan T, Gallego M, Kee C, Kay I, Lopez D, Waterer GW, DNA-Neumococo Study Group (2009) Severity of pneumococcal pneumonia associated with genomic bacterial load. Chest 136(3):832–840

Rodriguez A, Lisboa T, Blot S, Martin-Loeches I, Solé-Violan J, De Mendoza D, Rello J, Community-Acquired Pneumonia Intensive Care Units (CAPUCI) Study Investigators (2009) Mortality in ICU patients with bacterial community-acquired pneumonia: when antibiotics are not enough. Intensive Care Med 35(3):430–438

Romo H, Amaral AC, Vincent JL (2004) Effect of patient sex on intensive care unit survival. Arch Intern Med 164(1):61–65

Rosolem M, Rabello L, Leal J et al (2010) Understanding the PIRO concept: from theory to clinical practice – Part 2. Rev Bras Ter Intensiva 21(4):425–431

Veesenmeyer JL, Hauser AR, Lisboa T, Rello J (2009) Pseudomonas aeruginosa virulence and therapy: evolving translational strategies. Crit Care Med 37(5):1777–1786

Vidaur L, Gualis B, Rodriguez A et al (2005) Clinical resolution in patients with suspicion of ventilator-associated pneumonia: a cohort study comparing patients with and without acute respiratory distress syndrome. Crit Care Med 33(6):1248–1253

Vidaur L, Planas K, Sierra R et al (2008) Ventilator-associated pneumonia: impact of organisms on clinical resolution and medical resources utilization. Chest 133(3):625–632, Epub 2008 Jan 15

Vincent JL (2009) PIRO: the key of success? In: Rello J, Diaz E, Rodríguez A (eds) Management of sepsis: the PIRO approach. Springer, New York, pp 1–9

Vincent JL, de Mendonça A, Cantraine F, Moreno R, Takala J, Suter PM et al (1998) Use of the SOFA score to assess the incidence of organ dysfunction/failure in intensive care units: results of a multicenter, prospective study. Working group on "sepsis-related problems" of the European Society of Intensive Care Medicine. Crit Care Med 26(11):1793–1800

Vincent JL, Opal S, Torres A, Bonten M, Cohen J, Wunderink R (2003a) The PIRO concept: I is for infection. Crit Care 7(3):252–255

Vincent JL, Wendon J, Groeneveld J, Marshall JC, Streat S, Carlet J (2003b) The PIRO concept: O is for organ dysfunction. Crit Care 7(3):260–264

Vincent JL, Sakr Y, Sprung CL, Ranieri VM, Reinhart K, Gerlach H, Moreno R, Carlet J, Le Gall JR, Payen D, Sepsis Occurrence in Acutely Ill Patients Investigators (2006) Sepsis in European intensive care units: results of the SOAP study. Crit Care Med 34(2):344–353

Wichmann MW, Inthorn D, Andress HJ, Schildberg FW (2000) Incidence and mortality of severe sepsis in surgical intensive care patients: the influence of patient gender on disease process and outcome. Intensive Care Med 26(2):167–172

PIRO-Based Approach for Sepsis in Immunocompromised Patients: What's Different?

5

Jorge I.F. Salluh, Fernando Augusto Bozza, André Miguel Japiassu, and Márcio Soares

The frequency of immunocompromised patients has increased dramatically over the last decades because of the appearance of human immunodeficiency virus (HIV)-related opportunistic infections since the 1980s and the increasing number of patients with cancer receiving aggressive antineoplastic treatments, solid organ and bone marrow transplantations, newer immunosuppressive therapies (e.g., anti-TNF) for rheumatic and inflammatory bowel diseases, and other sources of immunosuppression, such as sepsis-associated immunosuppression. This major epidemiologic trend has also produced a significant impact on the critical care population. Presently, a wide array of immunocompromised patients are being admitted to intensive care mainly because of severe infections, but also routinely for other reasons such as postoperative care, monitoring for treatment-related toxicity and other associated medical causes (i.e.,-cardiovascular diseases). They represent a group of patients whose admission to the intensive care unit (ICU) is associated with significant morbidity and mortality not only as a result of the primary reason for the ICU stay, but

J.I.F. Salluh (✉) • M. Soares
Postgraduate Program, Instituto Nacional de Câncer,
Rio de Janeiro, RJ, Brazil

D'Or Institute for Research and Education,
Rio de Janeiro, RJ, Brazil
e-mail: jorgesalluh@yahoo.com.br

F.A. Bozza
D'Or Institute for Research and Education
Rio de Janeiro, RJ, Brazil

ICU, Instituto de Pesquisa Evandro Chagas,
Rio de Janeiro, RJ, Brazil

A.M. Japiassu
D'Or Institute for Research and Education,
Rio de Janeiro, RJ, Brazil

J. Rello (eds.), *Sepsis Management*,
DOI 10.1007/978-3-642-03519-7_5, © Springer-Verlag Berlin Heidelberg 2012

also because of the high susceptibility to hospital-acquired complications, especially nosocomial infections.

Despite the recent evidence demonstrating improved outcomes in critically ill cancer and HIV/AIDS patients (Japiassu et al. 2010; Soares et al. 2010a, b; Azoulay et al. 2001; Coquet et al. 2010), the care of these patients remains a major challenge for intensivists and infectious disease consultants. Notwithstanding the significant advances in prophylactic regimens, better hematologic support, use of granulocyte colony-stimulating factors for the reversion of neutropenia and the use of highly active antiretroviral therapies (HAART) for HIV, ICU admission still represents a major burden with high morbidity, mortality rates, length of stay and associated costs. Since most of the disease burden in these patients is associated with the occurrence of severe infections, appropriate diagnosis as well as risk assessment combined with prompt initiation of adequate broad-spectrum anti-infective therapies is the cornerstone for their management. Evidently, the superimposition of multiple sources of immunosuppression, such as disease-related immune defects, use of corticosteroids or other immunosuppressive agents, neutropenia and critical illness-related immunodeficiency make the diagnostic and therapeutic efforts troublesome. Therefore, the development of systematic approaches to evaluate these patients prompting the early and correct initiation of anti-infective treatment should be sought.

In this chapter, we present a review of the current epidemiology and management of sepsis in patients with cancer or HIV-related immunosuppression, aiming to provide a systematic approach for the assessment of these patients at bedside.

5.1 Sepsis in HIV/AIDS Patients

5.1.1 Epidemiology

The improvement of HIV/AIDS management has led to changes in the observed clinical manifestations and outcomes of these patients in ICUs, with a decreasing trend in admissions due to opportunistic infections, while an opposing trend has been observed for other infectious and metabolic diseases (Pacheco et al. 2009). Severe sepsis has emerged as a common cause of hospital admission for those living with HIV/AIDS (Afessa and Green 2000; Huang et al. 2006; Casalino et al. 2004). A cohort of critically ill HIV/AIDS patients started in 1981 has clearly demonstrated that the incidence of acute respiratory failure as the main cause of ICU admission (for example, caused by *Pneumocystis jiroveci* pneumonia) has been reducing since the 1990s, while admission for sepsis has been consistently increasing, mainly in the period of 2000–2003 (Huang et al. 2006). In addition, studies demonstrate that bacterial infections are becoming increasingly prevalent in patients with HIV admitted to the ICU, irrespective of HAART use (Table 5.1) (Rosen and Narasimhan 2006; Davaro and Thirumalai 2007; Grinsztejn et al. 2009).

Table 5.1 Characteristics of studies with critically ill septic HIV/AIDS patients

First author (year)	N	Inclusion period	Study design	Sepsis on admission (%)	Sepsis criteria	Mortality (%)
Afessa (2000)	169	1995–1999	Prospective cohort	15	Bone et al. (1992)	30
Morris (2002)	354	1996–1999	Retrospective longitudinal	12	Not specified	29
Narasimhan (2004)	63	2001	Retrospective	16	Not specified	29
Casalino (2004)	230	1995–1999	Prospective cohort	22	Bone et al. (1992)	20
Vincent (2004)	236	1995–1996 1998–2000	Retrospective and prospective concurrent cohorts	28	Septic shock; Not specified	25
Khouli (2005)	259	1997–1999	Retrospective longitudinal	13	Bone et al. (1992)	39
Palacios (2006)	49	1990–2003	Retrospective longitudinal	2	Not specified	57
Dickson (2007)	102	1999–2005	Retrospective longitudinal	9	Not specified	23
Powell (2009)	311	2000–2004	Retrospective longitudinal	20	Not specified	31
Croda (2009)	278		Retrospective cohort	31	Not specified	55
Barbier (2009)	147	1996–2006	Retrospective cohort	Not shown	–	20
Coquet (2010)	284	1996–2005	Retrospective	24	Not specified	14
Japiassú (2010)	88	2006–2008	Prospective cohort	20	Severe sepsis; Bone et al. (1992)	49

Fig. 5.1 Survival up to 28 days (**a**) and 6 months (**b**) is significantly affected by the presence of severe sepsis/septic shock in critically ill HIV/AIDS patients (Adapted from Japiassu et al. (2010))

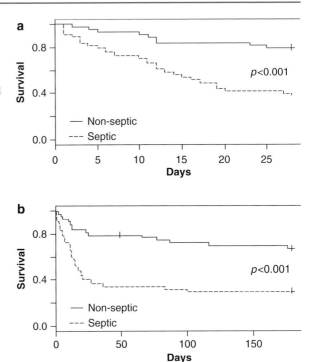

Epidemiological studies have shown that up to 10% of septic patients are individuals with HIV/AIDS, with a wide variation according to regional differences in the prevalence of HIV infection and ICU admission practices (Angus et al. 2001; Martin et al. 2003; Annane et al. 2003; Brun-Buisson et al. 2004; Andreu Ballester et al. 2008; Blanco et al. 2008; Khwannimit and Bhurayanontachai 2009; Beale et al. 2009). Even with the known greater incidence of sepsis in the HIV/AIDS population, an analysis of a large US database of septic patients showed that the septic HIV patients had lower rates of ICU admission compared to non-HIV groups (Mrus et al. 2005). However, such observations may be influenced by potential selection biases, as septic HIV/AIDS patients had lower chances of being admitted to the ICU, even when compared to other septic subpopulations with worse outcomes, such as severe hepatic disease and metastatic cancer. Moreover, severe sepsis is a major determinant of short- and medium-term outcomes in the HIV/AIDS population admitted to the ICU (Japiassu et al. 2010), whereas HIV-related factors, such as time since AIDS diagnosis, CD4 cell count and the use of HAART, are mainly related to long-term mortality (Fig. 5.1) (Coquet et al. 2010; Davis et al. 2008). In a cohort of mechanically ventilated HIV/AIDS patients with acute lung injury, lower tidal volume ventilation was associated with reduced mortality, whereas the use of HAART had no impact on the outcome (Davis et al. 2008). Another retrospective study showed that comorbidities and organ dysfunctions, but not HIV-related variables (newly diagnosed AIDS, CD4 cell count, viral load, previous opportunistic infections), were associated with hospital mortality (Coquet et al. 2010).

5.1.2   Predisposing Factors and Characteristics of Infection in Critically Ill HIV/AIDS Patients

HIV-related factors, and the consequent immunodeficiency, are implicated in the predisposition to bacterial, viral, fungal and parasitic infections. Low levels of CD4 cell count and high levels of viral load correlate with the degree of immunodeficiency. It is known that CD4 cell counts lower than $200/mm^3$ are associated with increased incidence of opportunistic infections, such as *P. jiroveci* pneumonia, neurotoxoplasmosis and cytomegalovirus infections, and common bacterial infections as well. In a randomized controlled trial evaluating cost-saving strategies of HAART, stopping treatment when the CD4 count was higher than 350 cells per mm^3 was associated with increased morbidity (Danel et al. 2006). In that study, the most frequent severe events were attributed to invasive bacterial diseases. Therefore, even HIV/AIDS patients with moderately diminished CD4 cell counts are more prone to serious bacterial infections. Conversely, the use of HAART has increased the lifespan of HIV/AIDS patients in the long term. Interestingly, in HIV patients maintaining a CD4 count higher than 500 cells/mm^3, mortality rates were comparable to the general population after the 6th year after HAART initiation (Lewden et al. 2007). But when patients receiving HAART are admitted to the hospital and to the ICU, this relative protection of HAART disappears, as demonstrated in recent studies (Coquet et al. 2010).

In a general view, even other HIV-related variables (CD4 count and viral load) have a smaller impact on the short and medium-term outcomes of the hospitalized HIV/AIDS population (Japiassu et al. 2010; Coquet et al. 2010; Davis et al. 2008). Since the introduction of HAART, the incidence of bacteremia in HIV patients has decreased significantly (Tumbarello et al. 2000; Meynard et al. 2003). In patients receiving cotrimoxazole prophylaxis against opportunistic *P. jiroveci* infection, there is protection against community-acquired bacteremia, as this antibiotic is effective against some pathogens (e.g., *Salmonella sp*, methicillin-sensitive *Staphylococcus sp* and pneumococci). Although these strategies are effective against community-acquired infections, there are no specific pharmacological measures to prevent hospital-acquired infections in this population. HIV/AIDS hospitalized patients are especially susceptible to nosocomial infections, mainly pneumonia and catheter-related bloodstream infections (Japiassu et al. 2010; Tumbarello et al. 2000; Meynard et al. 2003; Lambotte et al. 2000). Pneumonia is the most common nosocomial infection associated with sepsis in the HIV/AIDS population, and it is generally caused by the same hospital-acquired bacteria as in non-HIV hospitalized patients: *Pseudomonas aeruginosa*, *Enterobacteriaceae*, *Staphylococcus aureus* and *Staphylococcus epidermidis* (Japiassu et al. 2010; Mrus et al. 2005). The occurrence of bacteremia is also common in the hospitalized HIV/AIDS population, and it is derived from invasive peripheral or central venous catheters, but they can be diagnosed as primary bacteremias. Chronic HIV infection and AIDS themselves can predispose to intestinal bacterial translocation, as suggested by the presence of high serum lipopolysaccharide both in a simian model of immunodeficiency virus infection and in HIV-infected individuals (Brenchley et al. 2006). Indeed, the prevalence of bacteremia in the HIV/AIDS hospitalized population

Table 5.2 PIRO factors possibly related to HIV/AIDS patients

PIRO system	
Predisposing factors	HIV related factors: advanced AIDS diagnosis, low CD4 cell count, high viral load, HAART, prolonged hospitalization
Infection characteristics	Pneumonia; bacteremia/fungemia; opportunistic organisms (*P. jiroveci*, Mycobacteria, *Histoplasma sp.*, *Cryptococcus neoformans*, Cytomegalovirus); antibiotic-resistant microorganisms (CA-MRSA, *Pseudomonas sp.*, ESBL-producing Enterobacteriaceae)
Response of the host to the infection	Fever; leucopenia; C reactive protein; procalcitonin
Organ dysfunctions	Acute lung injury; thrombocytopenia; renal insufficiency; elevated total bilirrubin

HIV human immunodeficiency virus, *AIDS* acquired immunodeficiency syndrome, *HAART* highly active antiretroviral therapy, *CA-MRSA* community-acquired methicilin-resistant *Staphylococcus aureus, ESBL* extended spectrum beta-lactamase

is exceedingly high (around 40%) both as catheter-related bacteremia and associated with another site of infection (Japiassu et al. 2010) (Table 5.2).

Other microorganisms associated with pneumonia, bacteremia and severe sepsis are also detected in HIV/AIDS patients. Although there is predominance of gram-negative and gram-positive bacteria causing severe invasive infections, *Mycobacterium tuberculosis*, *Histoplasma capsulatum* and *Cryptococcus neoformans* can occur in a subset of AIDS patients with lower CD4 cell counts (Bianchi et al. 2000; Sivasangeetha et al. 2007; Taniguchi et al. 2010). *M. tuberculosis*, which is a highly prevalent infective agent in developing countries, has also been described as a cause of bacteremia in AIDS patients (Japiassu et al. 2010; Grinsztejn et al. 2009; Arthur et al. 2001; Waddell et al. 2001).

5.1.3 Response to Infection in HIV-Infected Patients and the Development of Organ Dysfunctions

Biomarkers have been studied in the HIV/AIDS population. HIV infection itself is able to activate the production of cytokines during the chronic infection. A comparison study between HIV and control subjects revealed that the levels of TNF-alpha, IL-6, myeloperoxidase, soluble vascular cell adhesion molecule-1 and C reactive protein (CRP) were significantly higher in HIV-infected patients (Ross et al. 2009). In HIV-infected patients, slightly elevated concentrations of CRP are associated with long-term mortality (Tien et al. 2010). When HIV patients present acute infections, there is also a significant increase in CRP and procalcitonin, mainly when bacterial pathogens are implicated. In a study comparing HIV- and non-HIV-infected children with lower respiratory tract infections, CRP could help to identify the presence of bacteremia. Studies have proposed that procalcitonin may be a more specific marker of bacterial sepsis in HIV-infected patients, as no increase in other secondary infections, such as fungal, mycobacterial and viral organisms, was detected.

Schleicher et al. have also demonstrated that procalcitonin and CRP help in the differentiation of etiologic agents involved in community-acquired pneumonia, being higher for pneumococcal infections as compared to tuberculosis (Schleicher et al. 2005). Also considered as a marker of an acute pulmonary distress, the measurement of lactate dehydrogenase (LDH) is very useful in HIV/AIDS patients, since its levels are increased above 500–600 U/L when they present with pneumonia (mainly by *P. jiroveci*). LDH levels can guide physicians to proceed to the respiratory infection diagnosis and evaluation, which is the main source of severe sepsis in HIV-infected patients. LDH levels are increased not only by *P. jiroveci* pneumonia (when LDH levels are very high), but also bacterial pneumonia and tuberculosis.

In a retrospective cohort of HIV/AIDS critically ill patients in the post HAART era, ICU mortality was mainly associated with the presence of acute organ dysfunctions, such as shock, renal and liver failure (Coquet et al. 2010). In a multivariate analysis, initial neurological dysfunction (OR, 2.73; 95% CI, 1.16–6.46) and acute renal failure during the ICU stay (OR, 4.21; 95% CI, 1.63–10.92) were associated with increased mortality.

Respiratory dysfunction occurs frequently and is by far the leading reason for ICU admission in the HIV/AIDS population (Nickas and Wachter 2000; Morris et al. 2002; Powell et al. 2009). However, the severity of respiratory dysfunction is not well characterized in most studies. Nonetheless, it is quite clear that *P. jiroveci* and bacterial pneumonia are responsible for the majority of respiratory dysfunction cases requiring intensive care (Japiassu et al. 2010; Pacheco et al. 2009; Afessa and Green 2000; Huang et al. 2006; Morris et al. 2002; Powell et al. 2009). Acute lung injury was also present in 35% of 7,638 septic HIV-infected patients in a large retrospective American study (Mrus et al. 2005). Besides, the presence of a previous opportunistic infection may be most strongly predictive of hospital mortality among HIV-positive patients with acute lung injury (Mendez-Tellez et al. 2010). Thus, respiratory dysfunction must be promptly and carefully evaluated and treated in this population.

Besides lung injury, other aspects of organ dysfunction seem to play a special role in HIV patients. Decreases in platelet count are usually considered as a surrogate marker for hematological dysfunction in critically ill patients and can be an early sign of sepsis in the HIV/AIDS population. There is substantial clinical evidence that platelets are activated in chronic HIV infection and AIDS (Torre and Pugliese 2008). Platelets have a direct interaction with HIV-1 itself, playing a role in host defense during HIV-1 infection by limiting viral spread and probably by inactivating viral particles. Platelets may also play a role in endothelial dysfunction of HIV-1 infection, as the interaction between platelets and endothelial cells is involved in the pathogenesis of atherosclerosis in HIV/AIDS patients (Torre and Pugliese 2008). There is scarce evidence. The incidence of hematological dysfunction in septic HIV/AIDS patients seems to be more common than in non-HIV populations, and platelet counts below the threshold of 150,000/mm^3 in those patients is independently associated with hospital mortality (Jacob et al. 2009). Therefore, subsequent epidemiological studies exploring the nature and evolution of organ dysfunctions in critically ill HIV/AIDS patients are needed to allow better risk assessment and resource allocation for this patient population.

5.2   Sepsis in Cancer Patients

5.2.1   Epidemiology

As previously stated, patients with cancer are at increased risk for sepsis as a consequence of multiple mechanisms of immunosuppression imposed by the disease
itself and by aggressive treatments, including combined regimens of chemo-, radia-
tion- and immunotherapy, as well as high doses of steroids and hematopoietic stem
cell transplantation (HSCT) (Fox et al. 2010; Thirumala et al. 2010). Epidemiological
estimates of sepsis in cancer patients have been published in the previous decade
providing valuable information regarding this frequently lethal condition. In 1999,
there was a reported a rate of 1,640 cases of severe sepsis per 100,000 cancer patients
in the US (Williams et al. 2004). Subsequently, Danai et al. evaluated 854,000,000
hospitalizations occurring from 1979 and 2001 in the US, of which 1,784,445 were
cases of sepsis in cancer patients (Danai et al. 2006). In this large database, they
could demonstrate that the prevalence of cancer increased during the study period,
and so did sepsis prevalence.

In large studies, up to one in five patients admitted to ICUs with sepsis have
cancer (Angus et al. 2001; Annane et al. 2003; Vincent et al. 2009; Taccone et al.
2009), and, along this line, sepsis is a leading reason for ICU admission in patients
with cancer in tertiary hospitals and specialized cancer centers (Soares et al. 2010a;
Williams et al. 2004; Taccone et al. 2009). Angus et al. demonstrated that one in
every six patients with severe sepsis had an associated diagnosis of cancer and that
these patients have a 30% higher risk of death as compared to non-cancer patients
(Angus et al. 2001). Williams et al., evaluating more than 600,000 cancer-related
hospitalizations in a US six-state database, could show that up to one-third of them
were sepsis-related (Williams et al. 2004). When compared to non-cancer hospitalized patients, cancer patients with severe sepsis were older, had a higher proportion
of co-morbid conditions (31.8% vs. 28%) and were more likely to receive intensive
care (48% vs. 14.8%). Overall mortality was also higher (38% vs. 25%). Moreover,
when a national estimate was produced, it could be inferred that there are a 126,000
cases of severe sepsis each year in the cancer population, only in the US resulting in
almost 47,000 deaths. The study by Williams et al. also evaluated the resource use
and costs, demonstrating that severe sepsis cancer length of stay was significantly
longer (17 vs. 6.7 days, $p < 0.0001$), and so were hospital costs (\$27,400 USD vs.
\$8,700 USD). This translated to national cancer estimated costs of \$3.4 billion USD
in 1999 (Williams et al. 2004). Danai et al. showed similar results in another large
US database (Danai et al. 2006). These authors also showed that GI malignancies
were the most common (24%), followed by lung cancer (20%) and lymphoma
(14%), probably reflecting a combination of cancer type prevalence, age and immunosuppressive and aggressive surgical treatments. Interestingly, the source of infection was most often associated with the tumor site. Therefore, lung cancer patients
had predominantly pulmonary infections (42%), whereas prostate, gastrointestinal
and female reproductive cancer was associated with urinary or surgical site sepsis.
As expected, hematological malignancies, namely lymphoma, had higher rates of

blood stream infections (39%). Actually, among cancer patients, those with hematologic malignancies seem to have a significantly (up to 15 times) increased risk of severe sepsis (Williams et al. 2004; Danai et al. 2006) and a higher risk of death (Williams et al. 2004; Taccone et al. 2009; Benoit et al. 2003).

Cancer patients clearly present an elevated risk of death when diagnosed with severe sepsis, and this risk is significantly higher compared to non-cancer patients (Williams et al. 2004; Danai et al. 2006). ICU physicians are currently more optimistic as recent studies show that survival rates for these patients seem to be increasing (Taccone et al. 2009; Pene et al. 2008). Nonetheless, despite improvements in the outcomes over the last years, sepsis in these patients is still associated with high morbidity, mortality, costs and use of ICU resources (Williams et al. 2004; Benoit et al. 2003; Pene et al. 2008; Maschmeyer et al. 2003; Regazzoni et al. 2004; Larche et al. 2003).

5.2.2 Predictors of Sepsis Mortality in Cancer Patients

There are numerous studies evaluating clinical factors associated with short- and long-term mortality in cancer patients (Soares et al. 2005, 2006a, b, 2007a, b, 2008, 2010a, c; Azoulay et al. 2001; Darmon and Azoulay 2009). In these studies, mostly performed in specialized cancer centers, the factors often associated with the worst outcomes were: the severity and number of organ dysfunctions, a medical diagnosis at admission (as compared to surgical status), age and the presence of comorbidities. The diagnosis of cancer encompasses a wide array of diseases with diverse clinical characteristics and biological behavior. Designing studies to evaluate specific groups of critically ill patients with cancer can be a difficult task. Traditionally, patients have been grouped in two large categories: solid tumors and hematological malignancies. Solid tumors are usually staged according to disease extension as locoregional or metastatic disease. Conversely, the classification and staging of hematological malignancies is much more complex; most authors choose to separate them into large categories such as multiple myeloma, Hodgkin's disease, leukemia and non-Hodgkin's lymphoma. Despite its diversity, several common cancer-related factors may adversely affect the outcomes of patients with sepsis.

Not surprisingly, cancer-related factors are usually identified as strong predictors of adverse outcomes, mainly performance status and active cancer. Interestingly, studies in the last decade showed that neutropenia (of short duration) was no longer associated with worse outcomes. These predictive factors were observed over different cohorts of ICU cancer patients, including those who were mechanically ventilated and those with acute kidney injury, many of whom had been admitted to the ICU because of severe sepsis. Therefore, it is clear that several cancer-related factors may contribute to the decreased survival chance of these patients (Larche et al. 2003; Darmon and Azoulay 2009; Velasco et al. 2009). We believe the knowledge of such characteristics may help improve patient selection, providing adequate resource allocation and allowing early treatment to patients who will potentially benefit from intensive care (Soares et al. 2010a; Thiery et al. 2005; Soares and Azoulay 2009). In addition, a careful review of the prognostic impacts should be performed from time to time as they may lose their strength as a result of changes and improvements in clinical practice and patient care.

Interestingly, recent evidence shows that starting chemotherapy in the ICU can be life-saving for patients with a first presentation of a malignancy even when a severe infection is present (Vandijck et al. 2008). This is especially valid as the use of granulocyte colony-stimulating factors has reduced both the risk and duration of neutropenia in patients receiving chemotherapy.

Pene et al. have demonstrated that better patient selection and improvements in care and management of sepsis correlated with survival gains in patients with cancer and severe sepsis (Pene et al. 2008). In that study, 238 consecutive cancer patients admitted to the ICU with septic shock were evaluated, and the authors showed that mortality in recent years had actually dropped from 47% to 27.8% with the incorporation of sepsis protocols.

5.2.3 What Are the Pathogens We Should Look for and Treat in Cancer-Related Sepsis?

Although cancer patients are, as acknowledged, at increased risk of severe infections, the knowledge of the usual pathogens is helpful in guiding the initial management (Table 5.3). In the past years changes in the microbiology of cancer were reported; these significant changes have certainly changed the current therapeutic guidelines. Danai et al. demonstrated a significant increase in gram-positive sepsis from 26% in the early 1980s to 53% in 2001 (Danai et al. 2006). Other recent evidence of change is related to the significant role that *Stenotrophomonas maltophilia* infection may play. This pathogen, traditionally associated with non-severe infections, has been also implicated in a wider spectrum of serious infectious complications, including pneumonia, bloodstream, urinary and soft tissue-related sepsis (Safdar and Rolston 2007; Aisenberg et al. 2007). The frequency of *S. maltophilia* infections seems to be increasing, and previous carbapenem exposure is a major risk factor for its acquisition. Also, in ICU-acquired sepsis, the risk of multidrug-resistant pathogens is elevated (Vincent et al. 2009), and thorough knowledge of the local antimicrobial resistance patterns as well as patients' risk factors and previous exposure to antibiotics will aid in the choice of the empiric regimen to be started.

Table 5.3 Microbiology of sepsis in immunocompromised hosts

	Gram-positive bacteria	Gram-negative bacteria	Mycobacteria and Listeria	CMV and herpes viruses	Candida	Aspergillus and molds
Neutropenia	++	+++	–	–	+++	++
HSCT	+	+	+	+++	++	+++
Corticosteroids	+	+	++	+	++	++
HIV/AIDS	++	++	++	+	++	++

HSCT hematopoietic stem cell transplant, *CMV* cytomegalovirus, – not significant, + occasionally increased, ++ significant, +++ major concern

Nonetheless, despite the observation that bacterial infections are still associated with elevated mortality, studies show better outcomes in critically ill patients with infections caused by such agents when compared to sepsis due to other pathogens such as invasive fungal or viral infections (Benoit et al. 2003).

Many specific opportunistic infectious diseases may occur with the use of immunosuppressive regimens (Gea-Banacloche et al. 2004). Perhaps the use of systemic corticosteroids is the most classic and reported association. Corticosteroids are frequently employed in cancer patients for numerous reasons, such as in association with chemotherapy regimens, to diminish nausea, as an adjuvant therapy for rapidly growing and swelling tumors as well as brain metastasis. The effects on the immune system are numerous, including the reduction of chemokine and cytokine production, T-cell suppression and induction of apoptosis (Japiassu et al. 2009). The risk for opportunistic infections is particularly higher in patients receiving prolonged courses of corticosteroids or doses ≥0.5 mg/kg/day of prednisone. There is an increased risk of bacterial infections, but also of less common pathogens such as *Nocardia, P. Jirovecci*, mycobacteria, *Cryptococcus, Aspergillus* and *Stronglyloides,* even in previously immunocompetent patients. *Stronglyloides* infection may ensue even after a single dose of corticosteroids, but is more frequent with high, sustained doses in hematological patients where the disseminated form may be associated with typical (albeit rare) periumbilical cutaneous purpura and carries a high mortality (Salluh et al. 2005). *Aspergillus* infection has been more commonly identified in ICU patients (Vandewoude et al. 2006), probably as a consequence of the potential immunosuppression that follows severe sepsis (Benjamim et al. 2005), but it is still classically associated with the prolonged duration of neutropenia that follows myeloablative regimens. Furthermore, cytoreductive agents, anti-TNF and mycophenolate also induce immune dysfunction and are associated with an increased risk for opportunistic infections (Table 5.4). The knowledge of such risk factors is essential in order to have a perspective on the possible implicated pathogens and the most effective empirical anti-infective therapy to start for the patient.

There is a risk of respiratory and systemic viral infections in cancer patients, the most frequent agents being herpes (HHV), cytomegalovirus (CMV), Epstein-Barr

Table 5.4 Immunosuppressive drugs and susceptibility to infection

Drug	Immunosuppressive pattern	Infection
Corticosteroids	Inhibition of phagocytosis, T cell suppression	Bacterial, fungal, herpes and Strongyloides
Cyclosporine/Tacrolimus	Inhibits lymphocyte proliferation	No specific association
Cyclophosphamide	Inhibits lymphocyte proliferation	Bacterial, VZV
Azathioprine	Inhibits lymphocyte proliferation	Bacterial
Micofenolate	Antilymphoproliferative agent	CMV, VZV
Methotrexate	Inhibits lymphocyte proliferation	Listeria, Histoplasma, Pneumocystis
Fludarabine	Inhibits DNA synthesis	Listeria, Herpesvirus, Cryptococcus

CMV cytomegalovirus, *VZV* varicella-zoster virus

(EBV), adenovirus and influenza viruses. The use of corticosteroids and HSCT represent the main immunosuppressive risk factors. Although always challenging, a diagnosis of viral infection should be pursued in the flu season or when risk factors are present and patients feature severe respiratory failure without usual signs of bacterial infections at initial presentation.

5.2.4 A PIRO-Based Approach for Patients with Cancer or HIV/AIDS and Sepsis

Refinements in the information about the epidemiology, outcomes and risk-stratification of these patients are essential for future research, for assisting clinicians in decision-making, and for counseling patients and families. In the 2001 International Sepsis Definitions Conference, the PIRO concept was forged as a hypothetical framework for staging sepsis to improve the characterization of patients with sepsis in terms of Predisposition (i.e., predisposing factors and premorbid conditions), the nature and characteristics related to the underlying Infection, host Response and Organ dysfunctions (Angus et al. 2003). As acknowledged by the authors, the PIRO concept was conceived as a work in progress rather than a model to be immediately adopted, thus requiring extensive clinical investigation for its validation and for the identification of refinement opportunities. Seven years after the report of the revised criteria and definitions for sepsis, studies evaluating the PIRO concept remain scarce (Rubulotta et al. 2010; Rello et al. 2009; Lisboa et al. 2008). All above-mentioned arguments about the particularities of patients with cancer and immunosuppression help with this evaluation.

An interesting and intuitive utility for the PIRO approach is the structured patient evaluation based on this concept at the bedside. This PIRO-based approach could allow an individual evaluation, taking into account patient-specific characteristics, and should be further evaluated in clinical practice in the ICU.

In this sense, there is a lesson to be learned from studies that applied good stratification strategies in infectious diseases to guide therapeutic interventions. In the 1980s, long before the PIRO system was conceived, patients with *P. jirovecci* pneumonia and AIDS were stratified to receive steroids according to a PIRO-based approach. Then, patients with a T-cell type immunodeficiency (Predisposition), with *P. jirovecci*, the same infectious microorganism (Infection), presenting with hypoxemia (Response) and respiratory failure (Organ dysfunction) were considered eligible to receive adjunctive corticosteroids. This approach was successful and remains so even decades after its initial proposal.

In a similar approach, bringing together data on the PIRO domains could be conceptually useful to shed light on the challenging task of diagnosing and treating sepsis in cancer patients. The predisposing factors (i.e., specific immune defects, previous antimicrobial or immunosuppressive exposure), Infection (i.e., microbiologic data or clinical features related to specific pathogens), Response (i.e., biomarkers, chest CT findings,) and Organ failure (i.e., main site of clinical expression of disease and/or associated organ dysfunction representing higher severity of illness) constitute the framework for therapeutic tailoring. Nevertheless, to the best of our knowledge, no study on patients with cancer or HIV patients has been performed. Although it is tempting to perform such studies using retrospective databases, we believe that despite the improvement in the current knowledge on the PIRO concept, the methodological approach used in the available studies evaluating the PIRO concept is similar to those used in the development of traditional prognostic scores. Although selecting variables according to each of the PIRO domains is a most likely way to identify outcome predictors, this is also a potential limitation. Actually, to move forward applying this new concept, we should choose a new methodological approach. There is enough evidence from the literature to show that clinical scores are inappropriate for risk stratification on an individual basis and should not be used either as a criterion for patient enrollment into clinical trials or for treatment decisions (Vincent et al. 2010). In addition, as sepsis is a dynamic and heterogeneous process, the development of databases for future studies should take into account this notion for all PIRO domains. The assessment of patterns of variation in organ dysfunctions (Levy et al. 2005) and biomarkers (Bozza et al. 2007; Salluh et al. 2011; Povoa 2008) is useful to assess individual outcomes in sepsis. Such an approach has been proposed in the context of theragnostics. The PIRO concept was conceived taking into consideration the use of the TNM classification to stratify patients with solid tumors. Again we can learn with oncologists about some successful experiences using theragnostics. This involved the expansion of TNM staging to include molecular and genetic patterns to guide specific therapeutic interventions. Successful examples are now applied as the standard for breast and lung cancer and also hematological malignancies. Therefore, despite the significant advances in the past decade, we should be aware that the PIRO concept is a work in progress rather than a model to be immediately adopted. The understanding of sepsis as a nonlinear biological system and its interaction with the specific immune changes in cancer and HIV patients is a major challenge. To face this we will require improved study designs, use of new statistical and mathematical modeling, and extensive clinical investigation for its validation before clinical implementation.

Acknowledgments
Financial support: Dr. Soares and Dr. Bozza are supported in part by individual research grants from CNPq.
Conflicts of interest: None.

References

Afessa B, Green B (2000) Clinical course, prognostic factors, and outcome prediction for HIV patients in the ICU. The PIP (pulmonary complications, ICU support, and prognostic factors in hospitalized patients with HIV) study. Chest 118(1):138–145

Aisenberg G, Rolston KV, Dickey BF, Kontoyiannis DP, Raad II, Safdar A (2007) Stenotrophomonas maltophilia pneumonia in cancer patients without traditional risk factors for infection, 1997–2004. Eur J Clin Microbiol Infect Dis 26(1):13–20

Andreu Ballester JC, Ballester F, Gonzalez Sanchez A, Almela Quilis A, Colomer Rubio E, Penarroja Otero C (2008) Epidemiology of sepsis in the Valencian Community (Spain), 1995–2004. Infect Control Hosp Epidemiol 29(7):630–634

Angus DC, Linde-Zwirble WT, Lidicker J, Clermont G, Carcillo J, Pinsky MR (2001) Epidemiology of severe sepsis in the United States: analysis of incidence, outcome, and associated costs of care. Crit Care Med 29(7):1303–1310

Angus DC, Burgner D, Wunderink R, Mira JP, Gerlach H, Wiedermann CJ et al (2003) The PIRO concept: P is for predisposition. Crit Care 7(3):248–251

Annane D, Aegerter P, Jars-Guincestre MC, Guidet B (2003) Current epidemiology of septic shock: the CUB-Rea Network. Am J Respir Crit Care Med 168(2):165–172

Arthur G, Nduba VN, Kariuki SM, Kimari J, Bhatt SM, Gilks CF (2001) Trends in bloodstream infections among human immunodeficiency virus-infected adults admitted to a hospital in Nairobi, Kenya, during the last decade. Clin Infect Dis 33(2):248–256

Azoulay E, Alberti C, Bornstain C, Leleu G, Moreau D, Recher C et al (2001) Improved survival in cancer patients requiring mechanical ventilatory support: impact of noninvasive mechanical ventilatory support. Crit Care Med 29(3):519–525

Barbier F, Coquet I, Legriel S, Pavie J, Darmon M, Mayaux J, Molina JM, Schlemmer B, Azoulay E (2009) Etiologies and outcome of acute respiratory failure in HIV-infected patients. Intensive Care Med 35(10):1678–1686

Beale R, Reinhart K, Brunkhorst FM, Dobb G, Levy M, Martin G et al (2009) Promoting Global Research Excellence in Severe Sepsis (PROGRESS): lessons from an international sepsis registry. Infection 37(3):222–232

Benjamim CF, Lundy SK, Lukacs NW, Hogaboam CM, Kunkel SL (2005) Reversal of long-term sepsis-induced immunosuppression by dendritic cells. Blood 105(9):3588–3595

Benoit DD, Vandewoude KH, Decruyenaere JM, Hoste EA, Colardyn FA (2003) Outcome and early prognostic indicators in patients with a hematologic malignancy admitted to the intensive care unit for a life-threatening complication. Crit Care Med 31(1):104–112

Bianchi M, Robles AM, Vitale R, Helou S, Arechavala A, Negroni R (2000) The usefulness of blood culture in diagnosing HIV-related systemic mycoses: evaluation of a manual lysis centrifugation method. Med Mycol 38(1):77–80

Blanco J, Muriel-Bombin A, Sagredo V, Taboada F, Gandia F, Tamayo L et al (2008) Incidence, organ dysfunction and mortality in severe sepsis: a Spanish multicentre study. Crit Care 12(6):R158

Bozza FA, Salluh JI, Japiassu AM, Soares M, Assis EF, Gomes RN et al (2007) Cytokine profiles as markers of disease severity in sepsis: a multiplex analysis. Crit Care 11(2):R49

Bone RC, Balk RA, Cerra FB, Dellinger RP, Fein AM, Knaus WA, Schein RM, Sibbald WJ (1992) Chest 101(6):1644–1655

Brenchley JM, Price DA, Schacker TW, Asher TE, Silvestri G, Rao S et al (2006) Microbial translocation is a cause of systemic immune activation in chronic HIV infection. Nat Med 12(12): 1365–1371

Brun-Buisson C, Meshaka P, Pinton P, Vallet B (2004) EPISEPSIS: a reappraisal of the epidemiology and outcome of severe sepsis in French intensive care units. Intensive Care Med 30(4):580–588; Epub 2004 Mar 2

Casalino E, Wolff M, Ravaud P, Choquet C, Bruneel F, Regnier B (2004) Impact of HAART advent on admission patterns and survival in HIV-infected patients admitted to an intensive care unit. AIDS 18(10):1429–1433

Coquet I, Pavie J, Palmer P, Barbier F, Legriel S, Mayaux J et al (2010) Survival trends in critically ill HIV-infected patients in the highly active antiretroviral therapy era. Crit Care 14(3):R107

Croda J, Croda MG, Neves A, De Sousa dos Santos S (2009) Crit Care Med 37(5):1605–1611

Danai PA, Moss M, Mannino DM, Martin GS (2006) The epidemiology of sepsis in patients with malignancy. Chest 129(6):1432–1440

Danel C, Moh R, Minga A, Anzian A, Ba-Gomis O, Kanga C et al (2006) CD4-guided structured antiretroviral treatment interruption strategy in HIV-infected adults in west Africa (Trivacan ANRS 1269 trial): a randomised trial. Lancet 367(9527):1981–1989

Darmon M, Azoulay E (2009) Critical care management of cancer patients: cause for optimism and need for objectivity. Curr Opin Oncol 21(4):318–326

Davaro RE, Thirumalai A (2007) Life-threatening complications of HIV infection. J Intensive Care Med 22(2):73–81

Davis JL, Morris A, Kallet RH, Powell K, Chi AS, Bensley M et al (2008) Low tidal volume ventilation is associated with reduced mortality in HIV-infected patients with acute lung injury. Thorax 63(11):988–993

Dickson SJ, Batson S, Copas AJ, Edwards SG, Singer M, Miller RF (2007) Thorax 62(11): 964–968. Epub 2007 May 21

Fox AC, Robertson CM, Belt B, Clark AT, Chang KC, Leathersich AM et al (2010) Cancer causes increased mortality and is associated with altered apoptosis in murine sepsis. Crit Care Med 38(3):886–893

Gea-Banacloche JC, Opal SM, Jorgensen J, Carcillo JA, Sepkowitz KA, Cordonnier C (2004) Sepsis associated with immunosuppressive medications: an evidence-based review. Crit Care Med 32(11 Suppl):S578–S590

Grinsztejn B, Veloso VG, Friedman RK, Moreira RI, Luz PM, Campos DP et al (2009) Early mortality and cause of deaths in patients using HAART in Brazil and the United States. AIDS 23(16):2107–2114

Huang L, Quartin A, Jones D, Havlir DV (2006) Intensive care of patients with HIV infection. N Engl J Med 355(2):173–181

Jacob ST, Moore CC, Banura P, Pinkerton R, Meya D, Opendi P et al (2009) Severe sepsis in two Ugandan hospitals: a prospective observational study of management and outcomes in a predominantly HIV-1 infected population. PLoS One 4(11):e7782

Japiassu AM, Salluh JI, Bozza PT, Bozza FA, Castro-Faria-Neto HC (2009) Revisiting steroid treatment for septic shock: molecular actions and clinical effects–a review. Mem Inst Oswaldo Cruz 104(4):531–548

Japiassu AM, Amancio RT, Mesquita EC, Medeiros DM, Bernal HB, Nunes EP et al (2010) Sepsis is a major determinant of outcome in critically ill HIV/AIDS patients. Crit Care 14(4):R152

Khouli H, Afrasiabi A, Shibli M, Hajal R, Barrett CR, Homel P (2005) Outcome of critically ill human immunodeficiency virus–infected patients in the era of highly active antiretroviral therapy. J Intensive Care Med 20:279–285

Khwannimit B, Bhurayanontachai R (2009) The epidemiology of, and risk factors for, mortality from severe sepsis and septic shock in a tertiary-care university hospital setting. Epidemiol Infect 137(9):1333–1341

Lambotte O, Lucet JC, Fleury L, Joly-Guillou ML, Bouvet E (2000) Nosocomial bacteremia in HIV patients: the role of peripheral venous catheters. Infect Control Hosp Epidemiol 21(5): 330–333

Larche J, Azoulay E, Fieux F, Mesnard L, Moreau D, Thiery G et al (2003) Improved survival of critically ill cancer patients with septic shock. Intensive Care Med 29(10):1688–1695

Levy MM, Macias WL, Vincent JL, Russell JA, Silva E, Trzaskoma B et al (2005) Early changes in organ function predict eventual survival in severe sepsis. Crit Care Med 33(10):2194–2201

Lewden C, Chene G, Morlat P, Raffi F, Dupon M, Dellamonica P et al (2007) HIV-infected adults with a CD4 cell count greater than 500 cells/mm³ on long-term combination antiretroviral therapy reach same mortality rates as the general population. J Acquir Immune Defic Syndr 46(1):72–77

Lisboa T, Diaz E, Sa-Borges M, Socias A, Sole-Violan J, Rodriguez A et al (2008) The ventilator-associated pneumonia PIRO score: a tool for predicting ICU mortality and health-care resources use in ventilator-associated pneumonia. Chest 134(6):1208–1216

Martin GS, Mannino DM, Eaton S, Moss M (2003) The epidemiology of sepsis in the United States from 1979 through 2000. N Engl J Med 348(16):1546–1554

Maschmeyer G, Bertschat FL, Moesta KT, Hausler E, Held TK, Nolte M et al (2003) Outcome analysis of 189 consecutive cancer patients referred to the intensive care unit as emergencies during a 2-year period. Eur J Cancer 39(6):783–792

Mendez-Tellez PA, Damluji A, Ammerman D, Colantuoni E, Fan E, Sevransky JE et al (2010) Human immunodeficiency virus infection and hospital mortality in acute lung injury patients. Crit Care Med 38(7):1530–1535

Meynard JL, Guiguet M, Fonquernie L, Lefebvre B, Lalande V, Honore I et al (2003) Impact of highly active antiretroviral therapy on the occurrence of bacteraemia in HIV-infected patients and their epidemiologic characteristics. HIV Med 4(2):127–132

Morris A, Creasman J, Turner J, Luce JM, Wachter RM, Huang L (2002) Intensive care of human immunodeficiency virus-infected patients during the era of highly active antiretroviral therapy. Am J Respir Crit Care Med 166(3):262–267

Mrus JM, Braun L, Yi MS, Linde-Zwirble WT, Johnston JA (2005) Impact of HIV/AIDS on care and outcomes of severe sepsis. Crit Care 9(6):R623–R630

Narasimhan M, Posner AJ, DePalo VA, Mayo PH, Rosen MJ (2004) Intensive care in patients with HIV infection in the era of highly active antiretroviral therapy. Chest 125:1800–1804

Nickas G, Wachter RM (2000) Outcomes of intensive care for patients with human immunodeficiency virus infection. Arch Intern Med 160(4):541–547

Pacheco AG, Tuboi SH, May SB, Moreira LF, Ramadas L, Nunes EP et al (2009) Temporal changes in causes of death among HIV-infected patients in the HAART era in Rio de Janeiro, Brazil. J Acquir Immune Defic Syndr 51(5):624–630

Palacios R, Hidalgo A, Reina C, de la Torre MV, Márquez M, Santos J (2006) Effect of antiretroviral therapy on admissions of HIV-infected patients to an intensive care unit. HIV Med 7:193–196

Pene F, Percheron S, Lemiale V, Viallon V, Claessens YE, Marque S et al (2008) Temporal changes in management and outcome of septic shock in patients with malignancies in the intensive care unit. Crit Care Med 36(3):690–696

Povoa P (2008) Serum markers in community-acquired pneumonia and ventilator-associated pneumonia. Curr Opin Infect Dis 21(2):157–162

Powell K, Davis JL, Morris AM, Chi A, Bensley MR, Huang L (2009) Survival for patients With HIV admitted to the ICU continues to improve in the current era of combination antiretroviral therapy. Chest 135(1):11–17

Regazzoni CJ, Irrazabal C, Luna CM, Poderoso JJ (2004) Cancer patients with septic shock: mortality predictors and neutropenia. Support Care Cancer 12(12):833–839

Rello J, Rodriguez A, Lisboa T, Gallego M, Lujan M, Wunderink R (2009) PIRO score for community-acquired pneumonia: a new prediction rule for assessment of severity in intensive care unit patients with community-acquired pneumonia. Crit Care Med 37(2):456–462

Rosen MJ, Narasimhan M (2006) Critical care of immunocompromised patients: human immunodeficiency virus. Crit Care Med 34(9 Suppl):S245–S250

Ross AC, Rizk N, O'Riordan MA, Dogra V, El-Bejjani D, Storer N et al (2009) Relationship between inflammatory markers, endothelial activation markers, and carotid intima-media thickness in HIV-infected patients receiving antiretroviral therapy. Clin Infect Dis 49(7): 1119–1127

Rubulotta F, Ramsay D, Williams MD (2010) PIRO score for community-acquired pneumonia: a new prediction rule for assessment of severity in intensive care unit patients with community-acquired pneumonia. Crit Care Med 38(4):1236; author reply −7

Safdar A, Rolston KV (2007) Stenotrophomonas maltophilia: changing spectrum of a serious bacterial pathogen in patients with cancer. Clin Infect Dis 45(12):1602–1609

Salluh JI, Bozza FA, Pinto TS, Toscano L, Weller PF, Soares M (2005) Cutaneous periumbilical purpura in disseminated strongyloidiasis in cancer patients: a pathognomonic feature of potentially lethal disease? Braz J Infect Dis 9(5):419–424

Salluh JI, Soares M, Coelho LM, Bozza FA, Verdeal JC, Castro-Faria-Neto HC et al (2011) Impact of systemic corticosteroids on the clinical course and outcomes of patients with severe community-acquired pneumonia: a cohort study. J Crit Care 26(2):193–200

Schleicher GK, Herbert V, Brink A, Martin S, Maraj R, Galpin JS et al (2005) Procalcitonin and C-reactive protein levels in HIV-positive subjects with tuberculosis and pneumonia. Eur Respir J 25(4):688–692

Sivasangeetha K, Harish BN, Sujatha S, Parija SC, Dutta TK (2007) Cryptococcal meningoencephalitis diagnosed by blood culture. Indian J Med Microbiol 25(3):282–284

Soares M, Azoulay E (2009) Critical care management of lung cancer patients to prolong life
    without prolonging dying. Intensive Care Med 35(12):2012–2014
Soares M, Salluh JI, Ferreira CG, Luiz RR, Spector N, Rocco JR (2005) Impact of two different
    comorbidity measures on the 6-month mortality of critically ill cancer patients. Intensive Care
    Med 31(3):408–415
Soares M, Salluh JI, Carvalho MS, Darmon M, Rocco JR, Spector N (2006a) Prognosis
    of critically ill patients with cancer and acute renal dysfunction. J Clin Oncol 24(24):
    4003–4010
Soares M, Carvalho MS, Salluh JI, Ferreira CG, Luiz RR, Rocco JR et al (2006b) Effect of age on
    survival of critically ill patients with cancer. Crit Care Med 34(3):715–721
Soares M, Darmon M, Salluh JI, Ferreira CG, Thiery G, Schlemmer B et al (2007a)
    Prognosis of lung cancer patients with life-threatening complications. Chest 131(3):
    840–846
Soares M, Salluh JI, Toscano L, Dias FL (2007b) Outcomes and prognostic factors in patients with
    head and neck cancer and severe acute illnesses. Intensive Care Med 33(11):2009–2013, Epub
    2007 Jul 10
Soares M, Salluh JI, Torres VB, Leal JV, Spector N (2008) Short- and long-term outcomes
    of critically ill patients with cancer and prolonged ICU length of stay. Chest 134(3):
    520–526
Soares M, Caruso P, Silva E, Teles JM, Lobo SM, Friedman G et al (2010a) Characteristics and
    outcomes of patients with cancer requiring admission to intensive care units: a prospective
    multicenter study. Crit Care Med 38(1):9–15
Soares M, Depuydt PO, Salluh JI (2010b) Mechanical ventilation in cancer patients: clinical
    characteristics and outcomes. Crit Care Clin 26(1):41–58
Soares M, Silva UV, Teles JM, Silva E, Caruso P, Lobo SM et al (2010c) Validation of four prog-
    nostic scores in patients with cancer admitted to Brazilian intensive care units: results from a
    prospective multicenter study. Intensive Care Med 36(7):1188–1195
Taccone FS, Artigas AA, Sprung CL, Moreno R, Sakr Y, Vincent JL (2009) Characteristics and
    outcomes of cancer patients in European ICUs. Crit Care 13(1):R15
Taniguchi T, Ogawa Y, Kasai D, Watanabe D, Yoshikawa K, Bando H et al (2010) Three cases of
    fungemia in HIV-infected patients diagnosed through the use of mycobacterial blood culture
    bottles. Intern Med 49(19):2179–2183
Thiery G, Azoulay E, Darmon M, Ciroldi M, De Miranda S, Levy V et al (2005) Outcome of
    cancer patients considered for intensive care unit admission: a hospital-wide prospective study.
    J Clin Oncol 23(19):4406–4413
Thirumala R, Ramaswamy M, Chawla S (2010) Diagnosis and management of infectious compli-
    cations in critically ill patients with cancer. Crit Care Clin 26(1):59–91
Tien PC, Choi AI, Zolopa AR, Benson C, Tracy R, Scherzer R et al (2010) Inflammation and
    mortality in HIV-infected adults: analysis of the FRAM study cohort. J Acquir Immune Defic
    Syndr 55(3):316–322
Torre D, Pugliese A (2008) Platelets and HIV-1 infection: old and new aspects. Curr HIV Res
    6(5):411–418
Tumbarello M, Tacconelli E, Donati KG, Citton R, Leone F, Spanu T et al (2000) HIV-associated
    bacteremia: how it has changed in the highly active antiretroviral therapy (HAART) era.
    J Acquir Immune Defic Syndr 23(2):145–151
Vandewoude KH, Blot SI, Depuydt P, Benoit D, Temmerman W, Colardyn F et al (2006) Clinical
    relevance of Aspergillus isolation from respiratory tract samples in critically ill patients. Crit
    Care 10(1):R31
Vandijck DM, Benoit DD, Depuydt PO, Offner FC, Blot SI, Van Tilborgh AK et al (2008) Impact
    of recent intravenous chemotherapy on outcome in severe sepsis and septic shock patients with
    hematological malignancies. Intensive Care Med 34(5):847–855
Velasco E, Portugal RD, Salluh JI (2009) A simple score to predict early death in adult cancer
    patients with bloodstream infections. J Infect 59(5):332–336

Vincent B, Timsit JF, Auburtin M, Schortgen F, Bouadma L, Wolff M, Regnier B (2004) Characteristics and outcomes of HIV-infected patients in the ICU: impact of the highly active antiretroviral treatment era. Intensive Care Med. 30(5):859–866. Epub 2004 Feb 6.

Vincent JL, Rello J, Marshall J, Silva E, Anzueto A, Martin CD et al (2009) International study of the prevalence and outcomes of infection in intensive care units. JAMA 302(21):2323–2329

Vincent JL, Opal SM, Marshall JC (2010) Ten reasons why we should NOT use severity scores as entry criteria for clinical trials or in our treatment decisions. Crit Care Med 38(1):283–287

Waddell RD, Lishimpi K, von Reyn CF, Chintu C, Baboo KS, Kreiswirth B et al (2001) Bacteremia due to Mycobacterium tuberculosis or M. bovis, Bacille Calmette-Guerin (BCG) among HIV-positive children and adults in Zambia. AIDS 15(1):55–60

Williams MD, Braun LA, Cooper LM, Johnston J, Weiss RV, Qualy RL et al (2004) Hospitalized cancer patients with severe sepsis: analysis of incidence, mortality, and associated costs of care. Crit Care 8(5):R291–R298

Intra-Abdominal Hypertension and MODS

6

Jan J. De Waele and Inneke De laet

6.1 Introduction

The pathophysiological mechanisms leading to organ dysfunction in septic shock are multiple and complex. Although the discovery of new pathways and mediators continuously improves our understanding of severe sepsis and septic shock, the search for new drugs targeting the inflammatory cascade has only rarely resulted in success or improved outcomes. The management in the intensive care unit (ICU) often is still focused on early removal of the infectious focus, appropriate antibiotic treatment and organ support when indicated.

Treatment of septic shock patients is often challenging, and complications – both short and long term – are frequent. It should be said that often these complications are the consequence of the treatment. Prevention and early recognition of these complications are therefore important.

Intra-abdominal hypertension (IAH) has recently been identified as a frequent problem in critically ill patients. Whereas initially considered relevant in patients admitted in a context of abdominal catastrophes such as ruptured aortic aneurysms or damage control laparotomy and when the patient presented with overt organ failure (or abdominal compartment syndrome, ACS), several authors have found IAH as frequently in medical patients as in surgical patients (Malbrain et al. 2005a).

J.J. De Waele (✉)
Department of Critical Care Medicine, Ghent University Hospital,
Ghent, Belgium
e-mail: jan.dewaele@ugent.be

I. De laet
Department of Critical Care Medicine, Ghent University Hospital
Ghent, Belgium

ICU, ZiekenhuisNetwerk Antwerpen, Campus Stuivenberg,
Antwerp, Belgium

J. Rello (eds.), *Sepsis Management*,
DOI 10.1007/978-3-642-03519-7_6, © Springer-Verlag Berlin Heidelberg 2012

In parallel, multiple animal and human studies have demonstrated that organ function is already affected when the intra-abdominal pressure is 12 mmHg or higher, making IAH a relevant problem before ACS develops.

Evidence is emerging that IAH is also a very common finding in patients with severe sepsis and septic shock. In a recent study, IAH was found in up to 85% of patients with septic shock during the first 3 days after admission (Regueira et al. 2008). A common finding in most of the recent literature is that fluid accumulation in this context is an important contributor to increasing IAP. As fluid resuscitation is an important aspect of the management of septic shock patients, more attention to the problem of IAH in this setting is urgently needed.

In this review, we will give an overview of the current understanding of IAH and ACS in general, and explore how it is relevant for severe sepsis patients and their treatment.

6.2   What is IAH?

IAH is defined as sustained or repeated IAP of 12 mmHg or more, and can be divided in four grades (Table 6.1). The clinical picture of a sustained IAP of 20 mmHg or more with the development of new organ dysfunction or failure has been named ACS. ACS has been divided into primary, secondary and recurrent ACS, where primary ACS refers to an intra-abdominal etiology, secondary ACS is

Table 6.1 Excerpt of consensus definitions regarding IAH and ACS

Definition 1	IAP is the steady-state pressure concealed within the abdominal cavity
Definition 7	IAH is defined by a sustained or repeated pathologic elevation of IAP$\geq$12 mmHg
Definition 8	IAH is graded as follows: • Grade I: IAP 12–15 mmHg • Grade II: IAP 16–20 mmHg • Grade III: IAP 21–25 mmHg • Grade IV: IAP>25 mmHg
Definition 9	ACS is defined as a sustained IAP>20 mmHg (with or without an APP<60 mmHg) that is associated with new organ dysfunction/failure
Definition 10	Primary ACS is a condition associated with injury or disease in the abdominal-pelvic region that frequently requires early surgical or interventional radiological intervention
Definition 11	Secondary ACS refers to conditions that do not originate from the abdominal-pelvic region
Definition 12	Recurrent ACS refers to the condition in which ACS redevelops following previous surgical or medical treatment of primary or secondary ACS

Adapted from Malbrain et al. (2006)
ACS abdominal compartment syndrome, *IAH* intra-abdominal hypertension, *IAP* intra-abdominal pressure, *APP* abdominal perfusion pressure

caused by an extra-abdominal etiology and recurrent ACS occurs after previous treatment for ACS (Malbrain et al. 2006).

IAP is determined by the intra-abdominal volume and the compliance of the abdominal wall. The most obvious contributor to IAH is increased volume in the abdominal domain, both within the peritoneal cavity and/or in the retro-peritoneum, but abdominal wall compliance is equally important. In patients with chronic liver failure, slowly increasing ascites volume causes a progressive elongation of the abdominal muscles, increasing the compliance and leading to better tolerance of acute increases of intra-abdominal volume. Similar to the situation in the skull, a pressure volume (PV) curve can be constructed with essentially two parts: when the abdominal wall is very compliant and at low intra-abdominal volumes, relatively large increases in volume will lead to only minor changes in IAP (Malbrain 2004); at higher volumes the abdominal wall compliance decreases and small volume changes can lead to large increases in IAP. This means both that a small increase in intra-abdominal volume can lead to clinically important effects on organ function and that relatively small decreases in volume can lower IAP significantly. This theoretical concept also offers options for treatment. The abdominal PV curve is shifted to the left in situations where the abdominal wall compliance is decreased because of hematoma, voluntary muscle activity, edema or other factors. The occurrence of IAH is usually associated with a situation that causes increased abdominal volume and decreased abdominal compliance, and often a combination of both of these factors. The WSACS published a list of conditions associated with these situations (Malbrain et al. 2006); these are summarized in Table 6.2.

Table 6.2 Conditions associated with IAH and ACS

(Predominant) Increased intra-abdominal volume
- GI tract dilatation: gastroparesis and gastric distention, ileus, volvulus, colonic pseudo-obstruction
- Intra-abdominal or retroperitoneal masses, e.g., abdominal tumor
- Ascites or hemoperitoneum
- Pneumoperitoneum , e.g., during laparoscopy

(Predominant) Decreased abdominal wall compliance
- Abdominal surgery, especially with tight abdominal closures
- Abdominal wall bleeding or rectus sheath hematomas
- Surgical correction of large abdominal hernias, gastroschisis or omphalocele

Combination of decreased abdominal wall compliance and increased intra-abdominal volume
- Obesity
- Sepsis, severe sepsis and septic shock
- Severe acute pancreatitis
- Massive fluid resuscitation
- Major burns (with or without abdominal eschars)
- Complicated intra-abdominal infection

Adopted from (Malbrain et al. 2006)

6.3   IAP Measurement

Surveys among clinicians show that many use clinical examination for the diagnosis of ACS (De Laet et al. 2007; Kimball et al. 2006). However, it was repeatedly demonstrated that clinical examination based on the abdominal perimeter, abdominal perimeter changes or palpation of the abdomen is using unreliable parameters to estimate IAP, and these should therefore not be used for screening or follow-up of IAP (Malbrain et al. 2009; Sugrue et al. 2002).

Reliable IAP measurement is the first step to the clinical management of patients with IAH or ACS.

Various methods for IAP measurement have been developed (Malbrain 2004); IAP can be measured either directly (using a needle puncture of the abdomen, during peritoneal dialysis or during laparoscopy) or indirectly (using the intravesicular pressure as measured via the Foley catheter or the gastric pressure via a balloon catheter), based on the principle that the abdominal cavity is a closed box (Malbrain et al. 2006). Therefore, the pressure measured at one point within this cavity reflects the pressure throughout the cavity, as its contents behave according to Pascal's law. From this it is assumed that IAP can be measured indirectly in all cavities within the abdomen. Transvesicular measurement of IAP is currently the most popular technique; several systems with or without the need for electronic equipment are available that also allow also IAP measurement in a non-ICU environment (De Waele et al. 2007). Per consensus, IAP is expressed in mmHg and measured at end expiration in the supine position in the absence of spontaneous muscle contractions. The mid-axillary line is used as the zero reference level for IAP measurement. Methods for continuous IAP measurement are also available, but are not yet widely used. A complete description of the different methods to measure IAP with the different pitfalls of each technique is outside the scope of this review; more information can be found in a number of recent articles (Balogh et al. 2007; Malbrain 2004; Malbrain et al. 2006) or at the website of the WSACS (www.wsacs. org). It is advised that IAP monitoring is based on a (site-specific) protocol, based on known risk factors, the monitoring equipment available and nursing staff experience, and should be linked directly to a local treatment protocol (De Waele et al. 2007). In our hospital, patients with any of the conditions associated with IAH (Table 6.2) are monitored using a transvesicular technique, at least every 4 h until IAP remains lower than 12 mmHg for at least 24 h in the absence of organ dysfunction.

Normal IAP is about 5–7 mmHg, but baseline levels are significantly higher in morbidly obese patients at about 9–14 mmHg (De Keulenaer et al. 2009), which may already affect organ function in other patients but appear to be tolerated in obese individuals. In children, normal IAP is generally lower (Ejike et al. 2007). In general, IAP readings must be interpreted relative to the individual patient's physiologic state.

6.4   How Does IAH Cause MODS?

ACS is diagnosed when the IAP is greater than 20 mmHg along with evidence of new end-organ dysfunction (Malbrain et al. 2005). However, organ dysfunction can also occur at levels of IAP previously deemed to be safe (Malbrain et al. 2006).

There is a "dose-dependent" relation between acute changes of IAP and the degree of organ dysfunction, but thresholds may differ from patient to patient. IAH has deleterious effects on organ function, both within and outside of the abdominal cavity. It is beyond the scope of this paper to give a complete overview of all pathophysiological mechanisms involved. We have focused on those pathologic observations that have direct implications on the clinical management of critically ill or injured patients. The effects of IAH on the kidney will be discussed more extensively in the next chapter.

Several factors account for the effects of IAH on the cardiovascular system (Cheatham and Malbrain 2006). Firstly, due to cranial displacement of the diaphragm during IAH, intrathoracic pressure increases during IAH. Animal and human experiments have shown that 20–80% of the IAP is transmitted to the thorax. This leads to compression of the heart and reduction of end-diastolic volume. Secondly, the cardiac preload decreases because of decreased venous return from the abdomen (and potentially the lower limbs), and the systemic afterload is initially increased because direct compression of vascular beds and vasoconstriction secondary to the activation of the renin-angiotensin-aldosteron system (Kashtan et al. 1981; Malbrain and Cheatham 2004; Richardson and Trinkle 1976). This leads to decreased cardiac output (CO). Mean arterial blood pressure may initially rise because of shunting of blood away from the abdominal cavity, but thereafter normalizes or decreases (Cheatham and Malbrain 2006). The cardiovascular effects are aggravated by hypovolemia and the application of PEEP (Burchard et al. 1985), whereas hypervolemia has a temporary protective effect (Bloomfield et al. 1997).

The increase in ITP also elevates all pressures measured in the thorax, including CVP, PAOP and pulmonary artery pressures, meaning that the values of these measurements may have different meaning than they would without IAH. This finding has important implications. The Surviving Sepsis Campaign guidelines targeting initial and ongoing resuscitation towards a CVP of 8–12 mmHg (Dellinger et al. 2004) should be interpreted and adjusted according to these findings – as was also addressed in the latest update of the guidelines. In patients with IAH higher targets should be used.

The transmission of IAP to the thorax also has an impact on the respiratory system (Pelosi et al. 2007). IAH decreases total respiratory system compliance by a decrease in chest wall compliance, whereas lung compliance remains virtually unchanged (Mutoh et al. 1991). This leads to increased inspiratory pressures or reduced tidal volumes depending on the mode of ventilation. Increased PEEP may be required to adequately oxygenate patients with IAH and ACS.

A direct relationship between IAP and intracranial pressure (ICP) has been observed in both animal and human studies (Citerio et al. 2001; Josephs et al. 1994). Several authors hypothesized that the increase in ICP secondary to IAH was caused by increased ITP, leading to increased CVP and decreased venous return from the brain and thus venous congestion and brain edema. This hypothesis gained acceptance when Bloomfield et al. demonstrated that the association between IAP and ICP could be abolished by performing a sternotomy and bilateral pleuropericardotomy in pigs (Bloomfield et al. 1997). The reduced systemic blood pressure associated with decreased cardiac preload and the increase in ICP will lead to a decrease in cerebral perfusion pressure (CPP). Some authors have even demonstrated successful treatment of refractory intracranial hypertension with abdominal decompression or neuromuscular blockers (Deeren et al. 2005; Josephs et al. 1994).

Obviously also intra-abdominal organs are affected: IAH causes diminished perfusion of all intra-abdominal organs, including the gut, liver and pancreas, and causes mucosal acidosis (Ivatury and Diebel 2006). ACS results in splanchnic hypoperfusion that may occur in the absence of hypotension or decreased cardiac output. This may lead to increased mucosal permeability and bacterial translocation, as has been shown in animal experiments, especially when combined with ischemia-reperfusion injury (Diebel et al. 1997; Doty et al. 2002; Yagci et al. 2005).

6.5   IAH in Sepsis

6.5.1   IAH in Severe Sepsis and Septic Shock

In the first epidemiological studies sepsis was not identified as a particular risk factor for the development of IAH (Malbrain et al. 2004), probably because of selection bias and the high cutoff levels used for the diagnosis of IAH. Subsequent studies proved otherwise. Malbrain et al. identified higher incidences of IAH in patients with sepsis, and more importantly, other conditions often associated with severe sepsis, such as massive fluid resuscitation, were associated with IAH (Malbrain et al. 2005).

Severe sepsis and septic shock were also the leading causes of secondary IAH in a single-center study of consecutive mechanically ventilated ICU patients, accounting for about 40% of the patients (Reintam et al. 2008). Similarly, in patients staying in the ICU for more than 24 h, IAH was found in 60% of patients who were admitted because of sepsis; sepsis was also the leading cause of IAH in medical patients (Vidal et al. 2008). In this study, fluid resuscitation, hypotension and mechanical ventilation were identified as risk factors associated with IAH, while infection per se was not. In another study from Italy in unselected patients admitted to the ICU for at least 24 h, it was found that sepsis was associated with IAH in logistic regression analysis (OR 2.11, 95% CI 1.01–3.78) (Dalfino et al. 2008). Again, shock and cumulative fluid balance were the most important determinants of IAH. From these studies, it appears that the treatment of septic shock rather than septic shock itself is associated with IAH. Nevertheless, IAH should be considered in all patients with severe sepsis and septic shock.

Data specifically coming from patients with septic shock confirm that the incidence of IAH in these patients is significant. In a prospective study, IAH was found in up to 76% of the patients in the first 72 h of septic shock, both in medical and surgical patients (although the incidence in surgical patients was the highest) (Regueira et al. 2008). Non-survivors had higher maximal IAP values (19.9 vs. 17.2 mmHg); patients with IAH had higher degrees of organ dysfunction across all organ systems. In survivors IAP had decreased to 13 mmHg at 72 h, whereas in non-survivors, IAP did not decrease with mean levels of 19 mmHg. Persistence of IAH therefore seems to be an important predictor of mortality and could serve as a therapeutic target. IAH also leads to lower APP values in non-survivors, and higher degrees of IAH were related to increased severity of kidney impairment.

6.5.2   IAH in Abdominal Sepsis

Apart from the above considerations, patients suffering from abdominal sepsis seem to be at particular risk for developing IAH. Often multiple other risk factors for IAH such as abdominal surgery, intra-abdominal fluid collections and pain are present, further increasing the risk of IAH. In epidemiological studies in critical care settings, IAI has been cited as the cause of IAH/ACS in 10–14% of the cases (Malbrain et al. 2005; Malbrain et al. 2004). Although not rare, IAI does not seem to be a major contributor to the incidence of IAH observed in the ICU, but this may strongly depend on the relative proportion of IAI in the ICU. In a recent study IAI was not found to be a risk factor for IAH (Vidal et al. 2008).

IAH may also contribute to the development of intra-abdominal infection. Bacterial translocation has been described in animal models of IAH (Diebel et al. 1997; Doty et al. 2002; Yagci et al. 2005). In patients with severe acute pancreatitis, a condition that is often associated with IAH in the early phase of the disease, bacteremia was a frequent finding in the first 2 weeks, with the same organisms often found in infected pancreatic necrosis at a later stage; unfortunately, IAP was not measured, and a direct connection between the two observations can only be suspected.

When IAP increases, the perfusion of a gastrointestinal anastomosis can also become compromised because of decreases in abdominal perfusion pressure further increasing the risk of subsequent leakage from the anastomosis. In two experimental studies, exposure to increased IAP led to impairment of different stages of the healing process, especially when exposed to prolonged duration of elevated IAP (Chaves et al. 2007; Kologlu et al. 1999).

6.6   Implications for Management

6.6.1   IAH as a Therapeutic Target

Although treatment options are available when ACS is diagnosed at a late, premortal stage, it is important to realize that prevention is better than cure, and therefore a low index of suspicion for the diagnosis of IAH in patients at risk is important. Whereas surgical decompression was once considered the only therapeutic option in patients with IAH or ACS, the contemporary management of IAH in the ICU consists of four different elements (Fig. 6.1).

Recognition of the problem is the first and essential step. IAP measurement is the key here, as organ dysfunction may not be prominent, and often attributed to other

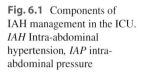

Fig. 6.1 Components of IAH management in the ICU. *IAH* Intra-abdominal hypertension, *IAP* intra-abdominal pressure

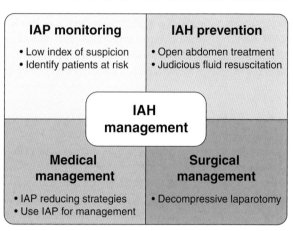

causes. IAP can be measured at the bedside or during an operation with relatively simple tools. Risk factors for the development have been described, but it has become clear that it may occur in any patient admitted to the ICU, and it is important to realize that this is not limited to surgical patients. With the increasing use of open abdomen strategies in emergency abdominal procedures, it is likely that ACS will become less frequent in the surgical ICU and more frequent in medical ICU patients.

Prevention of ACS can be done by treating IAH, the prelude to ACS. Treatment modalities do not include invasive surgery, and most of them use simple and widely available tools. They are aimed at either decreasing abdominal volume or increasing wall compliance, and have been summarized in the medical management algorithm from the World Society for the Abdominal Compartment Syndrome (WSACS), which is freely available to download from the society's website (www.wsacs.org). In this management algorithm, five different targets for intervention have been identified and a number of procedures advised in a stepwise fashion. These areas include evacuation of intraluminal contents, evacuation of intraperitoneal mass lesions and manipulation of the abdominal wall compliance, fluid balance and optimization of the regional perfusion.

Non-invasive removal of intraluminal contents by gastric tube placement and suctioning, rectal tube placement, enemas and, if indicated, endoscopic decompression should be attempted. Also, gastroprokinetics and/or colonoprokinetics may be used. Drainage of tense ascites most often results in a decrease in IAP. Paracentesis is the treatment of choice in burn patients with secondary ACS or any other patients who develop ascites after massive (usually crystalloid) fluid resuscitation. If intra-abdominal abscesses, hematomas or fluid collections are present, they should be drained as well. Also the use of neuromuscular blockers has to be considered. It was demonstrated that IAP can significantly be reduced, albeit that IAP was not completely normalized in patients with IAH. Fluid removal through diuresis or by means of ultrafiltration has been suggested to have a beneficial effect on IAP and possibly on organ function, e.g., compliance of the respiratory system. The institution of renal replacement therapy with fluid removal, if hemodynamically tolerated, should not be delayed in overresuscitated patients. In patients with borderline hemodynamic status, CVVH may be preferred over intermittent RRT to avoid hemodynamic instability.

If the attempts to lower the IAP are not effective, decompressive laparotomy (DL) should be considered. However, DL leaves the patient with an open abdomen, which can lead to extensive fluid losses, infection, enterocutaneous fistulae, ventral hernia and cosmetic dysfunction. Therefore, DL is mostly used today as a rescue therapy for patients with overt ACS who have not responded to medical treatment. It is important to bear in mind that the principles of medical management still apply after decompressive laparotomy. Application of this bundle of care leads to higher abdominal closure rates, shorter length of stay in the hospital and ICU, and decreased costs in a recent paper by Cheatham et al. The authors especially emphasize the importance of reducing bowel edema in order to avoid local complications in open abdomen management.

6.6.2   IAH and Treatment of Severe Sepsis and Septic Shock

Based on the above evidence, incorporation of IAH in the daily management of severe sepsis patients is advised. Especially in patients requiring fluid resuscitation, the need for IAP monitoring should be evaluated at admission and when organ dysfunction develops.

Fluid management is an important factor in both the treatment of sepsis and the development of IAH. There is overwhelming evidence that early and aggressive correction of hemodynamic disturbances and systemic perfusion is paramount in sepsis treatment. However, reports on the adverse effects of excess fluid loading are equally important and increasing in number. Positive fluid balance was identified as an independent risk factor for mortality in several large studies (Vincent et al. 2006). Increased IAP is probably one of the key factors connecting fluid administration to mortality. This observation has led the WSACS to incorporate optimization of fluid administration as one of the five main areas of focus for non-operative management of IAH. In a first step, it is important to avoid excessive fluid resuscitation and make efforts to achieve a zero to negative fluid balance by day 3. Bearing in mind that septic patients do need fluid resuscitation in the early stages of their disease, titrating fluid administration can be a difficult exercise in balance. It is also important to realize that urinary output is not a good target for resuscitation, especially in patients with IAH, since kidney injury occurs very early when IAP is increased, and if IAH induced oliguria leads to increased fluid administration, a vicious cycle of fluid loading, increased IAP and progressive oliguria follows. The aim should be to achieve the lowest intravascular volume status that will preserve end-organ perfusion and oxygenation. Since tissue oxygenation and microvascular organ perfusion cannot be measured routinely at the bedside (yet), clinicians are forced to rely mostly on crude hemodynamic parameters.

When interpreting centrally measured hemodynamic parameters such as central venous pressure (CVP) and pulmonary artery occlusion pressure (PAOP), it should be realized that IAH leads to an increase in all intrathoracic pressures, including CVP and PAOP. Patients with IAH will often have high CVP and PAOP yet still may be fluid responsive. Therefore, higher CVP and PAOP targets should be aimed for if these are used to guide fluid resuscitation. This was also added to the most recent update of the Surviving Sepsis Campaign guidelines.

Other measures of fluid responsiveness, such as SVV and PPV, may also be affected in IAH. Several studies have shown that stroke volume variation (SVV) and pulse pressure variation (PPV) are increased during IAH (Duperret et al. 2007; Renner et al. 2009). It is unclear whether this is the result of a measurement issue (meaning that cutoff values for triggering of fluid administration should be set higher) or a reflection of genuine increased fluid responsiveness. As other studies have shown that fluid loading can temporarily and partially protect the patient from IAH-induced organ dysfunction, the latter hypothesis seems to hold at least some truth. However, the association between fluid administration and increased IAP has been firmly established, and the authors feel that the focus of attention in a patient with IAH and increased SVV or PPV should be on decreasing IAP and less on fluid administration. Therefore, higher cutoff values for SVV and PPV in patients with IAH seem valid.

Another frequently used bedside parameter for fluid responsiveness is a passive leg-raising test. This is based on the observation of the hemodynamic effect of rais-ing the legs of the patient, creating autotransfusion. It is important to remember that venous return from the inferior vena cava may be impaired in patients with IAH and the effect of a passive leg raising maneuver may be blunted.

Volumetric hemodynamic parameters obtained via various techniques, such as LVEDV, RVEDV and GEDV, seem to be least affected by IAH, meaning that their value remains constant over a wide variety of IAP values. It may be preferable to titrate fluid administration according to such volumetric parameters in patients with IAH, although the other, previously mentioned parameters may also be used as long as their limitations and pitfalls in IAH are considered.

Whatever monitoring tools and parameters are used, the most important issue is to realize that fluid administration should be goal oriented and aimed at achieving the desired effect on oxygen transportation to the organs and tissues. Hypervolemic resuscitation does not contribute to this goal and is harmful to the patient. Even euvolemia might not be required.

A second step in the WSACS recommendations comprises the use of small volume resuscitation using hypertonic fluids and/or colloids and fluid removal through judicious diuresis. The debate on the use of colloids in septic shock is ongoing and lies beyond the scope of this chapter, but in terms of their effect on IAP, colloids have been used successfully in burn patients to reduce fluid admin-istration during the first post-burn 24 h, leading to a lesser increase in IAP and better organ function (O'Mara et al. 2005). Similar effects have been documented for hypertonic saline in burn patients (Oda et al. 2006). However, while burn shock is similar to septic shock in some ways, there are important differences as well, and the effect of colloid or hypertonic resuscitation on IAP in septic shock has not been studied so far. Nevertheless, the negative effects of excessive fluid resuscitation and positive fluid balance on mortality are clearly recognized, and we feel that all attempts should be made to avoid overresuscitation. Once fluid overload is present, the use of diuretics for fluid removal is recommended, although there is no direct evidence at this time that fluid removal in these patients improves outcome.

The third step in fluid management in patients with IAH calls for consideration of fluid removal through hemodialysis with ultrafiltration. There are several small series and reports that show that hemodialysis (both intermittent and continuous) can be used successfully to remove fluids, decrease IAP and improve organ function (Kula et al. 2008; Mullens et al. 2008). These studies were not specifically focused on septic patients, and it is conceivable that actively septic patients may not tolerate large volume fluid removal during RRT. Continuous RRT techniques might be better tolerated in this setting.

6.7   Conclusions

There appears to be a close link between IAH and severe sepsis and septic shock, with fluid resuscitation as one of the major contributors to elevated IAP. IAH adds to organ dysfunction in a dose-dependent manner, both in abdominal and extra-abdominal sepsis. IAP should be incorporated in the daily management of the patients as it influences commonly used hemodynamic monitoring parameters. Moreover, it can be used as a therapeutic target, as both medical management options and when necessary, surgical options are available.

References

Balogh Z, De Waele JJ, Malbrain ML (2007) Continuous intra-abdominal pressure monitoring. Acta Clin Belg Suppl (1):26–32

Bloomfield GL, Ridings PC, Blocher CR, Marmarou A, Sugerman HJ (1997) A proposed relationship between increased intra-abdominal, intrathoracic, and intracranial pressure. Crit Care Med 25:496–503

Burchard KW, Ciombor DM, McLeod MK, Slothman GJ, Gann DS (1985) Positive end expiratory pressure with increased intra-abdominal pressure. Surg Gynecol Obstet 161:313–318

Chaves N Jr, Magalhaes Lde T, Colleoni R, Del Grande JC (2007) Effects of increased intra-abdominal pressure on the healing process after surgical stapling of the stomach of dogs. Acta Cir Bras 22:379–386

Cheatham M, Malbrain M (2006) Cardiovascular implications of elevated intra-abdominal pressure. In: Ivatury R, Cheatham M, Malbrain M, Sugrue M (eds) Abdominal compartment syndrome. Landes Bioscience, Georgetown, pp 89–104

Citerio G, Vascotto E, Villa F, Celotti S, Pesenti A (2001) Induced abdominal compartment syndrome increases intracranial pressure in neurotrauma patients: a prospective study. Crit Care Med 29:1466–1471

Dalfino L, Tullo L, Donadio I, Malcangi V, Brienza N (2008) Intra-abdominal hypertension and acute renal failure in critically ill patients. Intensive Care Med 34:707–713

De Keulenaer BL, De Waele JJ, Powell B, Malbrain ML (2009) What is normal intra-abdominal pressure and how is it affected by positioning, body mass and positive end-expiratory pressure? Intensive Care Med 35:969–976

De Laet IE, Hoste EA, De Waele JJ (2007) Survey on the perception and management of the abdominal compartment syndrome among Belgian surgeons. Acta Chir Belg 107:648–652

De Waele JJ, De laet I, Malbrain ML (2007) Rational intraabdominal pressure monitoring: how to do it? Acta Clin Belg Suppl (1):16–25

Deeren D, Dits H, Malbrain MLNG (2005) Correlation between intra-abdominal and intracranial pressure in nontraumatic brain injury. Intensive Care Med 31:1577–1581

Dellinger RP, Carlet JM, Masur H, Gerlach H, Calandra T, Cohen J, Gea-Banacloche J, Keh D, Marshall JC, Parker MM, Ramsay G, Zimmerman JL, Vincent JL, Levy MM (2004) Surviving Sepsis Campaign guidelines for management of severe sepsis and septic shock. Intensive Care Med 30:536–555

Diebel LN, Dulchavsky SA, Brown WJ (1997) Splanchnic ischemia and bacterial translocation in the abdominal compartment syndrome. J Trauma 43:852–855

Doty JM, Oda J, Ivatury RR, Blocher CR, Christie GE, Yelon JA, Sugerman HJ (2002) The effects of hemodynamic shock and increased intra-abdominal pressure on bacterial translocation. J Trauma 52:13–17

Duperret S, Lhuillier F, Piriou V, Vivier E, Metton O, Branche P, Annat G, Bendjelid K, Viale JP (2007) Increased intra-abdominal pressure affects respiratory variations in arterial pressure in normovolaemic and hypovolaemic mechanically ventilated healthy pigs. Intensive Care Med 33(1):163–171, Epub 2006 Nov 11

Ejike JC, Humbert S, Bahjri K, Mathur M (2007) Outcomes of children with abdominal compartment syndrome. Acta Clin Belg Suppl (1):141–148

Ivatury R, Diebel L (2006) Intra-abdominal hypertension and the splanchnic bed. In: Ivatury R, Cheatham M, Malbrain M, Sugrue M (eds) Abdominal compartment syndrome. Landes Bioscience, Georgetown, pp 129–137

Josephs LG, Este-McDonald JR, Birkett DH, Hirsch EF (1994) Diagnostic laparoscopy increases intracranial pressure. J Trauma 36:815–818; discussion 818–819

Kashtan J, Green JF, Parsons EQ, Holcroft JW (1981) Hemodynamic effect of increased abdominal pressure. J Surg Res 30:249–255

Kimball EJ, Rollins MD, Mone MC, Hansen HJ, Baraghoshi GK, Johnston C, Day ES, Jackson PR, Payne M, Barton RG (2006) Survey of intensive care physicians on the recognition and management of intra-abdominal hypertension and abdominal compartment syndrome. Crit Care Med 34:2340–2348

Kologlu M, Sayek I, Kologlu LB, Onat D (1999) Effect of persistently elevated intraabdominal pressure on healing of colonic anastomoses. Am J Surg 178:293–297

Kula R, Szturz P, Sklienka P, Neiser J (2008) Negative fluid balance in patients with abdominal compartment syndrome–case reports. Acta Chir Belg 108:346–349

Malbrain ML (2004) Different techniques to measure intra-abdominal pressure (IAP): time for a critical re-appraisal. Intensive Care Med 30:357–371

Malbrain ML, Cheatham ML (2004) Cardiovascular effects and optimal preload markers in intra-abdominal hypertension. In: Vincent J-L (ed) Yearbook of intensive care and emergency medicine. Springer, Berlin, pp 519–543

Malbrain ML, Chiumello D, Pelosi P, Wilmer A, Brienza N, Malcangi V, Bihari D, Innes R, Cohen J, Singer P, Japiassu A, Kurtop E, De Keulenaer BL, Daelemans R, Del Turco M, Cosimini P, Ranieri M, Jacquet L, Laterre PF, Gattinoni L (2004) Prevalence of intra-abdominal hypertension in critically ill patients: a multicentre epidemiological study. Intensive Care Med 30:822–829

Malbrain ML, Chiumello D, Pelosi P, Bihari D, Innes R, Ranieri VM, Del Turco M, Wilmer A, Brienza N, Malcangi V, Cohen J, Japiassu A, De Keulenaer BL, Daelemans R, Jacquet L, Laterre PF, Frank G, de Souza P, Cesana B, Gattinoni L (2005a) Incidence and prognosis of intraabdominal hypertension in a mixed population of critically ill patients: a multiple-center epidemiological study. Crit Care Med 33:315–322

Malbrain ML, Deeren D, De Potter TJ (2005b) Intra-abdominal hypertension in the critically ill: it is time to pay attention. Curr Opin Crit Care 11:156–171

Malbrain ML, Cheatham ML, Kirkpatrick A, Sugrue M, Parr M, De Waele J, Balogh Z, Leppaniemi A, Olvera C, Ivatury R, D'Amours S, Wendon J, Hillman K, Johansson K, Kolkman K, Wilmer A (2006) Results from the International Conference of Experts on intra-abdominal hypertension and abdominal compartment syndrome. I. Definitions. Intensive Care Med 32:1722–1732

Malbrain ML, De laet I, Van Regenmortel N, Schoonheydt K, Dits H (2009) Can the abdominal perimeter be used as an accurate estimation of intra-abdominal pressure? Crit Care Med 37:316–319

Mullens W, Abrahams Z, Francis GS, Taylor DO, Starling RC, Tang WH (2008) Prompt reduction in intra-abdominal pressure following large-volume mechanical fluid removal improves renal insufficiency in refractory decompensated heart failure. J Card Fail 14:508–514

Mutoh T, Lamm WJ, Embree LJ, Hildebrandt J, Albert RK (1991) Abdominal distension alters regional pleural pressures and chest wall mechanics in pigs in vivo. J Appl Physiol 70: 2611–2618

Oda J, Ueyama M, Yamashita K, Inoue T, Noborio M, Ode Y, Aoki Y, Sugimoto H (2006) Hypertonic lactated saline resuscitation reduces the risk of abdominal compartment syndrome in severely burned patients. J Trauma 60:64–71

O'Mara MS, Slater H, Goldfarb IW, Caushaj PF (2005) A prospective, randomized evaluation of intra-abdominal pressures with crystalloid and colloid resuscitation in burn patients. J Trauma 58:1011–1018

Pelosi P, Quintel M, Malbrain ML (2007) Effect of intra-abdominal pressure on respiratory mechanics. Acta Clin Belg Suppl (1):78–88

Regueira T, Bruhn A, Hasbun P, Aguirre M, Romero C, Llanos O, Castro R, Bugedo G, Hernandez G (2008) Intra-abdominal hypertension: incidence and association with organ dysfunction during early septic shock. J Crit Care 23:461–467

Reintam A, Parm P, Kitus R, Kern H, Starkopf J (2008) Primary and secondary intra-abdominal hypertension–different impact on ICU outcome. Intensive Care Med 34:1624–1631

Renner J, Gruenewald M, Quaden R, Hanss R, Meybohm P, Steinfath M, Scholz J, Bein B (2009) Influence of increased intra-abdominal pressure on fluid responsiveness predicted by pulse pressure variation and stroke volume variation in a porcine model*. Crit Care Med 37(2): 650–658

Richardson JD, Trinkle JK (1976) Hemodynamic and respiratory alterations with increased intra-abdominal pressure. J Surg Res 20:401–404

Sugrue M, Bauman A, Jones F, Bishop G, Flabouris A, Parr M, Stewart A, Hillman K, Deane SA (2002) Clinical examination is an inaccurate predictor of intraabdominal pressure. World J Surg 26:1428–1431

Vidal MG, Ruiz Weisser J, Gonzalez F, Toro MA, Loudet C, Balasini C, Canales H, Reina R, Estenssoro E (2008) Incidence and clinical effects of intra-abdominal hypertension in critically ill patients. Crit Care Med 36:1823–1831

Vincent JL, Sakr Y, Sprung CL, Ranieri VM, Reinhart K, Gerlach H, Moreno R, Carlet J, Le Gall JR, Payen D, Sepsis Occurrence in Acutely Ill Patients Investigators (2006) Sepsis in European intensive care units: results of the SOAP study. Crit Care Med 34:344–353

Yagci G, Zeybek N, Kaymakcioglu N, Gorgulu S, Tas H, Aydogan MH, Avci IY, Cetiner S (2005) Increased intra-abdominal pressure causes bacterial translocation in rabbits. J Chin Med Assoc 68:172–177

Assessing Renal Dysfunction in Septic Patients

7

Gordon Y.S. Choi, Gavin M. Joynt, and Charles D. Gomersall

7.1   Introduction

Both sepsis and renal dysfunction are common in critically ill patients. A consensus definition for sepsis has existed for over 20 years, and more recently renal dysfunction has also been categorized by consensus into progressive grades and termed acute kidney injury (AKI). Of patients in the intensive care unit (ICU) who develop AKI, sepsis and septic shock have been estimated to be the likely cause in 11–50% of cases (Bagshaw et al. 2007a; Oh et al. 1993; Metnitz et al. 2002; Schwilk et al. 1997; Douma et al. 1997; Uchino et al. 2005). The incidence of AKI increases with the severity of sepsis, from approximately 19% in patients with moderate sepsis, to 23% in patients with severe sepsis, and 51% in patients with septic shock (Riedemann et al. 2003; Rangel-Frausto et al. 1995). AKI in septic patients, or septic AKI, is frequently associated with other organ failures. A retrospective analysis of over 120,000 patients in Australia and New Zealand, demonstrated that patients with septic AKI had greater physiological derangements with higher simplified acute physiology score II (SAPS II) and sequential organ failure (SOFA) scores, and a greater requirement for mechanical ventilation and infusion of vasoactive drugs, than non-septic AKI patients (Bagshaw et al. 2008). In this study septic AKI was associated with significantly higher covariate adjusted mortality in ICU (OR 1.60, 95% CI 1.5–1.7) and hospital mortality (OR 1.53, 95% CI 1.46–1.60) compared with non-septic AKI (Bagshaw et al. 2008).

The mortality of AKI in septic patients remains high (up to 70%) despite modern intensive care (Yegenaga et al. 2004; Neveu et al. 1996; Hoste et al. 2003). In a prospective observational study of over 1,700 critically ill patients in 54 hospitals in 73 countries, patients with septic AKI had a higher in-hospital case-fatality rate

G.Y.S. Choi • G.M. Joynt (✉) • C.D. Gomersall
Department of Anaesthesia and Intensive Care,
The Chinese University of Hong Kong, Prince of Wales Hospital,
Shatin, N.T, Hong Kong
e-mail: gavinmjoynt@cuhk.edu.hk

J. Rello (eds.), *Sepsis Management*,
DOI 10.1007/978-3-642-03519-7_7, © Springer-Verlag Berlin Heidelberg 2012

Table 7.1 A comparison of RIFLE and AKI definition and classification for AKI

	Serum creatinine criteria	Urinary output criteria
RIFLE classification (Bellomo et al. 2004)		
Risk	≥1.5-fold increase from baseline serum creatinine or decrease in GFR ≥25%	<0.5 mL/kg/h for ≥6 h
Injury	≥2.0-fold increase from baseline serum creatinine or decrease in GFR ≥50%	<0.5 mL/kg/h for ≥12 h
Failure	≥3.0-fold increase from baseline serum creatinine or decrease in GFR ≥75% or absolute serum creatinine ≥4.0 mg/dL (354 μmol/L) with an acute rise ≥0.5 mg/dL (44 μmol/L)	<0.3 mL/kg/h for ≥24 h or anuria ≥12 h
Loss	Need for renal replacement for ≥ 4 weeks	
End-stage kidney disease	Need for dialysis ≥ 3 months	
AKIN classification (Mehta et al. 2007)		
Stage 1	Acute rise of ≥0.3 mg/dL (26.4 μmol/L) serum creatinine or ≥150–200% increase from baseline serum creatinine	<0.5 mL/kg/h for ≥6 h
Stage 2	>200–299% increase from baseline serum creatinine	<0.5 mL/kg/h for ≥12 h
Stage 3	≥300% increase from baseline serum creatinine or absolute serum creatinine ≥4.0 mg/dL (354 lmol/L) with an acute rise ≥0.5 mg/dL (44 μmol/L) or initiation of RRT	<0.3 mL/kg/h for ≥24 h or anuria ≥12 h

compared with those who had non-septic AKI (70.2% vs. 51.8%; $P<0.001$). After adjustment for covariates, septic AKI remained associated with higher odds for death (1.48; 95% confidence interval 1.17–1.89; $P=0.001$). When stratified by RIFLE categories, patients with septic AKI had a higher ICU and hospital mortality. Moreover, septic AKI patients had a longer duration of stay in both ICU and hospital than non-septic AKI patients (Bagshaw et al. 2007a).

7.2 Definition

As is true for all disease processes, it is important to establish a common and clear definition of septic AKI. Until recently, there has been no agreed definition of acute renal failure or the various states of renal dysfunction that commonly precede renal failure. The Acute Dialysis Quality Initiative (ADQI) developed a consensus definition of AKI with the acronym of RIFLE (Bellomo et al. 2004a). More recently, minor modifications have been proposed by the Acute Kidney Injury Network (AKIN) group, however the definitions are broadly similar (Table 7.1) (Mehta et al. 2007).

Table 7.2 Consensus definitions of infection and sepsis

Infection	A pathologic process caused by the invasion of normally sterile tissue or fluid by pathogenic or potentially pathogenic microorganisms
Sepsis	The presence of infection, documented or strongly suspected, with a systemic inflammatory response, as indicated by the presence of two or more of the following criteria: 1. Temperature >38°C or <36°C 2. Heart rate > 90 beats/min 3. Respiratory rate > 20 breaths/min or $PaCO_2$ < 32 Torr (<4.3kPa) 4. WBC > 12.000 cells/mm³, <4.000 cells/mm³, or >10% immature (band) forms
Sepsis induced hypotension	A systolic blood pressure of <90 mmHg or a reduction of >40 mmHg from baseline in the absence of other causes for hypotension
Severe sepsis	Sepsis associated with organ dysfunction, hypoperfusion or hypotension. Hypoperfusion and perfusion abnormalities may include, but are not limited to, lactic acidosis, oliguria, or an acute alteration in mental status
Septic shock	Sepsis with hypotension, despite adequate fluid resuscitation, along with the presence of perfusion abnormalities that may include, but are not limited to, lactic acidosis, oliguria, or an acute alteration in mental status. Patients who are on inotropic or vasopressor agents may not be hypotensive at the time that perfusion abnormalities are measured
Multiple Organ Dysfunction Syndrome	Presence of altered organ function in an acutely ill patient such that homeostasis cannot be maintained without intervention

Adapted from (Bone et al. 1992)

In conjunction with the now widely accepted definition of sepsis, (Bone et al. 1992) the term septic AKI can be defined by the simultaneous presence of either the RIFLE or AKIN criteria for AKI, together with the consensus criteria for sepsis (Table 7.2), and the absence of other clear and established, non–sepsis-related etiologies (e.g., radiocontrast exposure, ischaemic injury, other nephrotoxins) (Bagshaw et al. 2007a; Mehta et al. 2007; Bellomo et al. 2004a).

The RIFLE classification is divided into three levels of renal dysfunction and two levels of clinical outcomes, the latter being represented by "Loss" and "End-stage kidney disease." More recently, the AKIN proposed refinements to the RIFLE criteria. In particular, the AKIN group sought to increase the sensitivity of the RIFLE criteria by recommending that a smaller change in serum creatinine ($\geq$26.2 μmol/L) be used as a threshold to define the presence of AKI and identify patients with Stage 1 AKI (analogous to RIFLE-Risk). Secondly, changes in serum creatinine are determined within a time window of 48 h instead of referring to a baseline value. Finally, any patients receiving renal replacement therapy (RRT) are to now be classified as Stage 3 AKI (RIFLE-Failure). Differences in nomenclature and classifications of AKI based on RIFLE and AKIN criteria are highlighted in (Table 7.1). It is currently unknown whether discernible advantages of one approach over the other exist, as previous comparative studies were either performed retrospectively or inclusion criteria used were significantly heterogeneous (Lopes et al. 2008; Ostermann et al. 2008; Bagshaw et al. 2008a). Nevertheless, the degree of severity AKI whether classified by either RIFLE or AKIN is associated with a proportional increased in hospital mortality (Joannidis et al. 2009).

Despite minor differences in the interpretation of the two criteria currently available, and the likelihood that there will be ongoing refinement of both definitions with time and the accrual of new knowledge, there is a general acceptance of the need to identify and classify AKI by recognized consensus definitions, both to improve diagnostic accuracy and to facilitate research (Ostermann et al. 2008; Ricci et al. 2008).

7.3 Pathogenesis

Despite a moderate reduction in the mortality of patients with sepsis in recent years, mortality from those with septic AKI requiring renal replacement therapy remains high (Levy et al. 2010; Uchino et al. 2005; Bagshaw et al. 2007). Unfortunately, the pathogenesis and pathology of septic AKI is not well understood at present and this may, at least in part, explain why therapeutic advances for AKI have been limited. We will briefly review recent studies that have attempted to elucidate mechanisms of renal dysfunction and damage. The results of such studies are likely to be important in future attempts to identify measures to diagnose renal pathology, assess function, predict progression and outcome, and assist formulation of targeted therapeutic intervention strategies.

Important potential factors related to the pathogenesis of septic AKI include both disturbances in systemic or regional renal blood flow, as well as renal cellular and tissue damage caused by the direct action of septic mediators or the micro-vascular complications of sepsis.

7.3.1 Systemic and Regional Blood flow Abnormalities

The classic theory of renal pathogenesis is that sepsis induces systemic vasodilation that is associated with regional renal vasoconstriction resulting in progressive hypoperfusion and ischemia of the kidneys (Fig. 7.1a). Persistent hypoperfusion ultimately causes acute tubular necrosis (ATN) (Lameire et al. 2005; Langenberg et al. 2006; Schrier and Wang 2004). This apparently paradoxical regional renal vasoconstriction is explained by observations that increased levels of catecholamine and activation of the rennin-angiotensin-aldosterone system occur in sepsis and septic shock as part of the central neurological response to vasodilatory induced hypotension (Schrier and Wang 2004). This model derives largely from the results of animal models investigating septic hypodynamic shock with reduced cardiac output (Udy et al. 2010). However it has more recently been observed that when basic principles of fluid and vasopressor resuscitation for septic ICU patients are implemented as a normal part of modern critically ill management, a hyperdynamic septic state with an increased cardiac output generally results and therefore potentially increased regional renal perfusion may also occur (Rivers et al. 2001). In view of this, the explanatory animal models of hypodynamic septic AKI leading to ATN have recently been challenged (Wan et al. 2008; Mathiak et al. 2000). For example, Langenberg et al. in an attempt to quantify the progression to ATN, reviewed histopathology data from 184 septic AKI patients, and found that only 22% had evidence of ATN (Langenberg et al. 2008). Newer septic animal models, for example those incorporating an animal model subjected to caecal ligation puncture (CLP), create a more clinically relevant haemodynamic pattern of a hyperdynamic circulation characterized by an elevated cardiac output (Mathiak et al. 2000; Koo et al. 2001; Villazón et al. 1975) and the use of appropriate fluid and vasopressor resuscitated

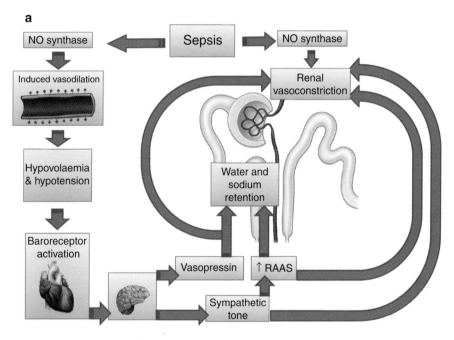

Fig. 7.1 (**a**) A simplified illustration of the traditional model of sepsis induced renal failure. Despite the vasodialtory effect of nitric oxide (*NO*) synthase, sepsis induced hypovolaemia and hypotension activates the sympathetic and renin-angiotensin-aldosterone system (*RAAS*) resulting in net renal vasoconstriction, decrease in glomerular filtration rate, and if severe and persistent enough, ischaemia induced tissue damage (ATN). (**b**) A simplified illustration of the proposed contemporary, resuscitated model of sepsis induced renal failure. Sepsis induced hypovolaemia and hypotension, when treated early and aggressively results in reduced activation the sympathetic and renin-angiotensin-aldosterone system (*RAAS*) causing less renal vasoconstriction. The net effect of vasodilatation from unopposed *NO* may result in a decrease in glomerular filtration rate because of the loss of afferent – efferent renal arteriolar control rather than decreased renal blood flow. Despite adequate renal blood flow, with time inflammatory mechanisms and apoptosis are likely to contribute to tissue damage. (**c**) A simplified diagram of inflammatory mechanisms potentially leading to endothelial and renal tissue damage

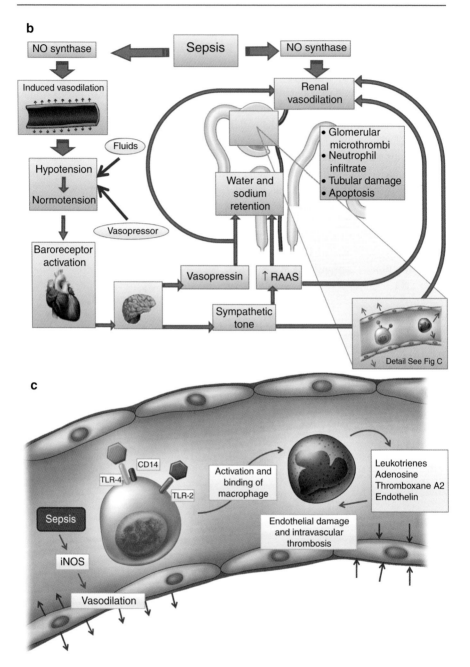

Fig. 7.1 (continued)

animal models to investigate the effect of sepsis on renal blood flow has revealed that renal blood flow is not necessarily reduced by sepsis. An experimental sheep model demonstrated that hyperdynamic sepsis with significantly increased cardiac output was associated with systemic and renal vasodilatation and a marked increase in renal blood flow (RBF) (Langenberg et al. 2006). Other experimental models of sepsis and septic shock have confirmed augmentation of renal blood flow and creatinine clearance (CrCl) when animals were resuscitated with normal saline and norepinephrine infusion (Wan et al. 2006; Di Giantomasso et al. 2003a). A recent multivariate analysis of 156 septic animal studies suggested that that renal blood flow responds primarily to cardiac output, such that, in the presence of a decreased cardiac output, RBF is typically decreased, whereas in the presence of a preserved or increased cardiac output, RBF is maintained or increased (Langenberg et al. 2005). These findings suggest that a reduction in renal blood flow is unlikely to be responsible for the functional changes and pathology of septic AKI in adequately resuscitated septic critically ill patients (Fig. 7.1b).

Glomerular filtration is an essential function of the kidney and assessment of glomerular filtration rate (GFR) is commonly used to assess renal function. GFR is primarily determined by the difference in arterial pressure between the afferent and efferent arterioles across the glomerular capillary bed (transcapillary filtration pressure). A complex set of interactions induced by septic mediators potentially influence changes in GFR during sepsis. The arterial vasodilatation that accompanies sepsis is mediated by cytokines that up-regulate the expression of inducible nitric oxide synthase and activate ATP-sensitive potassium channels. A deficiency of vasopressin over time may also contribute to changes in vascular reactivity both systemically and regionally (Landry and Oliver 2001). Animal studies suggest that in a resuscitated model of septic AKI, vasodilation is likely to affect regional renal vasculature in a similar way. In a well-resuscitated large mammal septic AKI model of hyperdynamic sepsis, RBF markedly increased while renal vascular resistance and GFR decreased, resulting in a reduction in glomerular filtration pressure. It was interesting that renal recovery from this form of septic AKI was associated with a decrease in cardiac output and RBF, but an increase in renal vascular resistance (Langenberg et al. 2006).

Other septic mediators may cause preferential glomerular afferent arteriolar constriction and these include leukotrienes, adenosine, thromboxane A2 and tumor necrosis factor induced endothelin (Kon and Badr 1991; Filep 2000). The effective reduction in the surface area for filtration as a local effect of vasoconstricting mediators within the afferent/efferent arteriolar system involved in sepsis has also been described (Ronco and Bellomo 1998).

These observations suggest that changes in regional renal vascular activity may be important in the loss of glomerular filtration pressure at least during the first 24–48 h of sepsis. Such dynamic fluctuations in glomerular filtration pressure in septic AKI in the setting of markedly increased RBF may represent a unique form of AKI. Which of the mechanisms discussed above is the predominant, how they interact or progress from one mechanism to another over time, how they are affected by systemic haemodynamic state (effect of resuscitation and vasopressor use), or whether the severity or type of septic insult affects the renal response is currently unknown.

It may be worth noting that current clinical methods of assessing renal function using parameters urine output and serum creatinine (SCr)/creatinine clearance (CrCl) may reflect functional and not necessarily intrinsic pathological changes to either cellular mechanisms or structure, particularly in the early stages of sepsis.

7.3.2 Renal Endothelial and Tissue Damage

Septic AKI most commonly occurs as part of the multiple organ dysfunction syndrome (MODS) complicating sepsis. The pathophysiology of sepsis and resulting MODS has been extensively reviewed elsewhere (Kohl and Deutschman 2006; Bone et al. 1992; Levy et al. 2003). In brief, the systemic hypermetabolic and inflammatory state occurs as a secondary response to the release of endogenous cytokines and other inflammatory mediators (Fig. 7.1c). Organs are affected as they respond to both the septic insult directly and as part of the systemic inflammatory process (Kohl and Deutschman 2006; Bone et al. 1992; Levy et al. 2003).

One of the most widely studied inflammatory pathways of sepsis is the interaction of Toll Like Receptors (TLRs) with their ligands, especially the release of the pro-inflammatory cytokine TNF-α and other chemokines, produced via the activation of NF-κB (Cohen 2002). Musson et al. demonstrated that systemic endotoxin has direct access to renal tissue and renal TLR4 increases endotoxin uptake by the kidney (Musson et al. 1978). Others have also demonstrated the presence of endotoxin intracellularly in the proximal tubules, and on both apical microvilli and intracellular organelles of tubular epithelial cells (Kang et al. 1995; El-Achkar et al. 2006).

In the kidney, sepsis is known to be associated with the generation of reactive oxygen species through the activity of tumor necrosis factor alpha (TNF-α) and other mediators. Reactive oxygen species are known to contribute to regional vasoconstriction and endothelial tissue damage. In non-septic states, endogenous scavengers of reactive oxygen species have been shown to attenuate these changes, however during endotoxaemia messenger RNA and extracellular superoxide dismutase protein molecules in blood vessels and the kidney are decreased, increasing the likelihood of endothelial and tissue damage from reactive oxygen species (Wang et al. 2003; Le Dorze et al. 2009). Other mechanisms that contribute to endothelial damage that may occur during sepsis include vascular obstruction from microthrombi that accompany the disseminated intravascular coagulation (DIC) associated with sepsis, or the increased concentration of von Willebrand factor in the circulation of septic patients (Reinhart et al. 2002).

There is also growing evidence to implicate apoptosis as another important mechanism of renal tubular injury during sepsis (Jo et al. 2002). Messmer et al. have shown that TNF-α and LPS elicit apoptotic cell death of cultured bovine glomerular endothelial cells in a time and concentration dependent manner (Messmer et al. 1999). In another recent CLP rat model, the expression of apoptosis regulator proteins such as bcl-2-associated x protein (bax) and caspase-8 protein were elevated significantly in a parallel fashion early in the course of sepsis and increases were associated with higher mortality (Messaris et al. 2008). A recent observational post-mortem study in humans demonstrated a higher percentage of apoptotic cells in the tubules of septic patients with AKI when compared with non-septic patients with AKI. Interestingly, intense infiltrates of glomeruli and interstitial capillaries by leucocytes was also noted in the septic AKI group (Lerolle et al. 2010).

Tissue ischaemia caused by one or a combination of vasoconstriction, thrombosis, endothelial dysfunction or endothelial damage, is frequently cited as a central mechanism explaining the tissue damage (or ATN) at times noted in septic AKI. Although there is some evidence to support this mechanism, cellular dysoxia secondary to sepsis-induced mitochondrial dysfunction has more recently been proposed as a major mechanism of cellular damage in sepsis and septic shock, challenging the concept that inadequate tissue oxygen delivery under ischaemic conditions is the prime cause of organ dysfunction, including septic AKI (Brealey and Singer 2003; Leverve 2007).

In summary, these observations suggest that direct cytotoxic and inflammatory mechanisms are important in mediating renal injury during sepsis and that hemodynamic factors do not operate in isolation, however, the relative contribution of these factors is poorly understood, and it is important that future research is conducted to evaluate these mechanisms in appropriate, clinically relevant, septic animal models of AKI.

7.4 Limitations of Conventional Definitions and Markers of Renal Function

It is important to have some understanding of the pathogenesis of septic AKI, despite its complexity and uncertainty, because methods of assessing AKI should ideally reflect the realities of the underlying pathophysiological abnormalities. Diagnosing and assessing the progress of AKI in the clinical setting is currently dependent on relatively crude measures of change in renal function such as urine output, and urea or creatinine concentrations in serum and urine (Mehta et al. 2007; Bellomo et al. 2004). These parameters are readily available, easy to measure and relatively cheap to acquire, however an understanding of their limitations, in the context of known pathogenesis, is critical to their proper interpretation.

The use of serum urea to diagnose AKI is no longer recommended, but in patients who require hemodialysis, serum urea concentration has been used to evaluate dialysis adequacy. http://www.kidney.org However, in the critically ill septic patient, a number of common factors such as reduction of effective circulating volume, increased dietary protein, gastrointestinal bleeding, and drugs (e.g., corticosteroids and tetracyclines) may give rise to an elevation of urea independent of changes of GFR and make interpretation more difficult. Of course, fever, trauma, burns and sepsis itself has been shown to cause an elevation of urea limiting its utility as a measure of renal function (Bellomo et al. 2004; Levey 1990).

Creatinine is an amino acid compound derived from skeletal muscle (Stevens and Levey 2005). Unfortunately, creatinine is often an unreliable indicator during acute changes in kidney function for a number of reasons: most of the total body creatine pool (98%) is in skeletal muscle, and baseline serum creatinine (SCr) levels can vary widely with age, gender, lean muscle mass, dietary intake, and muscle metabolism; changes in SCr are insensitive to renal dysfunction and are not detectable until about 50% of kidney function has been lost; and at lower rates of glomerular filtration, the increase tubular secretion of creatinine results in overestimation of renal function (Bellomo et al. 2004b). After acute changes in glomerular filtration, SCr does not accurately depict kidney function until steady-state equilibrium has been reached, a process that may require several days (Shemesh et al. 1985). Furthermore, in many centers, correct interpretation of SCr concentrations is also hampered by the variation in calibration of the different creatinine assays in different centers (Coresh et al. 2002; Delanghe 2002). Importantly, however, SCr is easily and cheaply measured, widely available and changes from baseline (including the rate of change) do correlate acceptably with changes in GFR. Therefore, despite the drawbacks, its measurement has been widely accepted, and included as the method of choice for GFR estimation in recent consensus definitions of acute kidney injury (Mehta et al. 2007; Bellomo et al. 2004b).

Due to its convenience, creatinine clearance is also commonly used as a marker to determine GFR directly. While measurements of the clearance of inulin or radio-labeled compounds such as iothalamate, DTPA, or EDTA provide a highly accurate assessment of GFR, (Brändström et al. 1998) these tests are not routinely available. A more practical and most commonly used approach is by determination a 24 h urine creatinine clearance, which should allow quantification of glomerular filtration once when a steady state is reached. However, even when collection is complete, the accuracy of creatinine clearance is limited because as GFR falls tubular creatinine secretion is increased, thus resulting in a potentially large overestimation of the GFR (by as much as a twofold difference) when creatinine clearance is very low (Kim et al. 1969; Stevens and Levey 2009). A shorter duration of urinary creatinine collection (8 and 12 h) has been used to determine the GFR in critically ill patients (Wells and Lipman 1997a, b). An ultra short collection time of 2 h has also been investigated and found to provide similar results to a 24 h collection (Sladen et al. 1987; Herrera-Gutiérrez et al. 2007). However, given the dynamic nature of development of sepsis, septic shock, and multiple organ dysfunction, controversy exists over the most useful duration of specimen collection. Furthermore, since patients are not likely to be in steady state during acute sepsis, urine creatinine clearance will not accurately reflect GFR.

Urine output is an easily and routinely measured parameter in the ICU. The trend in urine flow has the potential to provide a continuous estimation of renal function and is potentially more sensitive to changes in renal function than biochemical markers. However, it is affected by so many factors other than renal dysfunction that it is of limited value, except when severely decreased or absent. The associated volume depletion and hypotension, as commonly occurs in sepsis, are also profound stimuli for vasopressin secretion and may induce a centrally mediated decrease in urine output in the absence of renal dysfunction or AKI. Occasionally, satisfactory urine output may even be present in those with tubular damage and loss of concentrating ability (i.e., non-oliguric renal failure) (Kellum 2008).

In an attempt to distinguish possible causes for changes in urine output or the mechanism or stage of AKI, biochemical examination of urine (often interpreted in the context of serum biochemistry in the form of derived indices) is frequently practiced. Numerous tests of urinary biochemistry (e.g., osmolality [Uosm], sodium concentration [U_{Na}], fractional excretion of sodium [FeNa], fractional excretion of urea [FeU], fractional excretion of uric acid [FeUr], excretion of litium [FeLi]) have been described as surrogates of renal tubular cell function and traditionally used to aid clinicians in the detection and classification of early AKI into pre-renal (appropriate functional renal response under stressed conditions) and renal failure (acute tubular necrosis (ATN) or other actual tissue damage) (Brändström et al. 1998; Lameire et al. 2008). Unfortunately these well known tests have either been inadequately investigated or shown to be insensitive and nonspecific. A recent systematic review by Bagshaw et al. has demonstrated the lack of evidence to support the clinical utilities of urinary indices in patients with septic AKI. Specifically, U_{Na} level, Urine to Plasma (U/P) creatinine ratio, Uosm, U/P osmolality ratio, and serum urea-creatinine ratio have been inadequately studied in patients with sepsis and their diagnostic accuracy is unknown. Even FeNa, the most widely cited urinary biochemical index, has questionable diagnostic accuracy, and did not consistently predict the need for renal replacement therapy or renal recovery in patients with septic AKI (Bagshaw et al. 2006). There are also few data describing the progression of urinary markers following the onset of septic AKI, or changes in response to therapeutic interventions. Some studies suggest that early septic shock may be characterized by a sodium-avid state marked by low U_{Na} and FeNa, however, with time this pattern may change with progressively increasing urinary sodium losses. Therefore depending on the time of the first measurement in septic AKI, U_{Na} and FeNa results may vary widely (Lam and Kaufman 1985; Vaz 1983).

Urine microscopy has traditionally been used to identify tubular damage and distinguish pre-renal dysfunction from ATN. The distinguishing features for sediment in ATN being coarse granular or mixed cellular casts. Unfortunately little data supports the diagnostic accuracy of this approach in critically ill patients or septic AKI. Nevertheless urine analysis remains important to distinguish certain specific forms of renal disease such as glomerular disease or allergic interstitial nephritis (Bagshaw et al. 2006).

7.5 Newer Approaches to Assessing Dysfunction and Damage – Biomarkers

While serum urea, creatinine (SCr), urine output, urine biochemistry, and various indices derived from these parameters are commonly used to assess renal function, others such as urine microscopy attempt to assess renal cellular damage. As has been shown above, all currently used methods have relatively poor diagnostic and

Table 7.3 Potential candidates for future biomarkers of acute kidney injury (AKI)

Low molecular weight peptides/proteins

    s-Cystatin and u-Cystatin

    s-Neutrophil gelatinase-associated lipocalin (NGAL), u-NGAL

    u-$\beta2$-Microglobulin ($\beta2$-M)

    u-$\alpha1$-Microglobulin ($\alpha1$-M)

    u-Adenosine deaminase binding protein (ABP)

    u-Retinol binding protein (RBP)

    u-Proximal renal tubular epithelial antigen *(HRTE-1)*. Urinary

Urinary enzymes

    u-Alanine Aminopeptidase (AAP)

    u-Alkaline Phosphatase (ALP)

    u-N-acetyl-β-glucosaminidase (NAG)

    u-Lactate dehydrogenase (LDH)

    u-α-glutathione S-transferase (α-GST)

    u-π-glutathione S-transferase (π-GST)

    u-γ-glutamyl transpeptidase (γ-GT).

Urinary cytokines

    u-Platelet activating factor *(PAF)*

    u-Interleukin-18 *(IL-18)*

Miscellaneous biomarkers

    u-*Kidney injury molecule-1 (KIM-1)* -a type 1 transmembrane glycoprotein

    u-*Na+/H + exchanger isoform 3 (NHE3)*- sodium transporter in renal tubule

predictive ability. In clinical practice, the diagnosis of glomerular filtration failure is made late in the progression of the condition – only after endogenous filtration markers such as SCr have accumulated in the blood and/or oliguria or anuria has developed. This often occurs days after the injury, and then only when function has dramatically diminished. Better markers of early dysfunction or tissue damage may therefore: improve diagnostic ability (identify the anatomical location and type of injury); pathogenesis of the injury (septic, ischaemic or toxic); allow early and precise prediction of future deterioration (stratification of severity and outcome prediction). Improving the assessment of these factors is essential not only to guide the development of appropriate preventive measures, but also the development of specific therapeutic interventions.

Recently, several biomarkers, measured in both serum (s-) and urine (u-), have been identified that may be capable of identifying renal cellular damage or dysfunction (Table 7.3). Although few clinical studies have investigated the use of biomarkers in septic AKI, there have been limited investigations in critically ill patients and some potentially useful future markers for septic AKI have been identified.

Renal epithelial enzymes such as such as N-acetyl-b-D-glucosaminidase (NAG), brush border enzymes including g-glutamyl transferase (gGT) and alkaline phosphatase, as well as cytosolic proteins such as a-glutathione S-transferase (a-GST) are potential, but unproved candidates. More recently, the use of human neutrophil gelatinase-associated lipocalin (NGAL) has been extensive investigated to be of a potential early marker of AKI. It is a 25 kDa protein covalently bound to gelatinase in neutrophil granules and is normally expressed at very low levels in several human tissues including the kidney. NGAL expression is markedly induced in injured epithelia, and NGAL protein is easily detected in the blood and urine soon after AKI (Mori and Nakao 2007; Xu and Venge 2000). In critically ill children, serum NGAL concentration increases progressively with severity of sepsis, and AKI (Wheeler et al. 2008). A similar association with sepsis severity has been observed in critically adults with AKI, and in one study was independently associated with mortality (Kümpers et al. 2010). In another observational study of AKI patients, septic AKI was associated with significantly higher s-NGAL (293 vs. 166 ng/mL) and u-NGAL (204 vs. 39 ng/mg creatinine) concentration at enrollment, 12 and 24 h compared with non-septic AKI ($p < 0.001$) (Bagshaw et al. 2010). This observation suggests that measurement of NGAL concentrations may potentially provide a method of distinguishing septic AKI from other forms of AKI in critically ill patients such as AKI secondary to nephrotoxic agents like drugs and contrast agents, or ischaemic hypoxic insults. In another prospective observational study that specifically examined a subgroup of patients with septic shock, u-NGAL was significantly higher in patients with AKI than in those without AKI, and high concentrations of u-NGAL (>68 ng/mg creatinine) were able to predict the onset of AKI within 12 h (AUC-ROC 0.86) (Mårtensson et al. 2010). Thus it seems that NGAL may have potential uses as a biomarker in sepsis and AKI, with s-NGAL possibly being more useful to define the presence of sepsis in AKI patients, and u-NGAL having greater utility in predicting or confirming AKI in patients with sepsis and septic shock.

Interleukin 18 (IL-18) is a pro-inflammatory cytokine induced and activated in the proximal renal tubules in response to kidney injury. Thus it has potential as a diagnostic marker (Parikh and Devarajan 2008). In one study, excretion was higher in septic than in non-septic AKI, suggesting it may also have potential to differentiate sepsis or inflammatory causes of AKI from others (Bagshaw et al. 2007). In a large observational study in patients with acute lung injury, urine IL-18 predicted deterioration in kidney function 24 h before SCr, and was an independent predictor of mortality, suggesting it may be useful as a marker for early diagnosis as well as risk stratification (Parikh et al. 2005).

Following proximal tubular kidney injury, the ectodomain of Kidney Injury Molecule (KIM-1) protein is lost into urine. It is an early, sensitive and specific indicator of proximal tubular injury (Waikar and Bonventre 2007; Vaidya et al. 2006). It may be more specific for ischaemic and nephrotoxic kidney injury and of value in differentiating injury subtypes, (Parikh and Devarajan 2008; Liangos et al. 2007) but its early predictive value for failure or mortality in ICU patients is unclear (Liangos et al. 2007).

Cystatin C is a protein produced by all nucleated cells. It has a low molecular weight and is freely filtered by the glomerulus, but is then is avidly reabsorbed and metabolized in the proximal tubule. Reduced GFR results in increased serum Cystatin C concentrations (Villa et al. 2005; Delanaye et al. 2004). It has been used as a marker of acute renal dysfunction and for estimation of GFR in ICU patients with moderate success. When compared to creatinine, Cystatin C concentrations may be less dependent on age, sex, race and muscle mass, but may be affected by malignancy, thyroid disease and glucocorticoid use. Unfortunately, elevation of s-Cystatin C poorly predicts the need for renal replacement therapy in ICU patients (Bagshaw et al. 2007a). A recent human observational study in 444 patients showed that u-Cystatin C was independently associated with each of sepsis, AKI and death. u-Cystatin C was also predictive of these three outcomes, however it's utility as a biomarker for AKI in the ICU remains uncertain because the confounding effect of sepsis has yet to be clearly quantified (Nejat et al. 2010).

An increasing number of possible new biomarkers for the assessment of AKI are being identified. It has also been suggested that several biomarkers could be measured simultaneously as a panel in the clinical setting in future to allow delineation of insult timing, and improve the sensitivity and specificity of individual markers (Parikh and Devarajan 2008). This is an interesting concept, unfortunately, to date testing to confirm the validity of these individual markers has so far been in only small patient samples, and clinical use is likely to be some way off.

7.6   Supra-Normal Renal Function in Critically Ill Patients

Although data is currently limited, in critically ill patients with early sepsis, GFR may be increased by sepsis and some of the therapeutic interventions that form part of modern intensive therapy. There is evidence demonstrating that the haemodynamic alterations associated with sepsis, together with fluid resuscitation, and the use of vasopressors as part of the management of sepsis, increase cardiac output in patients with resuscitated sepsis (Parrillo et al. 1990; Di Giantomasso et al. 2003). These systemic haemodynamic changes are likely to contribute to increased renal blood flow, associated increased glomerular filtration pressure and consequently an increased GFR. This condition has consequences for drug dosing and the term augmented renal clearance (ARC) has been used in this context (Udy et al. 2010). Additionally, the phenomenon of augmented renal blood flow and GFR may potentially prevent the early detection of AKI by measures such as urine output, SCr and creatinine clearance.

7.7   Conclusion

Epidemiological data suggests that sepsis is an important cause of AKI and patients with septic AKI have a high mortality despite modern intensive care support. Current methods of assessing AKI are relatively insensitive and non-specific, and are unable to separate functional abnormalities from pathological changes. Thus individual patients need to be assessed in context and with careful clinical judgment. Nevertheless, consensus definitions are important to ensure diagnostic and prognostic uniformity, and recent definitions utilizing commonly available markers of function have made progress in this regard. Therefore we recommend that assessment of septic AKI for diagnostic and prognostic purposes in the ICU be primarily based on either of the recent consensus guidelines for AKI diagnosis, combined with consensus criteria for the diagnosis of sepsis (Tables 7.1 and 7.2).

It is likely to be important to distinguish between dysfunction and tissue injury, as therapeutic interventions would be expected to be different. This is currently not possible on a routine clinical basis, but tissue markers may provide a mechanism to make this distinction in the future. Specific tissue markers may soon be able to reflect sub-types of damage or dysfunction, amenable to specific interventions. As current functional criteria only recognize failure of function relatively late in the course of the disease, markers of earlier dysfunction or damage may also assist in the development of appropriate preventive measures. The further elucidation of the pathogenesis of septic AKI remains important as it may allow the development of better diagnostic and assessment criteria, providing a basis for improved preventive and therapeutic measures.

References

Bagshaw SM, Langenberg C, Bellomo R (2006) Urinary biochemistry and microscopy in septic acute renal failure: a systematic review. Am J Kidney Dis 48:695–705

Bagshaw SM, Uchino S, Bellomo R et al (2007a) Septic acute kidney injury in critically ill patients: clinical characteristics and outcomes. Clin J Am Soc Nephrol 2:431–439

Bagshaw SM, Langenberg C, Haase M et al (2007b) Urinary biomarkers in septic acute kidney injury. Intensive Care Med 33:1285–1296

Bagshaw SM, George C, Bellomo R et al (2008a) A comparison of the RIFLE and AKIN criteria for acute kidney injury in critically ill patients. Nephrol Dial Transplant 23:1569–1574

Bagshaw SM, George C, Bellomo R et al (2008b) Early acute kidney injury and sepsis: a multicentre evaluation. Crit Care 12:R47

Bagshaw SM, Bennett M, Haase M et al (2010) Plasma and urine neutrophil gelatinase-associated lipocalin in septic versus non-septic acute kidney injury in critical illness. Intensive Care Med 36:452–461

Bellomo R, Kellum JA, Ronco C (2004a) Defining acute renal failure: physiological principles. Intensive Care Med 30:33–37

Bellomo R, Ronco C, Kellum JA et al (2004b) Acute renal failure – definition, outcome measures, animal models, fluid therapy and information technology needs: the Second International Consensus Conference of the Acute Dialysis Quality Initiative (ADQI) Group. Crit Care 8:R204–R212

Bone RC, Balk RA, Cerra FB et al (1992) Definitions for sepsis and organ failure and guidelines for the use of innovative therapies in sepsis. The ACCP/SCCM Consensus Conference Committee. American College of Chest Physicians/Society of Critical Care Medicine. Chest 101:1644–1655

Brändström E, Grzegorczyk A, Jacobsson L et al (1998) GFR measurement with iohexol and 51Cr-EDTA. A comparison of the two favoured GFR markers in Europe. Nephrol Dial Transplant 13:1176–1182

Brealey D, Singer M (2003) Mitochondrial dysfunction in sepsis. Curr Infect Dis Rep 5:365–371

Cohen J (2002) The immunopathogenesis of sepsis. Nature 420:885–891

Coresh J, Astor BC, McQuillan G et al (2002) Calibration and random variation of the serum creatinine assay as critical elements of using equations to estimate glomerular filtration rate. Am J Kidney Dis 39:920–929

Delanaye P, Lambermont B, Chapelle JP et al (2004) Plasmatic cystatin C for the estimation of glomerular filtration rate in intensive care units. Intensive Care Med 30:980–983

Delanghe J (2002) Standardization of creatinine determination and its consequences for the clinician. Acta Clin Belg 57:172–175

Di Giantomasso D, May CN, Bellomo R (2003a) Norepinephrine and vital organ blood flow during experimental hyperdynamic sepsis. Intensive Care Med 29:1774–1781

Di Giantomasso D, May CN, Bellomo R (2003b) Vital organ blood flow during hyperdynamic sepsis. Chest 124:1053–1059

Douma CE, Redekop WK, van der Meulen JH et al (1997) Predicting mortality in intensive care patients with acute renal failure treated with dialysis. J Am Soc Nephrol 8:111–117

El-Achkar TM, Huang X, Plotkin Z et al (2006) Sepsis induces changes in the expression and distribution of Toll-like receptor 4 in the rat kidney. Am J Physiol Renal Physiol 290: F1034–F1043

Filep JG (2000) Role for endogenous endothelin in the regulation of plasma volume and albumin escape during endotoxin shock in conscious rats. Br J Pharmacol 129:975–983

Herrera-Gutiérrez ME, Seller-Pérez G, Banderas-Bravo E et al (2007) Replacement of 24-h creatinine clearance by 2-h creatinine clearance in intensive care unit patients: a single-center study. Intensive Care Med 33:1900–1906

Hoste EA, Lameire NH, Vanholder RC et al (2003) Acute renal failure in patients with sepsis in a surgical ICU: predictive factors, incidence, comorbidity, and outcome. J Am Soc Nephrol 14:1022–1030

Jo SK, Cha DR, Cho WY et al (2002) Inflammatory cytokines and lipopolysaccharide induce Fas-mediated apoptosis in renal tubular cells. Nephron 91:406–415

Joannidis M, Metnitz B, Bauer P et al (2009) Acute kidney injury in critically ill patients classified by AKIN versus RIFLE using the SAPS 3 database. Intensive Care Med 35:1692–1702

Kang YH, Falk MC, Bentley TB et al (1995) Distribution and role of lipopolysaccharide in the pathogenesis of acute renal proximal tubule injury. Shock 4:441–449

Kellum JA (2008) Acute kidney injury. Crit Care Med 36:S141–S145

Kim KE, Onesti G, Ramirez O et al (1969) Creatinine clearance in renal disease. A reappraisal. Br Med J 4:11–14

Kohl BA, Deutschman CS (2006) The inflammatory response to surgery and trauma. Curr Opin Crit Care 12:325–332

Kon V, Badr KF (1991) Biological actions and pathophysiologic significance of endothelin in the kidney. Kidney Int 40:1–12

Koo DJ, Zhou M, Chaudry IH et al (2001) The role of adrenomedullin in producing differential hemodynamic responses during sepsis. J Surg Res 95:207–218

Kümpers P, Hafer C, Lukasz A et al (2010) Serum neutrophil gelatinase-associated lipocalin at inception of renal replacement therapy predicts survival in critically ill patients with acute kidney injury. Crit Care 14:R9

Lam M, Kaufman CE (1985) Fractional excretion of sodium as a guide to volume depletion during recovery from acute renal failure. Am J Kidney Dis 6:18–21

Lameire N, Van Biesen W, Vanholder R (2005) Acute renal failure. Lancet 365:417–430

Lameire N, Van Biesen W, Vanholder R (2008) Acute kidney injury. Lancet 372:1863–1865

Landry DW, Oliver JA (2001) The pathogenesis of vasodilatory shock. N Engl J Med 345:588–595

Langenberg C, Bellomo R, May C et al (2005) Renal blood flow in sepsis. Crit Care 9:R363–R374

Langenberg C, Bellomo R, May CN et al (2006a) Renal vascular resistance in sepsis. Nephron Physiol 104:1–11

Langenberg C, Wan L, Egi M et al (2006b) Renal blood flow in experimental septic acute renal failure. Kidney Int 69:1996–2002

Langenberg C, Bagshaw SM, May CN et al (2008) The histopathology of septic acute kidney injury: a systematic review. Crit Care 12:R38

Le Dorze M, Legrand M, Payen D et al (2009) The role of the microcirculation in acute kidney injury. Curr Opin Crit Care 15:503–508

Lerolle N, Nochy D, Guérot E et al (2010) Histopathology of septic shock induced acute kidney injury: apoptosis and leukocytic infiltration. Intensive Care Med 36:471–478

Leverve XM (2007) Mitochondrial function and substrate availability. Crit Care Med 35:S454–S460

Levey AS (1990) Measurement of renal function in chronic renal disease. Kidney Int 38:167–184

Levy MM, Fink MP, Marshall JC et al (2003) 2001 SCCM/ESICM/ACCP/ATS/SIS International Sepsis Definitions Conference. Crit Care Med 31:1250–1256

Levy MM, Dellinger RP, Townsend SR et al (2010) The Surviving Sepsis Campaign: results of an international guideline-based performance improvement program targeting severe sepsis. Intensive Care Med 36:222–231

Liangos O, Perianayagam MC, Vaidya VS et al (2007) Urinary N-acetyl-beta-(D)-glucosaminidase activity and kidney injury molecule-1 level are associated with adverse outcomes in acute renal failure. J Am Soc Nephrol 18:904–912

Lopes JA, Fernandes P, Jorge S et al (2008) Acute kidney injury in intensive care unit patients: a comparison between the RIFLE and the Acute Kidney Injury Network classifications. Crit Care 12:R110

Mårtensson J, Bell M, Oldner A et al (2010) Neutrophil gelatinase-associated lipocalin in adult septic patients with and without acute kidney injury. Intensive Care Med 36(8):1333–1340, Epub 2010 Apr 16

Mathiak G, Szewczyk D, Abdullah F et al (2000) An improved clinically relevant sepsis model in the conscious rat. Crit Care Med 28:1947–1952

Mehta RL, Kellum JA, Shah SV et al (2007) Acute Kidney Injury Network: report of an initiative to improve outcomes in acute kidney injury. Crit Care 11:R31

Messaris E, Memos N, Chatzigianni E et al (2008) Apoptotic death of renal tubular cells in experimental sepsis. Surg Infect (Larchmt) 9:377–388

Messmer UK, Briner VA, Pfeilschifter J (1999) Tumor necrosis factor-alpha and lipopolysaccharide induce apoptotic cell death in bovine glomerular endothelial cells. Kidney Int 55:2322–2337

Metnitz PG, Krenn CG, Steltzer H et al (2002) Effect of acute renal failure requiring renal replacement therapy on outcome in critically ill patients. Crit Care Med 30:2051–2058

Mori K, Nakao K (2007) Neutrophil gelatinase-associated lipocalin as the real-time indicator of active kidney damage. Kidney Int 71:967–970

Musson RA, Morrison DC, Ulevitch RJ (1978) Distribution of endotoxin (lipopolysaccharide) in the tissues of lipopolysaccharide-responsive and -unresponsive mice. Infect Immun 21: 448–457

Nejat M, Pickering JW, Walker RJ et al (2010) Urinary cystatin C is diagnostic of acute kidney injury and sepsis, and predicts mortality in the intensive care unit. Crit Care 14:R85

Neveu H, Kleinknecht D, Brivet F et al (1996) Prognostic factors in acute renal failure due to sepsis. Results of a prospective multicentre study. The French Study Group on Acute Renal Failure. Nephrol Dial Transplant 11:293–299

Oh TE, Hutchinson R, Short S et al (1993) Verification of the Acute Physiology and Chronic Health Evaluation scoring system in a Hong Kong intensive care unit. Crit Care Med 21:698–705

Ostermann M, Chang R, Riyadh ICU, Group PU (2008) Correlation between the AKI classification and outcome. Crit Care 12:R144

Parikh CR, Devarajan P (2008) New biomarkers of acute kidney injury. Crit Care Med 36: S159–S165

Parikh CR, Abraham E, Ancukiewicz M et al (2005) Urine IL-18 is an early diagnostic marker for acute kidney injury and predicts mortality in the intensive care unit. J Am Soc Nephrol 16:3046–3052

Parrillo JE, Parker MM, Natanson C et al (1990) Septic shock in humans. Advances in the understanding of pathogenesis, cardiovascular dysfunction, and therapy. Ann Intern Med 113: 227–242

Rangel-Frausto MS, Pittet D, Costigan M et al (1995) The natural history of the systemic inflammatory response syndrome (SIRS). A prospective study. JAMA 273:117–123

Reinhart K, Bayer O, Brunkhorst F et al (2002) Markers of endothelial damage in organ dysfunction and sepsis. Crit Care Med 30:S302–S312

Ricci Z, Cruz D, Ronco C (2008) The RIFLE criteria and mortality in acute kidney injury: a systematic review. Kidney Int 73:538–546

Riedemann NC, Guo RF, Ward PA (2003) The enigma of sepsis. J Clin Invest 112:460–467

Rivers E, Nguyen B, Havstad S et al (2001) Early goal-directed therapy in the treatment of severe sepsis and septic shock. N Engl J Med 345:1368–1377

Ronco C, Bellomo R (1998) Critical care nephrology. Kluwer Academic, Dordrecht

Schrier RW, Wang W (2004) Acute renal failure and sepsis. N Engl J Med 351:159–169

Schwilk B, Wiedeck H, Stein B et al (1997) Epidemiology of acute renal failure and outcome of haemodiafiltration in intensive care. Intensive Care Med 23:1204–1211

Shemesh O, Golbetz H, Kriss JP et al (1985) Limitations of creatinine as a filtration marker in glomerulopathic patients. Kidney Int 28:830–838

Sladen RN, Endo E, Harrison T (1987) Two-hour versus 22-hour creatinine clearance in critically ill patients. Anesthesiology 67:1013–1016

Stevens LA, Levey AS (2005) Measurement of kidney function. Med Clin North Am 89:457–473

Stevens LA, Levey AS (2009) Measured GFR as a confirmatory test for estimated GFR. J Am Soc Nephrol 20:2305–2313

Uchino S, Kellum JA, Bellomo R et al (2005) Acute renal failure in critically ill patients: a multinational, multicenter study. JAMA 294:813–818

Udy AA, Roberts JA, Boots RJ et al (2010) Augmented renal clearance: implications for antibacterial dosing in the critically ill. Clin Pharmacokinet 49:1–16

Vaidya VS, Ramirez V, Ichimura T et al (2006) Urinary kidney injury molecule-1: a sensitive quantitative biomarker for early detection of kidney tubular injury. Am J Physiol Renal Physiol 290:F517–F529

Vaz AJ (1983) Low fractional excretion of urine sodium in acute renal failure due to sepsis. Arch Intern Med 143:738–739

Villa P, Jiménez M, Soriano MC et al (2005) Serum cystatin C concentration as a marker of acute renal dysfunction in critically ill patients. Crit Care 9:R139–R143

Villazón SA, Sierra UA, López SF et al (1975) Hemodynamic patterns in shock and critically ill patients. Crit Care Med 3:215–221

Waikar SS, Bonventre JV (2007) Biomarkers for the diagnosis of acute kidney injury. Curr Opin Nephrol Hypertens 16:557–564

Wan L, Bellomo R, May CN (2006) The effect of normal saline resuscitation on vital organ blood flow in septic sheep. Intensive Care Med 32:1238–1242

Wan L, Bagshaw SM, Langenberg C et al (2008) Pathophysiology of septic acute kidney injury: what do we really know? Crit Care Med 36:S198–S203

Wang W, Jittikanont S, Falk SA et al (2003) Interaction among nitric oxide, reactive oxygen species, and antioxidants during endotoxemia-related acute renal failure. Am J Physiol Renal Physiol 284:F532–F537

Wells M, Lipman J (1997a) Measurements of glomerular filtration in the intensive care unit are only a rough guide to renal function. S Afr J Surg 35:20–23

Wells M, Lipman J (1997b) Pitfalls in the prediction of renal function in the intensive care unit. A review. S Afr J Surg 35:16–19

Wheeler DS, Devarajan P, Ma Q et al (2008) Serum neutrophil gelatinase-associated lipocalin (NGAL) as a marker of acute kidney injury in critically ill children with septic shock. Crit Care Med 36:1297–1303

Xu S, Venge P (2000) Lipocalins as biochemical markers of disease. Biochim Biophys Acta 1482:298–307

Yegenaga I, Hoste E, Van Biesen W et al (2004) Clinical characteristics of patients developing ARF due to sepsis/systemic inflammatory response syndrome: results of a prospective study. Am J Kidney Dis 43:817–824

Monitoring Myocardial Dysfunction as Part of Sepsis Management

8

Olfa Hamzaoui and Jean-Louis Teboul

Abbreviations

A	Peak Doppler velocity of late diastolic flow
BNP	B-type natriuretic peptide
CFI	Cardiac function index
cTnI	Cardiac troponin I
cTnT	Cardiac troponin T
E	Peak Doppler velocity of early diastolic flow
Ea	Early diastolic mitral annular velocity
GEDV	Global end-diastolic volume
LVEF	Left ventricular ejection fraction
NO	Nitric oxide
NT-proBNP	N terminal proBNP
PAC	Pulmonary artery catheter
PAOP	Pulmonary artery occlusion pressure
PEEP	Positive end-expiratory pressure
$ScvO_2$	Central venous blood oxygen saturation
SvO_2	Mixed venous blood oxygen saturation
VTIAo	Velocity-time integral of aortic blood flow

O. Hamzaoui
Service de réanimation médicale, Hôpital Antoine Béclère,
Assistance Publique–Hôpitaux de Paris, Université Paris-Sud 11,
Clamart, France

J.-L. Teboul (✉)
Service de réanimation médicale, Centre Hospitalier Universitaire de Bicêtre,
Le Kremlin-Bicêtre, Paris, France
e-mail: jean-louis.teboul@bct.aphp.fr

J. Rello (eds.), *Sepsis Management*,
DOI 10.1007/978-3-642-03519-7_8, © Springer-Verlag Berlin Heidelberg 2012

8.1   Introduction

Septic shock is a combination of hypovolemia, peripheral vascular dysfunction resulting in hypotension and abnormalities in the local/regional distribution of blood flow, cardiac failure and cell dysfunction.

Importantly, the hemodynamic profile differs from patient to patient at least regarding the macrocirculatory disturbances. Some septic patients experience a high degree of hypovolemia, others experience a high degree of impairment of vascular tone, and others experience severe cardiac failure. A variety of combinations can thus exist.

Sepsis-induced cardiac dysfunction occurs early and is both diastolic and systolic. Systolic cardiac dysfunction is related to a sepsis-induced impairment of ventricular contractility affecting the left as well as the right ventricles. Using radionuclide cineangiographic evaluation, Parker et al. reported the presence of early depression of the left ventricular ejection fraction (LVEF) in patients with septic shock in spite of normal or elevated cardiac output (Parker et al. 1984). This myocardial depression persisted for up to 4 days and returned to normal within 7–10 days in survivors (Parker et al. 1984). Diastolic dysfunction is characterized by a reduced biventricular distensibility related to myocardial interstitial edema. The degree of cardiac dysfunction is highly variable among septic patients. Using echocardiography, Vieillard-Baron et al. recently showed that in only 40% of patients was the LVEF higher than 45% during the time course of septic disease (Vieillard-Baron et al. 2008). Interestingly, in 39% of patients, the LVEF was lower than 45% at day 1 and returned to normal values at either day 2 or day 3, or after weaning of vasopressors. In 21% of patients, the LVEF was normal at day 1, but decreased below 45% at either day 2 or day 3, and eventually improved in survivors.

8.2   Mechanisms of Systolic Cardiac Dysfunction

Numerous mechanisms have been proposed to be responsible for sepsis-induced systolic cardiac dysfunction. Since they are well detailed elsewhere (Rabuel and Mebazaa 2006), we only briefly review the role of the major mechanisms.

8.2.1   Role of Circulating Myocardial Depressant Factors

A so-called "myocardial depressant factor" was shown to be present in the serum of patients with septic shock (Parrillo et al. 1985). Indeed, serum obtained from patients during the acute phase of sepsis was able to decrease the extent and the velocity of rat cardiomyocytes shortening, whereas serum obtained from nonseptic patients immediately restored the contractile force (Parrillo et al. 1985). Importantly, this phenomenon was transient and no longer persisted in the recovery phase. Cytokines such as tumor necrosis factor and interleukin 1 could play an important role in this mechanism (Kumar et al. 2007).

8.2.2   Role of Coronary Blood Flood

Coronary blood flow is generally not considered to be decreased in septic patients (Cunnion et al. 1986; Dhainaut et al. 1987). However, if diastolic arterial pressure is very low because of a marked decrease in vascular tone, myocardial ischemia could ensue since diastolic blood pressure is the driving pressure for the coronary blood flow of the left ventricle (Lamia et al. 2005).

8.2.3   Role of β_1-Adrenergic Receptor Hyporesponsiveness

The β_1-adrenergic receptor stimulation of cyclic adenosine monophosphate is impaired during septic shock (Silverman et al. 1993), especially at the early phase (Abi-Gerges et al. 1999), and this could partly explain why β_1-agonist agents such as dobutamine exert attenuated effects on patients with severe septic shock compared to patients with sepsis without shock (Silverman et al. 1993).

8.2.4   Role of Reduced Sensitivity of Myofilaments to Calcium

A decrease in the sensitivity of myofilaments to calcium also plays a crucial role in sepsis-induced cardiac dysfunction. Protein phosphorylation of tropinin I at the site where the calcium ion normally combines to the troponin complex may be involved in the reduced ability of calcium to activate the myofilament (Tavernier et al. 2001).

8.2.5   Role of Nitric Oxide (NO)

It is now thought that NO does not play an acute and direct role in septic cardiomyopathy since the inhibition of NO synthases could not be demonstrated to restore contractility (Lancel et al. 2004). It is instead assumed that cytotoxic peroxynitrite, a product of NO and superoxide, could play a more direct role (Lancel et al. 2004; Ferdinandy et al. 2000).

8.2.6   Role of Apoptosis

Increased activity of myocyte caspases, which are effectors of apoptosis, can play a role in sepsis-induced cardiac dysfunction (Lancel et al. 2005). However, the reversible nature of sepsis-induced cardiac dysfunction suggests that apoptosis plays a minor role.

8.3   How to Detect Sepsis-Induced Cardiac Dysfunction

8.3.1   Echocardiography

Doppler echocardiography is the reference method to indicate cardiac dysfunction during sepsis. Echocardiography provides important information about the systolic and diastolic function. Both transthoracic and transesophageal approaches can be used. The new generations of transthoracic imaging equipment provide good quality imaging, although there are still individuals with poor echogenicity in whom a transesophageal approach is required. Using the Simpson method, echocardiography allows measuring the LVEF, which is the key variable for diagnosing myocardial depression. It must be stressed that LVEF depends on left ventricular systolic function and not only on left ventricular contractility. In this regard, the LVEF must be interpreted in the function of systolic arterial pressure, which is considered as the afterload of the left ventricle. For example, a LVEF value of 40% indicates a mild depression of left ventricular contractility in case of normal systolic arterial pressure, but a marked myocardial depression in case of low systolic arterial pressure. Doppler echocardiography also allows assessing the degree of diastolic impairment using the determination of transmitral flow and Doppler tissue imaging. The analysis of transmitral flow allows measuring the peak Doppler velocities of early (E) and late diastolic flow (A). The E/A ratio has been proposed to estimate the left ventricular filling pressure (Vanoverschelde et al. 1995). Tissue Doppler imaging enables the measurement of the early diastolic mitral annular velocity (Ea), which has been shown to be a load-independent measure of myocardial relaxation (Nagueh et al. 1997). The combination of tissue Doppler imaging and pulsed Doppler transmitral flow allows calculating the E/Ea ratio, which is considered one of the best echocardiographic estimates of left ventricular filling pressure (Nagueh et al. 1997).

Doppler echocardiography also allows estimating left ventricular preload through easy measurement of the left ventricular end-diastolic area using the short axis, cross-sectional view. The stroke volume can be calculated as the product of the velocity-time integral of aortic blood flow (VTIAo) by the aortic valve area. Using the apical five-chamber view, the VTIAo is computed from the area under the envelope of the pulsed-wave Doppler signal obtained at the level of the aortic annulus. Using the parasternal long axis view, the diameter of the aortic orifice is measured at the insertion of the aortic cusp, and the aortic valve area is calculated (π diameter^2/4).

Echocardiography can also evaluate right ventricular function, which can be severely impaired during sepsis not only in relation to a specific myocardial depression, but also in relation to a marked increase in the right ventricular afterload either because of an associated lung injury or consequences of mechanical ventilation. The best way to assess right ventricular dysfunction is to measure the right ventricular size and specifically the right ventricular/left ventricular end-diastolic area ratio in the four-chamber view. A normal ratio is below 0.6 (Vieillard-Baron 2009). In addition, the presence of a paradoxical septal motion in systole reflects the presence of right ventricular systolic overload (Vieillard-Baron 2009).

Doppler echocardiography has two important limitations. It is an operator-dependent technique, which requires a long training period to be skilled enough to obtain reliable measurements. Importantly, Doppler echocardiography is the reference method to diagnose cardiac dysfunction. However, although it allows repetitive measurements, it cannot be considered as a continuous monitoring method.

8.3.2   Pulmonary Artery Catheter (PAC)

This is a traditional hemodynamic monitoring method in patients with septic shock. It can help to detect sepsis-related cardiac dysfunction by showing low cardiac output and elevated cardiac filling pressures (Dellinger et al. 2008). However, this definition is very questionable. Firstly, during sepsis cardiac output can be normal or even high in spite of the presence of cardiac dysfunction. Secondly, measurements of cardiac filling pressures are subjects to numerous pitfalls and measurement errors. In addition, cardiac filling pressures can be falsely elevated in patients receiving positive end-expiratory pressure (PEEP) ventilation or experiencing intrinsic PEEP. Although there are now methods that help to subtract the transmitted pressure induced by PEEP or intrinsic PEEP (Pinsky et al. 1991; Teboul et al. 2000), these methods are used too rarely. More generally, difficulties in measurements and interpretation of PAC data due to insufficient physician knowledge (Iberti et al. 1990; Gnaegi et al. 1997) are probably one of the reasons for the decline in PAC use (Wiener and Welch 2007) in addition to its high invasiveness.

In the setting of sepsis, PAC would be more helpful for making the decision to infuse inotropic drugs and monitoring their effects than for diagnosing sepsis-induced cardiac dysfunction. In this context, continuous monitoring of mixed venous blood oxygen saturation (SvO_2) can be particularly useful. A low SvO_2 value (<65–70%) can serve as a trigger for deciding to initiate inotropic therapy in the context of low cardiac output and high PAOP, or even better in the context of a low echocardiographic LVEF.

8.3.3   PiCCO System

PiCCO technology emerged 10 years ago as an advanced hemodynamic monitoring technology aimed at being an alternative to PAC. Contained in a single device, the PiCCO system consists of two different technologies, transpulmonary thermodilution and the pulse contour analysis. The patient is connected to the PiCCO monitor by a central venous catheter and a specific femoral artery catheter, which is equipped with a thermistor at its distal tip.

The thermistor measures the downstream temperature changes induced by the injection of a cold saline solution bolus in the superior vena cava. The PiCCO monitor calculates the cardiac output from the thermodilution curve using the Stewart-Hamilton algorithm. It also calculates the mean transit time and the exponential down slope time of the transpulmonary thermodilution curve. The product of the cardiac output and mean transit time, i.e., the distribution volume of the thermal indicator, is the intrathoracic thermal volume. The product of the cardiac output and exponential down slope time is the pulmonary thermal volume. The global end-diastolic volume (GEDV) is calculated automatically as the difference between the intrathoracic and pulmonary thermal volumes obtained. Since the GEDV represents the largest volume of blood contained in the four heart chambers, it is assumed to be a volumetric marker of cardiac preload. This was confirmed in a study we performed in septic shock patients where fluid loading and dobutamine both increased cardiac output by a similar extent, while only fluid loading increased the GEDV (Michard et al. 2003).

Another PiCCO parameter, called the cardiac function index (CFI), is particularly useful for assessing cardiac function. The CFI is automatically calculated using the transpulmonary thermodilution method as the ratio between the cardiac output and GEDV. In a study performed in critically ill patients, Combes et al. found that CFI correlated with left ventricular area contraction, measured using transesophageal echocardiography (Combes et al. 2004). They also found a good correlation between changes in CFI and changes in left ventricular area contraction. In a small series of septic shock patients, Ritter et al. found that CFI positively correlated with the left ventricular stroke work index and with cardiac power, both measured with a pulmonary artery catheter (Ritter et al. 2009). In a recent study that we performed in 48 patients with septic shock, we found that CFI increased by 29% with dobutamine (5 μg/kg/min), but did not change after 500 mL saline fluid infusion, confirming that CFI actually behaved as an accurate marker of cardiac systolic function (Jabot et al. 2009). We also found a good correlation between the 96 measurements of CFI and those of the LVEF measured using echocardiography. Importantly, a value of CFI<3.2 predicted a LVEF<35% with good accuracy (Jabot 2009). This suggests that a low value of CFI can alert the clinician and incite him/her to (re)perform an echocardiographic examination to confirm that cardiac systolic function is actually impaired and to explore the underlying mechanisms responsible for this cardiac dysfunction. We also reported that changes in CFI with dobutamine or fluid infusion correlated well with changes in the LVEF (Fig. 8.1) (Jabot 2009). This suggests that repetitive CFI measurements can be performed to appropriately follow the direct impact of inotropic therapy on left ventricular dysfunction during septic cardiomyopathy.

The PiCCO system also allows real-time monitoring of cardiac output using the pulse contour analysis principle. It is clear that pulse contour cardiac output monitoring allows following the real-time impact of inotropic therapy on systemic blood flow.

8.3.4 B-Type Natriuretic Peptides

Prohormone B-type natriuretic peptide (BNP) is synthesized by the ventricular myocytes in response to an increased myocardial stretch. In the circulation, the

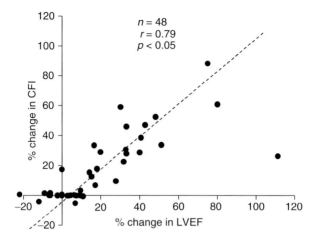

Fig. 8.1 Correlation between the changes in the cardiac function index (*CFI*) and changes in the left ventricular ejection fraction (*LVEF*) during therapeutic changes (fluid infusion and dobutamine infusion) (personal figure not shown in the paper by Jabot et al. 2009)

biologically active BNP hormone is separated from the N-terminal part of then pro-hormone, named NT-proBNP. The biologically active BNP is a 32-amino acid peptide with vasodilatory and natriuretic properties. Both systolic and diastolic dysfunction of the left ventricle can result in high circulating BNP and NT-proBNP levels. In this regard, elevated BNP plasma levels have been found in patients with myocardial infarction (Morita et al. 1993), nonischemic congestive heart failure (Yoshimura et al. 1993) and diastolic dysfunction (Yu et al. 1996). Elevated NT-proBNP levels also have been found in patients with congestive heart failure (Gardner et al. 2003) or with left ventricular diastolic dysfunction (Dahlström 2004).

In critically ill patients, such cardiac biomarkers are increasingly used as screening tools for ruling out cardiac dysfunction (McLean et al. 2008). Numerous studies have been undertaken to examine the significance of high levels of plasma BNP and/or NT-proBNP levels in the context of severe sepsis or septic shock. Variable findings have been reported. Some investigators reported a strong link between plasma BNP or NT-proBNP and prognosis, with higher levels in nonsurvivors (Charpentier et al. 2004; Ueda et al. 2006; Roch et al. 2005; Brueckmann et al. 2005). Others did not find such a link (McLean et al. 2007). Some studies showed that septic patients with myocardial depression had higher plasma BNP and/or NT-proBNP levels (Charpentier et al. 2004; Brueckmann et al. 2005; Roch et al. 2005), suggesting that BNP could be used to detect the presence of cardiac dysfunction in sepsis. However, some others showed that plasma BNP levels could be elevated during sepsis in spite of a normal LVEF (McLean et al. 2007; Maeder et al. 2006). In fact, in addition to myocardial stretch, other factors can contribute to elevating natriuretic peptides during sepsis. First, inflammatory mediators (e.g., pro-inflammatory cytokines) can impair the integrity of the cardiomyocyte membrane and thus result in an enhanced release of BNP and NT-proBNP in the blood. This potentially increases the plasma

BNP and NT-proBNP concentrations even in the absence of a marked increase in proBNP production secondary to increased myocardial stretch. Secondly, the BNP clearance pathway can be altered during septic shock. Neutral endopeptidase 24.11 is the enzyme responsible for the plasmatic degradation of BNP. The activity of this enzyme was recently shown to decrease more in patients with septic shock than in patients with sepsis, and it contributed to the higher levels of plasma BNP observed in the former when compared to the latter (Pirracchio et al. 2008).

Renal dysfunction, which is a common event during the course of severe sepsis/septic shock, can result in a reduced clearance of the natriuretic peptides and thus in elevated plasma BNP and NT-proBNP, even in the absence of a marked increase in proBNP production secondary to increased myocardial stretch.

In summary, during sepsis, divergent findings have been reported in terms of the identification of cardiac dysfunction with plasma BNP and NT-proBNP concentrations. It seems reasonable however, to state that low BNP levels should rule out severe cardiac dysfunction. On the other hand, the presence of high plasma BNP/NT-proBNP levels either on admission or during the course of the disease should rapidly prompt Doppler echocardiographic examination in order to check whether or not cardiac dysfunction has developed.

8.3.5   Cardiac Troponins

Cardiac troponins are regulatory proteins of the thin actin filaments of the cardiac muscle. Myocardial cell injury results in the release of cardiac troponin I and cardiac troponin T. The measurement of cTnI and cTnT levels in blood is a routine test for diagnosing myocardial ischemia. Cardiac troponin levels start to rise 3–4 h after the onset of myocardial damage and remain elevated for several days.

Several studies in severe sepsis patients found a relationship between elevated cardiac troponin levels and left ventricular dysfunction assessed by echocardiography (Fernandes et al. 1999; Ver Elst et al. 2000; Metha et al. 2004) and between elevated cardiac troponins and severity of the disease as assessed by global severity scores (Ver Elst et al. 2000; Metha et al. 2004) and short-term outcome (Spies et al. 1998; Ammann et al. 2003; Metha et al. 2004). Globally, elevated troponin levels in patients with sepsis indicate a higher severity of disease, the presence of myocardial dysfunction and a worse prognosis (Maeder et al. 2006).

The mechanisms contributing to elevate plasma troponin levels during sepsis are numerous. As mentioned earlier, coronary blood flow is generally maintained or even increased during sepsis (Cunnion et al. 1986; Dhainaut et al. 1987). However, in patients with prior coronary disease, high troponin levels due to myocardial ischemia may occur in relation to an increase in myocardial oxygen demand (tachycardia) and/or to a decrease in oxygen supply (anemia, hypoxemia, low diastolic arterial pressure). Microthombosis in the myocardium also may occur since severe sepsis is a procoagulant state. In addition, myocardial injury related to catecholamine toxicity must be considered as another possible mechanism contributing to increased troponin release. In this regard, Turner et al. reported a correlation between troponin levels and the maximal vasopressor doses administered. Finally, as pro-inflammatory mediators can alter the integrity of the cardiomyocyte membrane, release of troponins into the vascular compartment can be enhanced and can result in increased plasma troponins levels even in case of the absence of true myocardial necrosis.

In summary, during sepsis, cardiac troponin release indicates the presence of cardiomyocyte damage or loss of cell membrane integrity, and thus provides structural information. A great deal of evidence shows that elevated troponin levels in septic patients reflect higher disease severity and worse prognosis. It is therefore reasonable to recommend monitoring cardiac troponins during severe sepsis or septic shock to increase alertness to the presence of cardiac dysfunction in individual patients.

8.4 How the Effects of Treatment of the Sepsis-Induced Cardiac Dysfunction Can Be Monitored

Treating sepsis-induced myocardial depression is a matter of debate. Giving the patient inotropic drugs such as dobutamine is generally recommended only when the cardiac output remains low despite adequate volume resuscitation (Dellinger et al. 2008). However, dobutamine can be dangerous because of its potential adverse effects (tachycardia, arrhythmia, systemic vasodilation) that are particularly harmful in this specific context. On the other hand, β_1-agonist agents can be ineffective in case of marked impaired β-adrenergic receptor stimulation of cyclic adenosine monophosphate (Silverman et al. 1993). An alternative way would be to use a calcium sensitizer such as levosimendan, which still exerts inotropic effects even when dobutamine is no longer effective (Morelli et al. 2005).

It thus seems reasonable to assess the patient's cardiac function carefully before deciding to treat sepsis-induced myocardial depression. Indisputably, Doppler echocardiography is the best way to do so. Even when systolic cardiac dysfunction is well established (for example, LVEF<45%), the decision to treat is not straightforward. It seems to us and to others (Pottecher et al. 2006) that administration of dobutamine should be restricted to situations where the central venous oxygen saturation ($ScvO_2$) is quite low (< 65–70%). $ScvO_2$ can be obtained either from blood sampling through a central venous catheter or from continuous measurement using a fiberoptic probe.

Once the decision to administer dobutamine has been made, it is important to test its short-term effects in terms of efficacy as well as in tolerance. Indeed, probably because of a certain degree of β_1-receptor hyporesponsiveness, dobutamine therapy is not always effective enough to increase the LVEF and stroke volume as assessed by echocardiography (Kumar et al. 2008). As an alternative to echocardiography, the PiCCO system can be used to monitor the effects of dobutamine. In this regard, repetitive measurements of CFI can serve to assess the impact of inotropic therapy on cardiac contractility, while monitoring cardiac output (transpulmonary thermodilution or pulse contour analysis) can serve to measure its global impact on systemic blood flow. Obviously, if a PAC is already in place, it can be used to follow not only the changes in cardiac output and in cardiac filling pressures, but also the changes in SvO_2. Finally, the minimal way to check whether inotropic therapy is effective would be to follow the changes in SvO_2 using either repetitive blood sampling or continuous monitoring with a fiberpotic probe. Regarding the tolerance of dobutamine therapy, monitoring the heart rate and ECG is mandatory since this drug can induce tachycardia or arrhythmia. Careful blood pressure monitoring is also important since dobutamine can induce additional hypotension because of a specific vasodilation (through β_2-adrenergic receptor activation).

Clearly, repetitive assessment of the benefit/risk ratio of this treatment is important in order to make the decision to continue or stop the initial therapeutic strategy.

8.5 Conclusion

Sepsis-induced cardiac dysfunction occurs early in the course of septic shock. The degree of severity is variable from patient to patient. The mechanisms responsible for its development are complex and intricate. Doppler echocardiography is the best method to diagnose sepsis-induced cardiac dysfunction. The PiCCO system (CFI, cardiac output) and PAC (PAOP, cardiac output, SvO_2) can be used either to alert clinicians of the possibility of cardiac dysfunction or to monitor the effects of inotropic therapy. The real place of cardiac biomarkers is not well established. It seems reasonable to state that low BNP (or NT-proBNP) levels should rule out severe cardiac dysfunction. In contrast, high levels of natriuretic peptide do not allow diagnosing myocardial depression with certainty and should prompt the performance of an echocardiography examination. Administration of inotropic drugs, such as β_1-agonist agents, is a matter of debate and should be carefully monitored. The use of drugs that act on calcium sensitization is promising, but requires further evaluation before being definitively approved.

References

Abi-Gerges N, Tavernier B, Mebazaa A et al (1999) Sequential changes in autonomic regulation of cardiac myocytes after in vivo endotoxin injection in rat. Am J Respir Crit Care Med 160:1196–1204

Ammann P, Maggiorini M, Bertel O et al (2003) Troponin as a risk factor for mortality in critically ill patients without acute coronary syndromes. J Am Coll Cardiol 41:2004–2009

Brueckmann M, Huhle G, Lang S et al (2005) Prognostic value of plasma N-terminal pro-brain natriuretic peptide in patients with severe sepsis. Circulation 112:527–534

Charpentier J, Luyt CE, Fulla Y (2004) Brain natriuretic peptide: a marker of myocardial dysfunction and prognosis during severe sepsis. Crit Care Med 32:660–665

Combes A, Berneau JB, Luyt CE et al (2004) Estimation of left ventricular systolic function by single transpulmonary thermodilution. Intensive Care Med 30:1377–1383

Cunnion RE, Schaer GL, Parker MM et al (1986) The coronary circulation in human septic shock. Circulation 73:637–644

Dahlström U (2004) Can natriuretic peptides be used for the diagnosis of diastolic heart failure? Eur J Heart Fail 6:281–287

Dellinger RP, Levy MM, Carlet JM et al (2008) Surviving Sepsis Campaign: international guidelines for management of severe sepsis and septic shock. Crit Care Med 36:296–327

Dhainaut JF, Huyghebaert MF, Monsallier JF et al (1987) Coronary hemodynamics and myocardial metabolism of lactate, free fatty acids, glucose, and ketones in patients with septic shock. Circulation 75:533–541

Ferdinandy P, Danial H, Ambrus I et al (2000) Peroxynitrite is a major contributor to cytokine-induced myocardial contractile failure. Circ Res 87:241–247

Fernandes CJ Jr, Akamine N, Knobel E (1999) Cardiac troponin: a new serum marker of myocardial injury in sepsis. Intensive Care Med 25:1165–1168

Gardner RS, Ozalp F, Murday AJ et al (2003) N terminal pro-brain natriuretic peptide: a new gold standard in predicting mortality in patients with advanced heart failure. Eur Heart J 24: 1735–1743

Gnaegi A, Feihl F, Perret C (1997) Intensive care physicians' insufficient knowledge of right-heart catheterization at the bedside: time to act? Crit Care Med 25:213–220

Iberti TJ, Fischer EP, Leibowitz AB (1990) A multicenter study of physicians' knowledge of the pulmonary artery catheter. Pulmonary Artery Catheter Study Group. JAMA 264:2928–2932

Jabot J, Monnet X, Bouchra L et al. (2009) Cardiac function index provided by transpulmonary thermodilution behaves as an indicator of left ventricular systolic function. Crit Care Med 37:2913–8

Kumar A, Kumar A, Paladugu B et al (2007) Transforming growth factor-beta1 blocks in vitro cardiac myocyte depression induced by tumor necrosis factor-alpha, interleukin-1beta, and human septic shock serum. Crit Care Med 35:358–364

Kumar A, Schupp E, Bunnell E et al (2008) Cardiovascular response to dobutamine stress predicts outcome in severe sepsis and septic shock. Crit Care 12:R35

Lamia B, Chemla D, Richard C et al (2005) Clinical review: interpretation of arterial pressure wave in shock states. Crit Care 9:601–606

Lancel S, Tissier S, Mordon S et al (2004) Peroxynitrite decomposition catalysts prevent myocardial dysfunction and inflammation in endotoxemic rats. J Am Coll Cardiol 43:2348–2358

Lancel S, Joulin O, Favory R et al (2005) Ventricular myocyte caspases are directly responsible for endotoxin-induced cardiac dysfunction. Circulation 111:2596–2604

Maeder M, Fehr T, Rickli H et al (2006) Sepsis-associated myocardial dysfunction: diagnostic and prognostic impact of cardiac troponins and natriuretic peptides. Chest 129:1349–1366

McLean AS, Huang SJ, Hyams S et al (2007) Prognostic values of B-type natriuretic peptide in severe sepsis and septic shock. Crit Care Med 35:1019–1026

McLean AS, Huang SJ, Salter M (2008) Bench-to-bedside review: the value of cardiac biomarkers in the intensive care patient. Crit Care 12:215

Metha NJ, Khan IA, Gupta V et al (2004) Cardiac troponin predicts myocardial dysfunction and adverse outcome in septic shock. Int J Cardiol 95:13–17

Michard F, Alaya S, Zarka V et al (2003) Global end-diastolic volume as an indicator of cardiac preload in patients with septic shock. Chest 124:1900–1908

Morelli A, De Castro S, Teboul JL et al (2005) Effects of levosimendan on systemic and regional hemodynamics in septic myocardial depression. Intensive Care Med 31:638–644

Morita E, Yasue H, Yoshimura M et al (1993) Increased plasma levels of brain natriuretic peptide in patients with acute myocardial infarction. Circulation 88:82–91

Nagueh SF, Middleton KJ, Kopelen HA et al (1997) Doppler tissue imaging: a noninvasive technique for evaluation of left ventricular relaxation and estimation of filling pressures. J Am Coll Cardiol 30:1527–1533

Parker MM, Shelhamer JH, Bacharach SL et al (1984) Profound but reversible myocardial depression in patients with septic shock. Ann Intern Med 100:483–490

Parrillo JE, Burch C, Shelhamer JH et al (1985) A circulating myocardial depressant substance in humans with septic shock. Septic shock patients with a reduced ejection fraction have a circulating factor that depresses in vitro myocardial cell performance. J Clin Invest 76:1539–1553

Pinsky M, Vincent JL, De Smet JM (1991) Estimating left ventricular filling pressure during positive end-expiratory pressure in humans. Am Rev Respir Dis 143:25–31

Pirracchio R, Deye N, Lukaszewicz AC et al (2008) Impaired plasma B-type natriuretic peptide clearance in human septic shock. Crit Care Med 36:2542–2546

Pottecher T, Calvat S, Dupont H et al (2006) Hemodynamic management of severe sepsis: recommendations of the French Intensive Care' Societies (SFAR/SRLF) Consensus Conference, 13 October 2005, Paris, France. Crit Care 10:311

Rabuel C, Mebazaa A (2006) Septic shock: a heart story since the 1960s. Intensive Care Med 32:799–807

Ritter S, Rudiger A, Maggiorini M (2009) Transpulmonary thermodilution-derived cardiac function index identifies cardiac dysfunction in acute heart failure and septic patients: an observational study. Crit Care 13:R133

Roch A, Allardet-Servent J, Michelet P et al (2005) NH2 terminal pro-brain natriuretic peptide plasma level as an early marker of prognosis and cardiac dysfunction in septic shock patients. Crit Care Med 33:1001–1007

Silverman HJ, Penaranda R, Orens JB et al (1993) Impaired beta-adrenergic receptor stimulation of cyclic adenosine monophosphate in human septic shock: association with myocardial hyporesponsiveness to catecholamines. Crit Care Med 21:31–39

Spies C, Haude V, Fitzner R et al (1998) Serum cardiac troponin T as a prognostic marker in early sepsis. Chest 113:1055–1063

Tavernier B, Li JM, El-Omar MM et al (2001) Cardiac contractile impairment associated with increased phosphorylation of troponin I in endotoxemic rats. FASEB J 15:294–296

Teboul JL, Pinsky MR, Mercat A et al (2000) Estimating cardiac filling pressure in mechanically ventilated patients with hyperinflation. Crit Care Med 28:3631–3636

Ueda S, Nishio K, Akai Y et al (2006) Prognostic value of increased plasma levels of brain natriuretic peptide in patients with septic shock. Shock 26:134–139

Vanoverschelde JL, Robert AR, Gerbaux A et al (1995) Noninvasive estimation of pulmonary artery wedge pressure with Doppler transmitral flow velocity pattern in patients with known heart disease. Am J Cardiol 75:383–389

Ver Elst KM, Spapen HD, Nguyen DN et al (2000) Cardiac troponin I and T are biological markers of left ventricular dysfunction in septic shock. Clin Chem 46:650–657

Vieillard-Baron A (2009) Assessment of right ventricular function. Curr Opin Crit Care 15: 254–260

Vieillard-Baron A, Caille V, Charron C et al (2008) Actual incidence of global left ventricular hypokinesia in adult septic shock. Crit Care Med 36:1701–1706

Wiener RS, Welch HG (2007) Trends in the use of the pulmonary artery catheter in the United States, 1993–2004. JAMA 298:423–429

Yoshimura M, Yasue H, Okumura K et al (1993) Different secretion patterns of atrial natriuretic peptide and brain natriuretic peptide in patients with congestive heart failure. Circulation 87:464–469

Yu CM, Sanderson JE, Shum IO (1996) Diastolic dysfunction and natriuretic peptides in systolic heart failure. Higher ANP and BNP levels are associated with the restrictive filling pattern. Eur Heart J 17:1694–1702

The Lung in Multiorgan Failure

9

Rob Boots

9.1 Introduction

The acute respiratory distress syndrome (ARDS) initially described by Ashbaugh and colleagues encompasses the clinical signs of respiratory distress, hypoxemia, decreased pulmonary compliance and diffuse bilateral infiltrates on the chest X-ray, in the absence of fluid overload (Ashbaugh et al. 1967). Since then it has been described in pediatrics (Holbrook et al. 1980; Lyrene and Truog 1981), while a less severe clinical syndrome, acute lung injury (ALI), has also been reported (Bernard et al. 1994). Clinically it may represent an array of conditions, although pathologically, it is most commonly associated with diffuse alveolar damage. Increasingly it is recognized that there may be a genetic predisposition to the development of ARDS and that ventilatory strategies may also contribute to causing or worsening lung injury (Leikauf et al. 2001). ARDS and ventilatory strategies are also increasingly seen as potential drivers of multiorgan failure (Slutsky and Slutsky 2005).

9.2 Definitions of ARDS

ALI and ARDS have been estimated to affect 78.9 and 58.37 cases per 10^5 persons per year (Rubenfeld and Herridge 2007). This probably increases significantly where there are respiratory pandemics such as influenza or SARS. However, there is great variability in the reported incidence of ARDS of between 18 and 79 cases per 10^5 persons per year (Rubenfeld and Herridge 2007). This is most likely due to interpretation of the definition. The syndrome of respiratory failure characterized

R. Boots
Department of Intensive Care Medicine, Royal Brisbane and Women's Hospital,
The University of Queensland,
Herston, QLD, Australia
e-mail: rob_boots@health.qld.gov.au

J. Rello (eds.), *Sepsis Management*,
DOI 10.1007/978-3-642-03519-7_9, © Springer-Verlag Berlin Heidelberg 2012

Table 9.1 Definition of ALI/ARDS

Criteria (Bernard et al. 1994)
1. Acute onset illness
2. Bilateral infiltrates on frontal chest X-ray
3. Pulmonary artery wedge pressure ≤ 18 mmHg or no clinical evidence of pulmonary hypertension
4. $PaO_2/FiO_2 < 200$ mmHg (ARDS) or $PaO_2/FiO_2 < 300$ (ALI)

Table 9.2 ALI score (Murray score)

Parameter	Score
Number of quadrants of consolidation on chest X-ray	0–4
Hypoxemia score	
$\quad PaO_2/FiO_2 > 300$	0
$\quad PaO_2/FiO_2 = 225–229$	1
$\quad PaO_2/FiO_2 = 175–224$	2
$\quad PaO_2/FiO_2 = 100–174$	3
$\quad PaO_2/FiO_2 < 100$	4
PEEP Score (cmH_2O)	
$\quad \leq 5$ cmH_2O	0
$\quad 6–8$ cmH_2O	1
$\quad 9–11$ cmH_2O	2
$\quad 12–14$ cmH_2O	3
$\quad \geq 15$ cmH_2O	4
Compliance score (if measurable mLs/cmH_2O)	
$\quad \geq 80$	0
$\quad 60–79$	1
$\quad 40–59$	2
$\quad 20–39$	3
$\quad \leq 19$	4
Score = (sum of parameter values)/(number of parameters used)	
Maximal score 4	

Adapted from Murray et al. (1988)

clinically by an acute onset illness with impaired gas transfer of oxygen to the arterial blood, bilateral pulmonary infiltrates on the chest X-ray, and the absence of fluid overload or heart failure (a pulmonary capillary wedge pressure <18 mmHg) was described in 1994 in the American-European Consensus Conference (Bernard et al. 1994). At this time the term "Acute Lung Injury" was coined where the $PaO_2/FiO_2 < 300$ mmHg, while Acute Respiratory Distress Syndrome (ARDS) was used where the $PaO_2/FiO_2 < 200$ mmHg (Table 9.1). The recognized underlying pathology of this condition is generally accepted to be diffuse alveolar damage with hyaline membrane formation. However, pathological correlation with the clinical syndromes is rarely performed.

Table 9.3 GOCA scoring for ALI/ARDS

Letter	Meaning	Scale	Criteria
G	Gas exchange (a numeric descriptor in combination with a letter)	0	$PaO_2/FiO_2 \geq 301$
		1	PaO_2/FiO_2 200–300
		2	PaO_2/FiO_2 101–200
		3	$PaO_2/FiO_2 \leq 100$
		A	Spontaneously breathing – no PEEP
		B	PEEP 0–5 cmH_2O
		C	PEEP 6–10 cmH_2O
		D	PEEP >10 cmH_2O
O	Organ failure	A	Lung only
		B	Lung + 1 organ
		C	Lung + 2 organs
		D	Lung + ≥3 organs
C	Cause	1	Unknown
		2	Direct lung injury
		3	Indirect lung injury
A	Associated Diseases	0	No associated diseases that would cause death in the next 5 years
		1	Associated diseases that would cause death in the next 5 years
		2	Coexisting disease that would cause death in 6 months

Adapted from Artigas et al. (1998)

However, there are problems with this definition. Firstly, the meaning of acute is not specified, nor is the underlying pathology affecting the lung. As such, this definition would fit for a variety of interstitial and inflammatory lung diseases. However, Luhr found that patients requiring oxygen therapy on admission to the ICU who ultimately developed ARDS did so within the first 72 h following admission (Luhr et al. 1999). Secondly, the nature of the pulmonary infiltrates on the chest X-ray is not defined, which does not help characterize the differential diagnosis. Thirdly, the oxygenation index is significantly affected by positive end respiratory pressure (PEEP), which is not part of the definition. Fourthly, it can be difficult to fully differentiate cardiac from noncardiac pulmonary edema even using brain natriuretic peptide or the pulmonary artery catheter (Forfia et al. 2005; Rana et al. 2006). Finally, the often concurrent organ dysfunctions occurring at the time of lung injury are not specified (Abraham et al. 2000). All of the major criteria to diagnose ARDS clinically have been shown to have poor reliability (Rubenfeld 2003). As such, a clearer physiological definition was provided by Murray to describe more explicitly the degree of pulmonary dysfunction (Table 9.2) (Murray et al. 1988). The GOCA (gas exchange, organ failure, cause and associated diseases) is a stratification system for patients with ALI/ARDS, which attempts to provide a uniform stratification to describe patients consistently and succinctly for epidemiological comparisons. It is not designed as a clinical mortality scoring system (Artigas et al. 1998) (Table 9.3).

Table 9.4 Clinical conditions associated with ALI/ARDS

Prevalence	Direct insult	Indirect insult
Common	Aspiration pneumonia	Sepsis
	Pneumonia	Severe multitrauma
		Shock, any cause
Less common	Inhalation injury	Acute pancreatitis
	Pulmonary contusions	Transfusion related (TRALI)
	Fat emboli	Cardiopulmonary bypass
	Near drowning	Burns
	Reperfusion injury	Head injury/neurogenic pulmonary edema
		Drug overdose
		Disseminated intravascular coagulation
		Uremia
		Toxins/drugs, e.g., mitomycin C

Adapted from Atabai and Matthay (2002), Ferguson et al. (2004, 2005c), Ware (2005)

9.3 Clinical Presentation

Acute respiratory distress syndrome pathologically represents diffuse alveolar damage as a general overwhelming inflammatory reaction of the lung parenchyma to either direct injury or involvement of the lung in a systemic inflammatory process (Table 9.4).

Most frequently, ALI/ARDS is associated with sepsis, pneumonia, peritonitis and multi-/polytrauma (Atabai and Matthay 2002; Ferguson et al. 2005c; Frutos-Vivar et al. 2004; Ware 2005). Multiple potential insults (Pepe et al. 1982) and alcoholism (Moss et al. 2003) are associated with an increased risk of ARDS. Chronic alcohol ingestion has been associated with changes to the function of epithelial and endothelial cells as well as the production of surfactant in the lung, predisposing to malfunction of the alveolar-capillary barrier (Guidot and Roman 2002). Independent risk factors for the development of ARDS include peak airway pressure (OR 1.31), high fluid balance (OR 1.3), transfusion of plasma (OR 1.26), sepsis (OR 1.57) and tidal volume (OR 1.29) (Jia et al. 2008). Moss found that diabetes mellitus patients with sepsis rarely developed ARDS (OR 0.33) (Moss et al. 2000).

ALI/ARDS presents as a rapid onset pulmonary consolidation. The symptoms are non-specific, consisting of increasing dyspnea, hypoxemia and work of breathing associated with tachypnea and increased use of accessory muscles. Additional symptoms and signs relate to the primary cause of the ALI/ARDS in addition to associated organ dysfunction. Respiratory examination findings can be variable, but reflect pulmonary consolidation and possible associated pleural effusions.

The chest X-ray may initially be normal depending upon the primary cause of the ARDS (Caironi et al. 2006). Direct lung injury from pneumonia or aspiration may commence with a focal infiltrate. Progression typically occurs over 48 h to bilateral diffuse interstitial changes or alveolar shadows. Pleural effusions (exudates) are common and do not necessarily imply raised filling pressures. Radiological resolution may be rapid where the insult has not led to physical disruption of the alveolar membrane and the edema is rapidly cleared. This may be seen in neurogenic pulmonary edema or near drowning. However, if the fibroproliferative stage develops, particularly if the patient requires mechanical ventilation, pneumothoraces, pneumomediastinum and intrapulmonary pneumatocoeles may develop.

Computerized tomography of the lung has significantly increased our understanding of ALI/ARDS (Gattinoni et al. 2006b). The CT may initially be normal and maintain near normal appearances in the non-dependent lung regions. The infiltrate patterns include a ground-glass infiltrate in the mid-zones whereby the bronchial and vascular edges are preserved. Consolidation often with air bronchograms is seen in the dependent lung regions along with pleural effusions. There does not seem to be a difference in the nature of the infiltrates according to cause (Goodman et al. 1999; Puybasset et al. 2000). The changes in lung compliance are correlated with the amount of "normal" lung that is present, creating the notion of a small, rather than a stiff lung.

Resolution may result in a normal radiological appearance or severe fibrosis with honeycomb appearances (Caironi et al. 2006). A reticular pattern on resolution is commonly found in non-dependent lung regions (Desai et al. 1999). Persisting radiological abnormalities are associated with ventilation strategies producing peak inspiratory pressures greater than 30 mmHg and a requirement for more than 70% inspired oxygen (Nobauer-Huhmann et al. 2001). In surviving patients, pulmonary symptoms are generally mild (10% of patients) and do not correlate with radiological abnormalities (Nobauer-Huhmann et al. 2001). However, the reported frequency of respiratory symptoms may be as high as 55% (Ghio et al. 1989). Some 50% of patients have a persisting restrictive defect on lung function testing with 13% being severe (Ghio et al. 1989). Of those with persisting abnormalities on CT scanning, some 87% have parenchymal changes consistent with pulmonary fibrosis – thickened interlobular septa and localized non-septal lines, parenchymal bands and subpleural/intrapulmonary cysts. Ground-glass appearances may still be found if assessment is performed prior to 6 months from the acute illness. Evidence of pulmonary fibrosis occurs in <15% with localized distortion of architecture, consolidation, bronchiectasis and honeycombing. Ventral involvement is more pronounced (Nobauer-Huhmann et al. 2001).

The prevalence of ALI/ARDS in a general ICU population is 7–20% depending upon definitions and case mix at risk (Vincent et al. 2006). Mortality is generally described between 20% and 65% (Vincent et al. 2006) with less than 20% dying directly of their respiratory failure. Some 50% die as a result of sepsis and multiorgan failure (Ferring and Vincent 1997). Intensive care and hospital mortality is higher for ARDS (49% and 58%, respectively) than ALI (23% and 33%, respectively) (Brun-Buisson et al. 2004). The relatively high mortality rates of acute lung injury/acute respiratory distress syndrome are primarily related to the underlying disease, the severity of the acute illness and the degree of organ dysfunction. Table 9.5 outlines described prognostic factors for ALI/ARDS outcome.

Barotrauma (interstitial emphysema, pneumothorax, pneumomediastinum, pneumoperitoneum or subcutaneous emphysema) occurs in some 2.9% of mechanically

Table 9.5 Prognostic factors for ALI/ARDS

	ALI/ARDS	OR	Reference
Poor outcome factors	Metabolic acidosis occurring after the diagnosis of ARDS	4.7	Ferguson et al. (2005b)
	pH < 7.3 at ARDS onset	1.88	Brun-Buisson et al. (2004)
	Immunodeficiency	1.2–2.88	Luhr et al. (1999); Brun-Buisson et al. (2004)
	Air leak for 2 days	3.16	Brun-Buisson et al. (2004)
	Higher FiO_2/oxygenation index	1.05–1.77	Monchi et al. (1998); Ferguson et al. (2005b)
	PF > 100	0.74	Luhr et al. (1999)
	Renal failure occurring after the ARDS diagnosis	4.45	Ferguson et al. (2005b)
	Logistic organ dysfunction score	1.25	Brun-Buisson et al. (2004)
	ARDS developing after the onset of mechanical ventilation	1.1–2.09	Monchi et al. (1998); Ferguson et al. (2005c)
	SAPS II score	1.1–2.64	Monchi et al. (1998); Brun-Buisson et al. (2004); Ferguson, et al. (2005c)
	Age	1.09–1.98	Zilberberg and Epstein (1998); Luhr et al. (1999); Brun-Buisson et al. (2004); Ferguson et al. (2005c)
	CXR quadrants	1.14	Luhr et al. (1999)
	Respiratory acidosis occurring after the diagnosis of ARDS	2.94	Ferguson et al. (2005b)
	Right ventricular dysfunction	5.1	Monchi et al. (1998)
	Cirrhosis (ARDS)	27–1.75	Monchi, Bellenfant et al. (1998); Zilberberg and Epstein (1998) Doyle et al. (1995); Luhr et al. (1999)
	MODS >=8	8.7	Rocco et al. (2001)
	Direct lung injury	0.89–2.6	Monchi et al. (1998); Luhr et al. (1999)
	APS > 15	1.3	Luhr et al. (1999)
	LIS > 3	15.1	Rocco et al. (2001)
	LIS 2.76–3	2.8	
	Nonpulmonary organ dysfunction	8.1	Doyle et al. (1995)
	Sepsis	1.98–2.8	Doyle et al. (1995); Zilberberg and Epstein (1998)
	Transplant	2.8	Zilberberg and Epstein (1998)
	Comorbidities	4.0	Ferguson et al. (2005b)
	HIV	1.75	Zilberberg and Epstein (1998)
	Active malignancy	1.6	Zilberberg and Epstein (1998)
Protective factors	High PEEP	0.91	Ferguson et al. (2005a)

ventilated patients with ARDS and is most likely to occur within the first 3 days of mechanical ventilation (Anzueto et al. 2004). Surprisingly, levels of PEEP and inflation pressures were not predictors of the development of barotrauma, but rather the presence of asthma (relative risk 2.58), chronic interstitial lung disease (relative risk 4.23), previous ARDS (relative risk 2.70) and ARDS developing during mechanical ventilation (relative risk 2.53) (Anzueto et al. 2004).

9.4 Pathophysiology

9.4.1 Pathology

ARDS as diffuse alveolar damage can be described in three phases (Atabai and Matthay 2002; Frutos-Vivar et al. 2004).

1. A lung injury characterized by cellular and structural damage, alveolar edema and inflammation in an uneven distribution. This acute phase of ALI/ARDS is associated with disruption of the alveolar-capillary interface with leakage of protein-rich fluid into the interstitium and alveolar space. There is discontinuity of the type I epithelial cells with sometimes complete destruction in many areas. Type II cells are often preserved. Pulmonary and non-pulmonary insults result in inflammatory stimuli for neutrophil attraction via chemoattractants and cellular adhesion molecules.

   Neutrophil infiltration and release of inflammatory cytokines are the result of increased expression of adhesion molecules and chemoattractants such as integrin, ICAM-1 and interleukin (IL)-8. Inflammatory cytokines are increased, whereas anti-inflammatory cytokines such as IL-10, IL-1 receptor antagonist, soluble tumor necrosis factor (TNF) and IL-1 receptors are decreased. Nuclear factor kappa-beta (NF-KB) is a protein complex that directly affects the expression of many of the cytokine and adhesion molecule genes involved in the development of ARDS. The inflammatory process also increases the capillary leakiness. In established ARDS, the additional role of high oxygen concentrations is ill defined in worsening the inflammatory injury.

   Edema, reduced surfactant production and altered surfactant function from inflammatory exudates all promote unstable alveoli with alveolar collapse and ventilatory perfusion mismatching causing hypoxemia. The heavy edematous lung is the initial cause of reduced pulmonary compliance.

2. Tissue repair begins with clearing of edema and intra-alveolar debris. Functioning type II pneumocytes would appear to be important in this process of clearance (Olivera et al. 1995; Sznajder et al. 1995).

3. Recovery resulting in tissue restoration of extracellular matrix, revascularization and re-epithelization of alveolar surfaces. This later reparative phase is characterized by fibroproliferation and organization of lung tissue. The scaffold of inflammatory proteins such as fibronectin and fibrin maintain an interstitial structure to allow repair. Disordered collagen deposition occurs, leading to extensive lung scarring where resolution does not occur.

9.4.2 Genetic and Contributing Factors

Increasingly it is recognized that some patients do not seem to develop ALI/ARDS despite similar predisposing causes. Animal studies have shown different suscepti-bilities to environmental agents known to induce ALI/ARDS perhaps related to the expression of inflammatory agents (Leikauf et al. 2001). However, characterizing specific genetic predispositions is difficult because of the range of inciting causes of ALI and the large number of factors involved in the inflammatory cascade. A specific biomarker of the disease is lacking. There is an increasing range of genetic polymor-phisms being described in humans, which influence the functioning of innate and acquired immune systems including mannose-binding lectin and surfactant protein B, as well as the extent of inflammatory cytokines, such as IL-1 family, TNF, IL-6, IL-8, pre B cell colony-enhancing factor 1, macrophage inhibitory factor and vascu-lar endothelial growth factor (VEGF), which may influence responses to infection as well as the inflammatory response in the lung (Villar 2002; Christie 2004; Gao and Barnes 2009). Angiotensin-converting enzyme is rich in the lung, and genetic polymorphisms have been found to increase the risk and mortality of ARDS (Marshall et al. 2002) as well as susceptibility to meningococcal disease (Stuber 2002). Anti-inflammatory cytokine polymorphisms have included IL-10. Myosin-light chain kinase involved in the maintenance of epithelial cell cytoskeleton and bar-rier function has also been implicated, in addition to cell signaling, blood coagulation, oxidant-mediated systems and altered iron handling (Gao and Barnes 2009).

9.4.3 The Role of Mechanical Ventilation in the Development of ARDS and Multiorgan Failure

It is common for the ALI/ARDS to be part of a multi-organ failure (MOF). This condition is associated with systemic inflammation in which the lung is commonly the first organ compromised. However, in many patients the initiating cause for the progressive organ deterioration remains unclear. Such lung disease typically requires commencement of mechanical ventilation to support the progressive respiratory failure. A general outline of possible mechanisms contributing to multiorgan failure and the role of ventilator-induced lung injury is illustrated in Fig. 9.1.

Conditions morphologically, physiologically and radiologically indistinguish-able from ALI/ARDS are well described associated with the processes of mechan-ical ventilation (1999). The term ventilator-induced lung injury (VILI) refers to acute lung injury in animal models directly as a result of the ventilation strategy. Ventilator-associated lung injury is an acute lung injury similar to ARDS in patients receiving mechanical ventilation and may be associated with a pre-exist-ing pulmonary condition. However, whether "protective" ventilation of the normal lung causes lung damage and a systemic response is unclear (Wrigge et al. 2004; Plotz et al. 2002).

ARDS is an inhomogeneous disease process with near normal as well as collapsed and consolidated areas of lung (Gattinoni et al. 2006b). Conventional mechanical

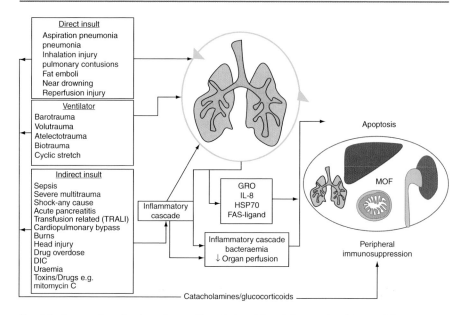

Fig. 9.1 Proposed mechanisms for ventilator-induced lung injury and multiorgan failure

ventilation tends to overinflate the near normal areas of lung while having little effect on recruiting the severely diseased lung. Injury can be caused by excessive pressures (barotrauma), volume (volutrauma), and the repeated cycling of opening and closing of collapsed alveoli (shear stress). Mechanisms contributing to lung trauma in mechanical ventilation are synergistic and not mutually exclusive. The processes contributing to VILI include (1) stress failure of the epithelial membrane, which may include necrosis; (2) failure under stress of the endothelial-epithelial barrier with loss of compartment integrity between the air and the interstitial-vascular compartments; (3) tissue overdistention without causing tissue destruction but promoting inflammatory and other cellular signaling (mechanotransduction); and (4) positive pressure ventilation raising the pressure in the pulmonary circulation promoting vascular shear stress, cellular signaling and mediator production from the endothelial cells (Uhlig 2002).

The non-homogeneous inflation of lung tissue results in shear forces that are much greater that the applied transalveolar pressure (Mead et al. 1970). Despite transalveolar pressures of 30 cmH$_2$O some 140 cmH$_2$O of shear force can be generated, potentially leading to disruption of the alveolar-capillary basement membrane. Opening and closing of alveoli during mechanical ventilation where surfactant is deficient exacerbate lung injury (Steinberg et al. 2004). In this model, histopathological evidence of injury only occurred in those alveoli that were demonstrated to be unstable. PEEP was shown to stabilize collapsing alveoli and reduce the severity of the lung injury. Preventing the repeated cycle of alveoli opening and collapse decreases lung injury (Ranieri et al. 1999).

High pressure, high volume ventilation in animals is associated with a diffuse alveolar injury similar to ALI/ARDS and exacerbates the injury of previously damaged lung (Pinhu et al. 2003). However, high pressure ventilation in the absence of high lung volumes does not necessarily result in VILI. High inflation pressures in rats of 40 cmH$_2$O causes ALI/ARDS, which is prevented by 10 cmH$_2$O of PEEP (Webb and Tierney 1974). High transalveolar pressures applied while preventing large tidal volumes by strapping of the chest avoid the ALI/ARDS, which develops as a result of either high pressure or high volume ventilation (Dreyfuss et al. 1988). PEEP was again demonstrated to limit the development of pulmonary edema.

However, despite an ARDSnet type strategy of low tidal volume (6 mLs/kg) and reducing plateau pressures <30 cmH$_2$O to minimize the risks of barotrauma and volutrauma, and the application of PEEP to limit shear stress, 30% of such ventilated patients with ARDS still demonstrate alveolar overdistention on CT scanning (Terragni et al. 2007). Evidence of overdistention was associated with an increase in inflammatory cytokines in the lung. A more individualized approach may be required because of the varied severity and heterogeneous distribution of the lung injury (Hager et al. 2005).

However, despite numerous studies to determine the best or optimal PEEP for the management of ARDS, a defined strategy remains unclear except for the improvement of oxygenation and avoiding hemodynamic compromise. For most patients, the most beneficial PEEP is a relatively narrow range with the ARDSnet strategy the only recommendations with a large body of evidence (Kallet and Branson 2007). Given the heterogeneity of the lung injury in ARDS, the individualized titration of PEEP could be based upon the respiratory-system pressure-volume curve, PEEP/tidal-volume titration grids or a recruitment maneuver with a PEEP decrement trial (Levy 2002).

Increasing the information available during mechanical ventilation may allow a less arbitrary application of PEEP. Transthoracic impedance tomography by allowing a visual image of lung volume at the bedside may in the future assist in the setting of PEEP (Bikker et al. 2009; Fagerberg et al. 2009). Use of esophageal pressure measurements as a surrogate for pleural pressure results in higher PEEP being applied compared to an ARDSnet protocol with a trend to a lower mortality (Talmor et al. 2008).

Where there are perturbations of excretion and function of surfactant resulting in increased surface tension at the air-alveolar interface, alveoli become unstable and collapse. Higher airway pressures are required to open these airspaces. There is also a resultant transmural pressure increase favoring fluid movement into the alveolar space. These abnormalities are common in ALI/ARDS. Mechanical ventilation has been shown to promote alveolar injury in these circumstances (Taskar et al. 1997). Ventilation with low tidal volumes and adequate PEEP has been shown to maintain function of surfactant aggregates in experimental models of ARDS (Ito et al. 1997).

Mechanical forces have been shown in the lung to induce cellular signal transduction (Riley et al. 1990), including the production of inflammatory mediators (dos Santos et al. 2004). Alveolar epithelial cells on gene expression microarray studies of cellular stretch alter their morphology and gene expression in a synergistic way when there is activation of an inflammatory cascade (dos Santos et al. 2004). Such mechanical forces would seem to be involved with alveolar epithelial cell signaling for membrane proteins, apoptosis as well as intracellular signal transduction. Large tidal volume mechanical ventilation has been demonstrated to result in physical fractures in both the alveolar epithelial and endothelial plasma membrane integrity. This triggers a proinflammatory cascade with increased cytokine concentration in the lung and systemic circulations (Vlahakis and Hubmayr 2005). This appears to be important in the generation of multiorgan failure. Protective strategies for mechanical ventilation with lung volume limitation result in a reduction in both pulmonary and systemic circulation cytokine levels and decreased organ dysfunction (Ranieri et al. 1999, 2000).

Bronchoalveolar lavage concentrations of neutrophils, IL-1β, IL-6 and IL-1 receptor antagonist, and plasma concentrations of tumor necrosis factor α, IL-6 and TNF-α receptors were significantly elevated over 36 h in ventilated patients with ARDS comparing a conventional with a volume-restricted strategy (Ranieri et al. 1999). Elevated platelet activating factor and thromboxane-B2 are also released by macrophages in saline lavage models of ARDS (Imai et al. 1994). Neutrophil priming appears important as granulocytopenic models of ARDS demonstrate less lung injury Kawano et al. 1987). Granulocyte-depleted animals maintained gas exchange with only a small protein leak and no hyaline membranes. Upon repletion with donor rabbit granulocytes, gas exchange deteriorates with hyaline membrane formation.

Improved oxygenation is described when inhaled nitric oxide (iNO) is administered at an early stage of ALI, but this has not translated into a mortality benefit (Adhikari et al. 2007). Lung injury is attenuated and alveolar-capillary membrane integrity is preserved with the administration of iNO at the beginning of reperfusion injury (Dong et al. 2009; Phillips et al. 2009; Sedoris et al. 2009). iNO attenuates ALI in a rabbit model in the early stages of ARDS through inhibition of NF-kB (Koh et al. 2001; Skerrett et al. 2004; Hu et al. 2007). It is considered that iNO has a protective role in oxidative lung capillary injury.

In patients receiving mechanical ventilation for ARDS, multi-organ failure scores increase significantly after 72 h of conventional mechanical ventilation when a lung protective strategy is not used (Ranieri et al. 2000). Renal failure was the predominant organ dysfunction. Multiorgan failure was significantly less in patients receiving a volume-limited strategy. The frequency of multiorgan failure was significantly correlated with plasma concentrations of IL-6, α-TNF, IL-1β and IL-8.

Heat shock proteins (HSP-70) have also been seen to be induced in lungs ventilated with low end expiratory pressures in ventilated models of ARDS (Ribeiro et al. 2001; Vreugdenhil et al. 2003). The application of PEEP attenuated this expression. In this setting, heat shock protein expression represents a response from the lung under stress to maintain structural and functional integrity of intracellular proteins. Heat shock protein expression in respiratory epithelial cells reduces inflammatory cytokine production by decreasing nuclear transcription factor κB activation (Yoo et al. 2000). It has been shown that HSP-70 expression decreases the severity of ARDS in experimental models (Weiss et al. 2002).

Inflammatory cytokines and chemokines have been shown to increase epithelial cell apoptosis. This contributes to multiorgan failure in patients dying of sepsis, trauma and shock (Hotchkiss et al. 1999; 2000; Cobb et al. 2000). Apoptosis refers to genetically controlled programmed cell death that is not the result of necrosis, whereby cells fragment and are phagocytosed by surrounding parenchymal or inflammatory cells (Papathanassoglou et al. 2000). Scarring usually does not occur. Specific receptor/ligand interactions activate a cascade of intracellular signaling pathways leading to DNA cleavage and apoptotic cell death. Cytokines IL-8, monocyte chemoattractant protein 1 (MCP-1), growth-regulated oncogene (GRO) and the Fas ligand are principle regulators and are produced during VILI and released into the plasma (Imai et al. 2003). Fas is a cell membrane receptor and soluble ligand that is a part of the tumor necrosis factor family of proteins that accumulates at sites of inflammation and promotes apoptosis of leukocytes, epithelial and parenchymal cells. The expression of the Fas ligand is regulated by such factors as surfactant protein A, angiotensin II, transforming growth factor β and a Fas ligand decoy receptor (Del Sorbo and Slutsky 2010). Inhibition of the soluble Fas ligand, which is released into the circulation during lung injury, decreases the apoptosis in organs distant to the lungs (Imai et al. 2003). High lung injury models cause type II cell necrosis in the lung rather than apoptosis.

Selective blocking of aspects of the inflammatory cascade produces less VILI in experimental models. The use of an interleukin-1 receptor antagonist decreased markers of the inflammatory response and histological evidence of lung injury (Narimanbekov and Rozycki 1995). IL-1 blockade had no effect on the decline in dynamic compliance and oxygenation, implying that given the great redundancy in the inflammatory cascade and multiple pathways, no one specific site of targeting therapy is likely to be successful.

The prone position in animals has been associated with a reduced apoptosis index in lung, diaphragm, liver, intestines and kidney (Nakos et al. 2006). Interestingly, the apoptotic index was highest in dorsal areas compared with ventral areas in both the prone and supine positions. Clinically, renal failure is less common in patients undergoing a protective lung strategy of mechanical ventilation (Ranieri et al. 2000). High frequency oscillation by reducing shear forces applied across the lung during mechanical ventilation in rabbit ARDS models reduces the production of neutrophils and inflammatory cytokines (Imai et al. 1994).

There is abnormal release and dysfunction of surfactant in ARDS. Surfactant is often used to improve oxygenation and lung function, especially in children. However, in experimental ventilated mouse ARDS models, the addition of surfactant augmented ventilator-induced release of TNF and IL-6, but not keto-PGF1α, despite improvement in oxygenation and pulmonary compliance (Stamme et al. 2002). The effect would seem to be due to improved "stretching" of the alveolar epithelial cells rather than an effect on alveolar macrophages. This may risk and increase in the risk of multiorgan failure, but this has not been described in studies of surfactant use in ARDS.

There is a body of evidence of suppression of inflammatory responses systemically outside of a local area of inflammation that may play a role in multiorgan failure. A local area of inflammation in the lung may result in a state of general immunosuppression whereby peripheral white cell response to cytokine stimulants is reduced. Such an effect may result from inflammation in the lung from injurious mechanical ventilation (Plotz et al. 2002). Also the β2 stimulation of the activation of the adrenergic nervous system in times of stress enhances the production of anti-inflammatory cytokines and down-regulates the production of inflammatory cytokines, which may contribute to suppression of the systemic immune response (Kavelaars et al. 1997).

Bacterial translocation from the lung is possible in the presence of low PEEP, high transalveolar pressure ventilation or prolonged inspiratory time (Ozcan et al. 2007). PEEP can ameliorate these effects even with persisting lung overdistention despite increased histological and gravimetric indices of lung injury in dependent lung regions (Nahum et al. 1997). Translocation of bacteria from the gut has also been implicated as a driver of multiorgan failure (Balzan et al. 2007). Ventilation with high airway pressures may diminish mesenteric blood flow and potentially impair the mucosal barrier of the gut. The effect of mechanical ventilation strategies may affect gut permeability (Guery et al. 1997) perhaps as a result of cytokine release (Imai et al. 2003).

9.5   Treatment

Treatment for ALI/ARDS is largely supportive in addition to treatment of the primary inciting condition. Although it is outside the scope of the chapter to give a detailed description of the complex mechanical ventilation options available, a general overview of principles is outlined. As a result of such supportive processes the survival rate has improved to around 70% (National Heart (2006a), Blood Institute Acute Respiratory Distress Syndrome Clinical Trials et al. 2006a). A general consideration of strategies is outlined in Table 9.6.

Table 9.6 Therapies commonly used in the management of ALI/ARDS

Therapies of value	Restrict tidal volumes < 6 mL/kg and plateau pressures < 30 cmH$_2$O (2000)
	Restrict positive fluid balances (aim neutral fluid balance, CVP < 4 cmH$_2$O if able) (National Heart, Blood Institute Acute Respiratory Distress Syndrome Clinical Trials et al. 2006)
	Extracorporeal membrane oxygenation (Peek et al. 2009)
Therapies of uncertain value	High frequency oscillatory ventilation (Imai and Slutsky 2005)
	Prone positioning of patient (Sud et al. 2008)
	High PEEP levels (Levy 2002)
	Corticosteroids (Tang et al. 2009)
	Recruitment maneuvers (Gattinoni et al. 2006a)
	Surfactant (Davidson et al. 2006; Duffett et al. 2007)
	Nitric oxide (Adhikari et al. 2007)
	Prostacyclin (Walmrath et al. 1996)
	Almitrine (Gillart et al. 1998)
Therapies best avoided	High FiO$_2$ (>0.6) to keep PaO$_2$ > 60 mmHg (Sinclair et al. 2004)
	Invasive monitoring (National Heart (2006b), Blood Institute Acute Respiratory Distress Syndrome Clinical Trials et al. 2006b)

9.5.1 Protective Lung Ventilation

9.5.1.1 Conventional Ventilation

Mechanical ventilation remains the mainstay of the management of ALI/ARDS. It provides support for the patient while awaiting the primary insult causing the lung injury to resolve. Progressively the tidal volumes and inspiratory pressures are reduced, and there are many ventilation methods used for the pressure and volume limit. Few have been rigorously assessed in large randomized trials. Increasingly combined modality approaches are being applied.

In an early trial of protective ventilation strategies, Amato reduced tidal volumes to less than 6 mL/kg with driving pressures of 20 cmH_2O above PEEP, PEEP set above the low inflection point of a static compliance curve and pressure limitation to 40 cmH_2O. This was compared to 12 mL /kg and the maintenance of normocapnia (Amato et al. 1998). A 32% absolute risk reduction for 28-day mortality, a 37% improvement in weaning rates and a 35% absolute risk reduction in clinical barotraumas was found. The difference in the PEEP was 16.4 versus 8.7 cmH_2O in the intervention compared to the conventional ventilation group. There was no difference in hospital survival.

The Acute Respiratory Distress Syndrome Network study in 2000 compared 12 mL/kg predicted body weight and an airway plateau pressure ≤50 cmH_2O to an initial tidal volume of 6 mL/kg predicted body weight and a plateau pressure ≤30 cm of water (2000). However, both groups used a complex PEEP-FiO_2 titration table with the aim to keep the SpO2 > 88%. The average PEEP in both groups was <10 cmH_2O. There was an 8.8% absolute risk reduction in hospital death or failure to wean by day 28 (31% compared to 39.8%), a 3-day reduction in non-pulmonary organ failures and a reduction in plasma IL-6 levels.

Whether other strategies to accomplish a limited tidal volume and limited pressure strategy, such as pressure control, airway pressure release, bilevel, inverse inspiratory:expiratory ratio and pressure-regulated volume control ventilation, offer an advantage or a refinement of these approaches remains to be tested.

9.5.1.2 Open Lung Strategies

Low tidal volume ventilation prevents alveolar but does not prevent shear injury from repeated opening and closing of alveoli. Such shear injury is reduced by PEEP. The open lung strategy involves the application of recruitment maneuvers of the short applications of increases in mean airway pressure to open collapsed alveoli and, when open, maintains this with higher levels of PEEP (Gattinoni et al. 2006a). This may be done as intermittent sighs, short duration increases in PEEP, stepwise increases in PEEP or sustained application of pressure to achieve total lung capacity (Marini 2001). Recruitment maneuvers are more effective when performed in the presence of PEEP (Foti et al. 2000), when the patients are paralyzed (Lim et al. 2001) or when a higher tidal volume is accomplished during the recruitment (Richard et al. 2001). The variability found in studies for the duration of the effectiveness of recruitment maneuvers possibly relates to the method of PEEP titration used and small studies of heterogeneous patients (Toth et al. 2007; Tugrul et al. 2003; Girgis et al. 2006). In general, the recruitment maneuvers are hemodynamically well tolerated (Toth et al. 2007).

9.5.1.3 High Frequency Oscillation

High frequency oscillation ventilation (HFOV) represents a technique where high mean inflation pressures are accomplished (around 30 cmH_2O) with CO_2 removal achieved by using high frequencies of ventilation (4–6 Hz). Small tidal volumes of around 1–5 mL are used, and the lower the ventilation frequency is, the higher the achieved tidal volume. This approach accomplishes alveolar recruitment, reduces shear injury and may provide a better lung volume for the effectiveness of adjunct therapies such as inhaled nitric oxide (Dobyns et al. 2002). It also has been shown to decrease the levels of systemic inflammatory markers (Imai et al. 2001; Imai and Slutsky 2005). Although better pulmonary outcomes have been demonstrated in children (Courtney et al. 2002), there has not been a clear mortality benefit (Derdak et al. 2002; Dobyns et al. 2002; David et al. 2003; Ferguson et al. 2005a).

9.5.1.4 Extracorporeal Membrane Oxygenation

Where the lungs are so severely damaged that it is not possible to oxygenate the patient with recruitment, high PEEP and high concentrations of oxygen, using an extracorporeal circuit and a membrane oxygenator is increasingly recognized as a salvage technique (Australia, New Zealand Extracorporeal Membrane Oxygenation Influenza Investigators 2009; Peek et al. 2009). It also allows CO_2 elimination. It can be used with veno-venous access to support gas exchange or with arterio-venous access to support both gas exchange and the systemic circulation. The lungs are rested on CPAP or low volume-low frequency ventilation, and anticoagulation is required. The major complications are bleeding, thrombosis and infection. The best outcome would appear to be from units that routinely perform the procedure. Many patients referred to such centers often avoid ECMO by further adjustment of conventional ventilation and attention to fluid balance (Peek et al. 2009). It is unclear whether the avoidance of mechanical ventilation by using CPAP and ECMO can reduce the degree of lung injury.

9.5.1.5 Liquid Ventilation

Full or partial ventilation with perflurocarbon (PFC) is not commercially available. By filling the functional residual capacity of the lung with PFC, oxygenation and lung mechanics are improved (Reickert et al. 2002). There may be an additional benefit to diluting the inflammatory process in the lung and assisting with the clearance of the inflammatory exudate. Partial liquid ventilation allows gas tidal volume breaths on top of a PFC-filled FRC. However, the technique has not been shown to improve mortality, but may be associated with worsening respiratory failure (Hirschl et al. 2002).

9.5.2 Fluid Management

Randomized controlled trials have demonstrated that a conservative approach to fluid management in ALI/ARDS to maintain an equal fluid balance rather than a liberal administration of fluids results in an improved oxygenation index with a reduction in ventilation time and intensive care stay by 2.5 days (National Heart (2006b), Blood Institute Acute Respiratory Distress Syndrome Clinical Trials et al. 2006b). Mortality, shock and renal failure prevalences were similar. There was however a difference in cumulative fluid balance of some 7 L. Importantly, the use of a pulmonary artery catheter (PAC) to guide fluid therapy in ALI/ARDS only causes catheter-related complications, even in the presence of shock, without improving mortality, ventilation or ICU length of stay or organ function (National Heart (2006a), Blood Institute Acute Respiratory Distress Syndrome Clinical Trials et al. 2006a). Interestingly fluid balance was similar despite the use of the PAC.

9.5.3 Prone Positioning

Prone positioning has been shown to regularly improve oxygenation, ventilation-perfusion matching, secretion clearance and chest wall mechanics. The resulting increase in secretion clearance, reduced lung compression from the abdomen and heart, redistribution of trans-alveolar forces and altered chest wall mechanics results in improved ventilation-perfusion matching and regional ventilation in addition to a reduction in ventilator-associated pneumonia (Guerin 2006; Sud et al. 2008). It may not be as effective when applied late in the course of respiratory failure. There are potential risks with accidental extubation, general care and decubitus pressure effects, including the eyes, when using such an approach, and the turns may be associated with hemodynamic instability. There has been no mortality benefit noted (Guerin 2006; Sud et al. 2008).

9.5.4 Avoiding High Oxygen Concentrations

Both animal and human experimental data confirm that high oxygen concentrations ($FiO_2 > 0.6$) are associated with the development of ALI/ARDS (Burrows and Edwards 1970; Glauser and Smith 1975; Nader-Djalal et al. 1997; Sinclair et al. 2004; Fisher and Beers 2008). It may potentially worsen the effects of VILI (Bailey et al. 2003). However, in the setting of already severe lung injury, it becomes unavoidable in some circumstances in order to maintain tissue oxygenation. All efforts should be used to recruit lung to avoid prolonged periods of a $FiO_2 > 0.6$ as a pragmatic recommendation.

9.5.5 Pharmacologic Approaches

9.5.5.1 Surfactant

The use of exogenous surfactant has predominantly found benefits in children (Duffett et al. 2007). No clear benefit has been demonstrated in adults despite an improvement in oxygenation regardless of whether artificial or bovine surfactant was used (Davidson et al. 2006). Dosing, mode of delivery, the composition of the surfactant as well as the degree of recruitment on the lung may be significant factors to explain the lack of efficacy. The meta-analysis by Duffett in children noted that the use of surfactant for ALI resulted in a relative risk reduction of 0.7, an increase in ventilator-free days of 2.5 days and a reduced duration of mechanical ventilation of 2.3 days (Duffett et al. 2007). In general it seems well tolerated with reported hypotension, transient hypoxemia and perhaps a reduction in the incidence of ventilator-associated pneumonia.

9.5.5.2 Glucocorticoids

Glucocorticoids have been used in the management of ARDS to try to dampen the fibroproliferative phase. The doses, type of corticosteroids and duration of treatment vary significantly in the studies. The meta-analysis by Tang reports an average dose of 140 mg of methylprednisolone or the equivalent used per day (Tang et al. 2009). Although neither cohort nor randomized controlled studies have demonstrated a mortality benefit, the combined relative risk was 0.62. The duration of mechanical ventilation was reduced by 4 days, with reduction in the severity scores for multiple organ dysfunction and lung injury in addition to improving oxygenation. Complications are uncommon, but include infection, neuropathy/myopathy and gastrointestinal bleeding, but do not seem to be increased over control groups.

9.5.5.3 Nitric Oxide

Inhaled nitric oxide (iNO) is used in doses up to 100 ppm to improve the pulmonary hypertension and oxygenation in ALI/ARDS. In general up to 10 ppm is used for the management of hypoxemia and more than this for the management of pulmonary hypertension. In addition to its effects as a pulmonary vasodilator (with a half-life of some 20 s due to its inactivation by binding with hemoglobin), iNO also has an antithrombotic effect (Gries et al. 1998). Its selectivity as a pulmonary vasodilator is due to having a localized effect of ventilation-perfusion matching achieved by being delivered by the inhaled route. In ARDS/ALI, iNO is associated with less neutrophil migration, reduced neutrophil and macrophage function and reduced lung parenchymal damage in experimental models, and has been shown to attenuate lung injury. Adequate lung recruitment seems important to its effects. There may be tachyphylaxis to its efficacy (Gerlach et al. 2003). It has been seen to be additive to the effects of prone positioning and high frequency oscillation. It potentially causes met-hemoglobinemia, and higher oxides of nitrogen are produced when combined with high concentrations of oxygen such as NO_2, which are corrosive to the lung. However, with modern mass flow controller delivery and monitoring, these issues are not a common problem. Commercially available nitric oxide is expensive to use. Despite the effects on oxygenation and pulmonary pressures, there has not been a mortality benefit demonstrated in adult patients (Dellinger et al. 1998; Lundin et al. 1999; Taylor et al. 2004).

9.5.5.4 Inhaled Prostacycline

Inhaled prostacycline is used as an alternative to iNO in doses up to 50 ng/kg/min. It also has local vasodilation effects improving oxygenation and pulmonary pressures in ALI/ARDS, as well as an antithrombotic effect. As it is aerosolized, its effectiveness may vary with the delivery system used. No mortality benefit has been reported (Walmrath et al. 1996; Dahlem et al. 2004).

9.6   Outcomes

The mortality rate from ALI/ARDS is around 30–40% with a falling case fatality rate accounted for by increasing rates of trauma (Stapleton et al. 2005). Death most commonly occurs from multiorgan failure (30–50%) rather than refractory hypoxemia (<20%). The mortality rate in sepsis patients with ARDS has not changed. Death less than 72 hours from the onset of ARDS represents 26–44% of the total mortality. There is great heterogeneity of outcome, but it is unclear whether this represents different mechanisms or responses to treatment (Dicker et al. 2004). Eisner reviewed the outcome of patients in the ARDSnet trial of low tidal volume ventilation (Eisner et al. 2001). Mortality was highest in patients with sepsis (43%) with pneumonia 36% and aspiration 37%, and lowest in trauma at 11%. Low tidal volume ventilation was equally beneficial in all primary causes of ARDS, and no difference was found in the rates of ventilation wean or the development of non-pulmonary organ failures. It is also possible to predict which patients with mild respiratory failure will deteriorate to having ARDS (Rubenfeld and Christie 2004).

The long-term morbidity of patients surviving ARDS is similar to that of any patient with multi-organ failure and a prolonged ICU stay. Persistent respiratory symptoms are common after recovery from ARDS/ALI. Most patients have a reduced diffusion capacity and a restrictive defect. Airways obstruction and reactive airways disease are also described. Importantly, the major morbidity for ARDS patients is not pulmonary disease. Principally, these are neuromuscular dysfunction including critical illness, polyneuropathy and myopathy, neurocognitive dysfunction and neuropsychological dysfunction, including depression, anxiety and post-traumatic stress disorder (Rubenfeld and Herridge 2007). Physical disorders are generally related to prolonged immobility such as joint contractures and calcification. There is increasing recognition of the costs of caregiver support and financial burdens to both families and the health care system (Rubenfeld and Herridge 2007).

Previous studies note that 12 months following illness some 60% of patients may not have returned to regular activity and that lung function remains stable after this time with between 50% and 60% having spirometry of less than 80% of the predicted value (Heyland et al. 2005). Lung function is strongly correlated to physical function. With the advent of lung rest strategies such as extracorporeal membrane oxygenation, 75% of patients are described as returning to their previous employment, and no patients required the use of supplementary oxygen (Linden et al. 2009). In general, functional outcome scores in this ECMO group were higher compared to previous studies (Davidson et al. 1999; Heyland et al. 2005; Groll et al. 2006).

In the meta-analysis of quality of life following ARDS by Dowdy assessed using the SF-36, it was uncommon for there to be improvement in functioning after 6 months from critical illness (Dowdy et al. 2006). Each of the eight scales of the SF-36 represents the weighted sums of the questions with each scale. Each scale is directly transformed into a 0–100 scale assuming that each question carries equal weight. For patients assessed more than 12 months from hospital discharge, on average there was a mean fall between 15 and 25 points from previous functioning for physical functioning, bodily pain, general health perceptions, vitality, social functioning and emotional role. Patient's physical role (a 40 point decrement) was the worst outcome with mental health deteriorating by 11 points. A sleep disorder in patients screened for sleeping problems after ARDS included chronic conditioned insomnia (71%), parasomnia (14%) and obstructive sleep apnea (14%), with 57% having periodic leg movements of uncertain clinical significance.

9.7   Summary

ALI/ARDS continues to represent diagnostic and therapeutic challenges in the intensive care unit. Increasingly it is recognized as part of the spectrum of multiorgan failure. In addition there is evidence that mechanical ventilation practices influence the severity of the illness and may also influence the degree of organ dysfunction. Preventative and therapeutic approaches will need to consider multiple modalities and approaches.

References

(1999) International consensus conferences in intensive care medicine: Ventilator-associated Lung Injury in ARDS. This official conference report was cosponsored by the American Thoracic Society, The European Society of Intensive Care Medicine, and The Societe de Reanimation de Langue Francaise, and was approved by the ATS Board of Directors, July 1999. Am J Respir Crit Care Med 160(6):2118–2124

(2000) Ventilation with lower tidal volumes as compared with traditional tidal volumes for acute lung injury and the acute respiratory distress syndrome. The Acute Respiratory Distress Syndrome Network. N Engl J Med 342(18):1301–1308

Abraham E, Matthay MA et al (2000) Consensus conference definitions for sepsis, septic shock, acute lung injury, and acute respiratory distress syndrome: time for a reevaluation. Crit Care Med 28(1):232–235

Adhikari NKJ, Burns KEA et al (2007) Effect of nitric oxide on oxygenation and mortality in acute lung injury: systematic review and meta-analysis. BMJ 334(7597):779

Amato MB, Barbas CS et al (1998) Effect of a protective-ventilation strategy on mortality in the acute respiratory distress syndrome. N Engl J Med 338(6):347–354

Anzueto A, Frutos-Vivar F et al (2004) Incidence, risk factors and outcome of barotrauma in mechanically ventilated patients. Intensive Care Med 30(4):612–619

Artigas A, Bernard GR et al (1998) The American-European Consensus Conference on ARDS, part 2: ventilatory, pharmacologic, supportive therapy, study design strategies, and issues related to recovery and remodeling. Acute respiratory distress syndrome. Am J Respir Crit Care Med 157(4 Pt 1):1332–1347

Ashbaugh DG, Bigelow DB et al (1967) Acute respiratory distress in adults. Lancet 2(7511):319–323

Atabai K, Matthay MA (2002) The pulmonary physician in critical care. 5: acute lung injury and the acute respiratory distress syndrome: definitions and epidemiology. Thorax 57(5):452–458

Australia and New Zealand Extracorporeal Membrane Oxygenation (ANZ ECMO) Influenza Investigators et al (2009) Extracorporeal membrane oxygenation for 2009 influenza A(H1N1) acute respiratory distress syndrome. JAMA 302(17):1888–1895

Bailey TC, Martin EL et al (2003) High oxygen concentrations predispose mouse lungs to the deleterious effects of high stretch ventilation. J Appl Physiol 94(3):975–982

Balzan S, de Almeida Quadros C et al (2007) Bacterial translocation: overview of mechanisms and clinical impact. J Gastroenterol Hepatol 22(4):464–471

Bernard GR, Artigas A et al (1994) The American-European Consensus Conference on ARDS. Definitions, mechanisms, relevant outcomes, and clinical trial coordination. Am J Respir Crit Care Med 149(3 Pt 1):818–824

Bikker IG, Leonhardt S et al (2009) Lung volume calculated from electrical impedance tomography in ICU patients at different PEEP levels. Intensive Care Med 35(8):1362–1367

Brun-Buisson C, Minelli C et al (2004) Epidemiology and outcome of acute lung injury in European intensive care units. Results from the ALIVE study. Intensive Care Med 30(1):51–61

Burrows FG, Edwards JM (1970) A pulmonary disease in patients ventilated with high oxygen concentrations. Br J Radiol 43(516):848–855

Caironi P, Carlesso E et al (2006) Radiological imaging in acute lung injury and acute respiratory distress syndrome. Semin Respir Crit Care Med 27(4):404–415

Christie JD (2004) Genetic epidemiology of acute lung injury: choosing the right candidate genes is the first step. Crit Care (Lond) 8(6):411–413

Cobb JP, Buchman TG et al (2000) Molecular biology of multiple organ dysfunction syndrome: injury, adaptation, and apoptosis. Surg Infect 1(3):207–213; discussion 214–205

Courtney SE, Durand DJ et al (2002) High-frequency oscillatory ventilation versus conventional mechanical ventilation for very-low-birth-weight infants. N Engl J Med 347(9):643–652

Dahlem P, van Aalderen WMC et al (2004) Randomized controlled trial of aerosolized prostacyclin therapy in children with acute lung injury. Crit Care Med 32(4):1055–1060

David M, Weiler N et al (2003) High-frequency oscillatory ventilation in adult acute respiratory distress syndrome. Intensive Care Med 29(10):1656–1665

Davidson TA, Caldwell ES et al (1999) Reduced quality of life in survivors of acute respiratory distress syndrome compared with critically ill control patients. JAMA 281(4):354–360

Davidson WJ, Dorscheid D et al (2006) Exogenous pulmonary surfactant for the treatment of adult patients with acute respiratory distress syndrome: results of a meta-analysis. Crit Care (Lond) 10(2):R41

Del Sorbo L, Slutsky AS (2010) Ventilatory support for acute respiratory failure: new and ongoing pathophysiological, diagnostic and therapeutic developments. Curr Opin Crit Care 16(1):1–7

Dellinger RP, Zimmerman JL et al (1998) Effects of inhaled nitric oxide in patients with acute respiratory distress syndrome: results of a randomized phase II trial. Inhaled Nitric Oxide in ARDS Study Group. Crit Care Med 26(1):15–23

Derdak S, Mehta S et al (2002) High-frequency oscillatory ventilation for acute respiratory distress syndrome in adults: a randomized, controlled trial. Am J Respir Crit Care Med 166(6): 801–808

Desai SR, Wells AU et al (1999) Acute respiratory distress syndrome: CT abnormalities at long-term follow-up. Radiology 210(1):29–35

Dicker RA, Morabito DJ et al (2004) Acute respiratory distress syndrome criteria in trauma patients: why the definitions do not work. J Trauma 57(3):522–526; discussion 526–528

Dobyns EL, Anas NG et al (2002) Interactive effects of high-frequency oscillatory ventilation and inhaled nitric oxide in acute hypoxemic respiratory failure in pediatrics. Crit Care Med 30(11):2425–2429

Dong BM, Abano JB et al (2009) Nitric oxide ventilation of rat lungs from non-heart-beating donors improves posttransplant function. Am J Transplant 9(12):2707–2715

dos Santos CC, Han B et al (2004) DNA microarray analysis of gene expression in alveolar epithelial cells in response to TNFalpha, LPS, and cyclic stretch. Physiol Genomics 19(3): 331–342

Dowdy DW, Eid MP et al (2006) Quality of life after acute respiratory distress syndrome: a meta-analysis. Intensive Care Med 32(8):1115–1124

Doyle RL, Szaflarski N et al (1995) Identification of patients with acute lung injury. Predictors of mortality. Am J Respir Crit Care Med 152(6 Pt 1):1818–1824

Dreyfuss D, Soler P et al (1988) High inflation pressure pulmonary edema. Respective effects of high airway pressure, high tidal volume, and positive end-expiratory pressure. Am Rev Respir Dis 137(5):1159–1164

Duffett M, Choong K et al (2007) Surfactant therapy for acute respiratory failure in children: a systematic review and meta-analysis. Crit Care (Lond) 11(3):R66

Eisner MD, Thompson T et al (2001) Efficacy of low tidal volume ventilation in patients with different clinical risk factors for acute lung injury and the acute respiratory distress syndrome. Am J Respir Crit Care Med 164(2):231–236

Fagerberg A, Stenqvist O et al (2009) Electrical impedance tomography applied to assess matching of pulmonary ventilation and perfusion in a porcine experimental model. Crit (Lond) 13(2):R34

Ferguson ND, Chiche J-D et al (2005a) Combining high-frequency oscillatory ventilation and recruitment maneuvers in adults with early acute respiratory distress syndrome: the Treatment with Oscillation and an Open Lung Strategy (TOOLS) Trial pilot study. Crit Care Med 33(3): 479–486

Ferguson ND, Frutos-Vivar F et al (2005b) Airway pressures, tidal volumes, and mortality in patients with acute respiratory distress syndrome (see comment). Crit Care Med 33(1):21–30

Ferguson ND, Frutos-Vivar F et al (2005c) Acute respiratory distress syndrome: underrecognition by clinicians and diagnostic accuracy of three clinical definitions. Crit Care Med 33(10): 2228–2234

Ferring M, Vincent JL (1997) Is outcome from ARDS related to the severity of respiratory failure? Eur Respir J 10(6):1297–1300

Fisher AB, Beers MF (2008) Hyperoxia and acute lung injury. Am J Physiol Lung Cell Mol Physiol 295(6):L1066; author reply L1067

Forfia PR, Watkins SP et al (2005) Relationship between B-type natriuretic peptides and pulmonary capillary wedge pressure in the intensive care unit. J Am Coll Cardiol 45(10):1667–1671

Foti G, Cereda M et al (2000) Effects of periodic lung recruitment maneuvers on gas exchange and respiratory mechanics in mechanically ventilated acute respiratory distress syndrome (ARDS) patients. Intensive Care Med 26(5):501–507

Frutos-Vivar F, Nin N et al (2004) Epidemiology of acute lung injury and acute respiratory distress syndrome. Curr Opin Crit Care 10(1):1–6

Gao L, Barnes KC (2009) Recent advances in genetic predisposition to clinical acute lung injury. Am J Physiol Lung Cell Mol Physiol 296(5):L713–L725

Gattinoni L, Caironi P et al (2006a) Lung recruitment in patients with the acute respiratory distress syndrome. N Engl J Med 354(17):1775–1786

Gattinoni L, Caironi P et al (2006b) The role of CT-scan studies for the diagnosis and therapy of acute respiratory distress syndrome. Clin Chest Med 27(4):559–570; abstract vii

Gerlach H, Keh D et al (2003) Dose-response characteristics during long-term inhalation of nitric oxide in patients with severe acute respiratory distress syndrome: a prospective, randomized, controlled study. Am J Respir Crit Care Med 167(7):1008–1015

Ghio AJ, Elliott CG et al (1989) Impairment after adult respiratory distress syndrome. An evaluation based on American Thoracic Society recommendations [Erratum appears in Am Rev Respir Dis 1989 Sep;140(3):862]. Am Rev Respir Dis 139(5):1158–1162

Gillart T, Bazin JE et al (1998) Combined nitric oxide inhalation, prone positioning and almitrine infusion improve oxygenation in severe ARDS. Can J Anaesth 45(5 Pt 1):402–409

Girgis K, Hamed H et al (2006) A decremental PEEP trial identifies the PEEP level that maintains oxygenation after lung recruitment. Respir Care 51(10):1132–1139

Glauser FL, Smith WR (1975) Pulmonary interstitial fibrosis following near-drowning and exposure to short-term high oxygen concentrations. Chest 68(3):373–375

Goodman LR, Fumagalli R et al (1999) Adult respiratory distress syndrome due to pulmonary and extrapulmonary causes: CT, clinical, and functional correlations. Radiology 213(2):545–552

Gries A, Bode C et al (1998) Inhaled nitric oxide inhibits human platelet aggregation, P-selectin expression, and fibrinogen binding in vitro and in vivo. Circulation 97(15):1481–1487

Groll DL, Heyland DK et al (2006) Assessment of long-term physical function in acute respiratory distress syndrome (ARDS) patients: comparison of the Charlson Comorbidity Index and the Functional Comorbidity Index. Am J Phys Med Rehabil 85(7):574–581

Guerin C (2006) Ventilation in the prone position in patients with acute lung injury/acute respiratory distress syndrome. Curr Opin Crit Care 12(1):50–54

Guery B, Neviere R et al (1997) Mechanical ventilation regimen induces intestinal permeability changes in a rat model (abstract). Am J Respir Crit Care Med 155:A505

Guidot DM, Roman J (2002) Chronic ethanol ingestion increases susceptibility to acute lung injury: role of oxidative stress and tissue remodeling. Chest 122(6 Suppl):309S–314S

Hager DN, Krishnan JA et al (2005) Tidal volume reduction in patients with acute lung injury when plateau pressures are not high. Am J Respir Crit Care Med 172(10):1241–1245

Heyland DK, Groll D et al (2005) Survivors of acute respiratory distress syndrome: relationship between pulmonary dysfunction and long-term health-related quality of life. Crit Care Med 33(7):1549–1556

Hirschl RB, Croce M et al (2002) Prospective, randomized, controlled pilot study of partial liquid ventilation in adult acute respiratory distress syndrome. Am J Respir Crit Care Med 165(6):781–787

Holbrook PR, Taylor G et al (1980) Adult respiratory distress syndrome in children. Pediatr Clin North Am 27(3):677–685

Hotchkiss RS, Schmieg RE Jr et al (2000) Rapid onset of intestinal epithelial and lymphocyte apoptotic cell death in patients with trauma and shock. Crit Care Med 28(9):3207–3217

Hotchkiss RS, Swanson PE et al (1999) Apoptotic cell death in patients with sepsis, shock, and multiple organ dysfunction. Crit Care Med 27(7):1230–1251

Hu X, Guo C et al (2007) Inhaled nitric oxide attenuates hyperoxic and inflammatory injury without alteration of phosphatidylcholine synthesis in rat lungs. Pulm Pharmacol Ther 20(1):75–84

Imai Y, Kawano T et al (1994) Inflammatory chemical mediators during conventional ventilation and during high frequency oscillatory ventilation. Am J Respir Crit Care Med 150(6 Pt 1):1550–1554

Imai Y, Nakagawa S et al (2001) Comparison of lung protection strategies using conventional and high-frequency oscillatory ventilation. J Appl Physiol 91(4):1836–1844

Imai Y, Parodo J et al (2003) Injurious mechanical ventilation and end-organ epithelial cell apoptosis and organ dysfunction in an experimental model of acute respiratory distress syndrome. JAMA 289(16):2104–2112

Imai Y, Slutsky AS (2005) High-frequency oscillatory ventilation and ventilator-induced lung injury. Crit Care Med 33(3 Suppl):S129–S134

Ito Y, Veldhuizen RA et al (1997) Ventilation strategies affect surfactant aggregate conversion in acute lung injury. Am J Respir Crit Care Med 155(2):493–499

Jia X, Malhotra A et al (2008) Risk factors for ARDS in patients receiving mechanical ventilation for > 48 h. Chest 133(4):853–861

Kallet RH, Branson RD (2007) Respiratory controversies in the critical care setting. Do the NIH ARDS Clinical Trials Network PEEP/FIO2 tables provide the best evidence-based guide to balancing PEEP and FIO2 settings in adults? Respir Care 52(4):461–475; discussion 475–467

Kavelaars A, van de Pol M et al (1997) Beta 2-adrenergic activation enhances interleukin-8 production by human monocytes. J Neuroimmunol 77(2):211–216

Kawano T, Mori S et al (1987) Effect of granulocyte depletion in a ventilated surfactant-depleted lung. J Appl Physiol 62(1):27–33

Koh Y, Kang JL et al (2001) Inhaled nitric oxide down-regulates intrapulmonary nitric oxide production in lipopolysaccharide-induced acute lung injury. Crit Care Med 29(6): 1169–1174

Leikauf GD, McDowell SA et al (2001) Functional genomics of oxidant-induced lung injury. Adv Exp Med Biol 500:479–487

Levy MM (2002) Optimal peep in ARDS. Changing concepts and current controversies. Crit Care Clin 18(1):15–33

Lim CM, Koh Y et al (2001) Mechanistic scheme and effect of "extended sigh" as a recruitment maneuver in patients with acute respiratory distress syndrome: a preliminary study. Crit Care Med 29(6):1255–1260

Linden VB, Lidegran MK et al (2009) ECMO in ARDS: a long-term follow-up study regarding pulmonary morphology and function and health-related quality of life. Acta Anaesthesiol Scand 53(4):489–495

Luhr OR, Antonsen K et al (1999) Incidence and mortality after acute respiratory failure and acute respiratory distress syndrome in Sweden, Denmark, and Iceland. The ARF Study Group. Am J Respir Crit Care Med 159(6):1849–1861

Lundin S, Mang H et al (1999) Inhalation of nitric oxide in acute lung injury: results of a European multicentre study. The European Study Group of Inhaled Nitric Oxide. Intensive Care Med 25(9):911–919

Lyrene RK, Truog WE (1981) Adult respiratory distress syndrome in a pediatric intensive care unit: predisposing conditions, clinical course, and outcome. Pediatrics 67(6):790–795

Marini JJ (2001) Recruitment maneuvers to achieve an "open lung"–whether and how? Crit Care Med 29(8):1647–1648

Marshall RP, Webb S et al (2002) Angiotensin converting enzyme insertion/deletion polymorphism is associated with susceptibility and outcome in acute respiratory distress syndrome. Am J Respir Crit Care Med 166(5):646–650

Mead J, Takishima T et al (1970) Stress distribution in lungs: a model of pulmonary elasticity. J Appl Physiol 28(5):596–608

Monchi M, Bellenfant F et al (1998) Early predictive factors of survival in the acute respiratory distress syndrome. A multivariate analysis. Am J Respir Crit Care Med 158(4): 1076–1081

Moss M, Guidot DM et al (2000) Diabetic patients have a decreased incidence of acute respiratory distress syndrome. Crit Care Med 28(7):2187–2192

Moss M, Parsons PE et al (2003) Chronic alcohol abuse is associated with an increased incidence of acute respiratory distress syndrome and severity of multiple organ dysfunction in patients with septic shock. Crit Care Med 31(3):869–877

Murray JF, Matthay MA et al (1988) An expanded definition of the adult respiratory distress syndrome [Erratum appears in Am Rev Respir Dis 1989 Apr;139(4):1065]. Am Rev Respir Dis 138(3):720–723

Nader-Djalal N, Knight PR et al (1997) Hyperoxia exacerbates microvascular lung injury following acid aspiration. Chest 112(6):1607–1614

Nahum A, Hoyt J et al (1997) Effect of mechanical ventilation strategy on dissemination of intra-tracheally instilled *Escherichia coli* in dogs. Crit Care Med 25(10):1733–1743

Nakos G, Batistatou A et al (2006) Lung and "end organ" injury due to mechanical ventilation in animals: comparison between the prone and supine positions. Crit Care (Lond) 10(1):R38

Narimanbekov IO, Rozycki HJ (1995) Effect of IL-1 blockade on inflammatory manifestations of acute ventilator-induced lung injury in a rabbit model. Exp Lung Res 21(2):239–254

National Heart, Lung, and Blood Institute Acute Respiratory Distress Syndrome (ARDS) Clinical Trials Network et al (2006a) Pulmonary-artery versus central venous catheter to guide treatment of acute lung injury. N Engl J Med 354(21):2213–2224

National Heart, Lung, and Blood Institute Acute Respiratory Distress Syndrome (ARDS) Clinical Trials Network et al (2006b) Comparison of two fluid-management strategies in acute lung injury. N Engl J Med 354(24):2564–2575

Nobauer-Huhmann IM, Eibenberger K et al (2001) Changes in lung parenchyma after acute respiratory distress syndrome (ARDS): assessment with high-resolution computed tomography. Eur Radiol 11(12):2436–2443

Olivera WG, Ridge KM et al (1995) Lung liquid clearance and Na, K-ATPase during acute hyperoxia and recovery in rats. Am J Respir Crit Care Med 152(4 Pt 1):1229–1234

Ozcan PE, Cakar N et al (2007) The effects of airway pressure and inspiratory time on bacterial translocation. Anesth Analg 104(2):391–396

Papathanassoglou ED, Moynihan JA et al (2000) Does programmed cell death (apoptosis) play a role in the development of multiple organ dysfunction in critically ill patients? a review and a theoretical framework. Crit Care Med 28(2):537–549

Peek GJ, Mugford M et al (2009) Efficacy and economic assessment of conventional ventilatory support versus extracorporeal membrane oxygenation for severe adult respiratory failure (CESAR): a multicentre randomised controlled trial. Lancet 374(9698):1351–1363

Pepe PE, Potkin RT et al (1982) Clinical predictors of the adult respiratory distress syndrome. Am J Surg 144(1):124–130

Phillips L, Toledo AH et al (2009) Nitric oxide mechanism of protection in ischemia and reperfusion injury. J Invest Surg 22(1):46–55

Pinhu L, Whitehead T et al (2003) Ventilator-associated lung injury. Lancet 361(9354):332–340

Plotz FB, Vreugdenhil HAE et al (2002) Mechanical ventilation alters the immune response in children without lung pathology. Intensive Care Med 28(4):486–492

Puybasset L, Gusman P et al (2000) Regional distribution of gas and tissue in acute respiratory distress syndrome. III. Consequences for the effects of positive end-expiratory pressure. CT Scan ARDS Study Group. Adult Respiratory Distress Syndrome. Intensive Care Med 26(9):1215–1227

Rana R, Vlahakis NE et al (2006) B-type natriuretic peptide in the assessment of acute lung injury and cardiogenic pulmonary edema. Crit Care Med 34(7):1941–1946

Ranieri VM, Giunta F et al (2000) Mechanical ventilation as a mediator of multisystem organ failure in acute respiratory distress syndrome. JAMA 284(1):43–44

Ranieri VM, Suter PM et al (1999) Effect of mechanical ventilation on inflammatory mediators in patients with acute respiratory distress syndrome: a randomized controlled trial. JAMA 282(1):54–61

Reickert CA, Rich PB et al (2002) Partial liquid ventilation and positive end-expiratory pressure reduce ventilator-induced lung injury in an ovine model of acute respiratory failure. Crit Care Med 30(1):182–189

Ribeiro SP, Rhee K et al (2001) Heat stress attenuates ventilator-induced lung dysfunction in an ex vivo rat lung model. Am J Respir Crit Care Med 163(6):1451–1456

Richard JC, Maggiore SM et al (2001) Influence of tidal volume on alveolar recruitment. Respective role of PEEP and a recruitment maneuver. Am J Respir Crit Care Med 163(7):1609–1613

Riley DJ, Rannels DE et al (1990) NHLBI Workshop Summary. Effect of physical forces on lung structure, function, and metabolism. Am Rev Respir Dis 142(4):910–914

Rocco TR Jr, Reinert SE et al (2001) A 9-year, single-institution, retrospective review of death rate and prognostic factors in adult respiratory distress syndrome. Ann Surg 233(3):414–422

Rubenfeld GD (2003) Epidemiology of acute lung injury. Crit Care Med 31(4 Suppl): S276–S284

Rubenfeld GD, Christie JD (2004) The epidemiologist in the intensive care unit. Intensive Care Med 30(1):4–6

Rubenfeld GD, Herridge MS (2007) Epidemiology and outcomes of acute lung injury. Chest 131(2):554–562

Sedoris KC, Ovechkin AV et al (2009) Differential effects of nitric oxide synthesis on pulmonary vascular function during lung ischemia-reperfusion injury. Arch Physiol Biochem 115(1):34–46

Sinclair SE, Altemeier WA et al (2004) Augmented lung injury due to interaction between hyperoxia and mechanical ventilation. Crit Care Med 32(12):2496–2501

Skerrett SJ, Liggitt HD et al (2004) Respiratory epithelial cells regulate lung inflammation in response to inhaled endotoxin. Am J Physiol Lung Cell Mol Physiol 287(1):L143–L152

Slutsky AS, Slutsky AS (2005) Ventilator-induced lung injury: from barotrauma to biotrauma. Respir Care 50(5):646–659

Stamme C, Brasch F et al (2002) Effect of surfactant on ventilation-induced mediator release in isolated perfused mouse lungs. Pulm Pharmacol Ther 15(5):455–461

Stapleton RD, Wang BM et al (2005) Causes and timing of death in patients with ARDS. Chest 128(2):525–532

Steinberg JM, Schiller HJ et al (2004) Alveolar instability causes early ventilator-induced lung injury independent of neutrophils. Am J Respir Crit Care Med 169(1):57–63

Stuber F (2002) Genomics and acute respiratory distress syndrome. Am J Respir Crit Care Med 166(5):633–634

Sud S, Sud M et al (2008) Effect of mechanical ventilation in the prone position on clinical outcomes in patients with acute hypoxemic respiratory failure: a systematic review and meta-analysis. Can Med Assoc J 178(9):1153–1161

Sznajder JI, Olivera WG et al (1995) Mechanisms of lung liquid clearance during hyperoxia in isolated rat lungs. Am J Respir Crit Care Med 151(5):1519–1525

Talmor D, Sarge T et al (2008) Mechanical ventilation guided by esophageal pressure in acute lung injury. N Engl J Med 359(20):2095–2104

Tang BMP, Craig JC et al (2009) Use of corticosteroids in acute lung injury and acute respiratory distress syndrome: a systematic review and meta-analysis. Crit Care Med 37(5): 1594–1603

Taskar V, John J et al (1997) Surfactant dysfunction makes lungs vulnerable to repetitive collapse and reexpansion. Am J Respir Crit Care Med 155(1):313–320

Taylor RW, Zimmerman JL et al (2004) Low-dose inhaled nitric oxide in patients with acute lung injury: a randomized controlled trial. JAMA 291(13):1603–1609

Terragni PP, Rosboch G et al (2007) Tidal hyperinflation during low tidal volume ventilation in acute respiratory distress syndrome. Am J Respir Crit Care Med 175(2):160–166

Toth I, Leiner T et al (2007) Hemodynamic and respiratory changes during lung recruitment and descending optimal positive end-expiratory pressure titration in patients with acute respiratory distress syndrome. Crit Care Med 35(3):787–793

Tugrul S, Akinci O et al (2003) Effects of sustained inflation and postinflation positive end-expiratory pressure in acute respiratory distress syndrome: focusing on pulmonary and extrapulmonary forms. Crit Care Med 31(3):738–744

Uhlig S (2002) Ventilation-induced lung injury and mechanotransduction: stretching it too far? Am J Physiol Lung Cell Mol Physiol 282(5):L892–L896

Villar J (2002) Genetics and the pathogenesis of adult respiratory distress syndrome. Curr Opin Crit Care 8(1):1–5

Vincent JL, Zambon M et al (2006) Why do patients who have acute lung injury/acute respiratory distress syndrome die from multiple organ dysfunction syndrome? Implications for management. Clin Chest Med 27(4):725–731, abstract x–xi

Vlahakis NE, Hubmayr RD (2005) Cellular stress failure in ventilator-injured lungs. Am J Respir Crit Care Med 171(12):1328–1342

Vreugdenhil HA, Haitsma JJ et al (2003) Ventilator-induced heat shock protein 70 and cytokine mRNA expression in a model of lipopolysaccharide-induced lung inflammation. Intensive Care Med 29(6):915–922

Walmrath D, Schneider T et al (1996) Direct comparison of inhaled nitric oxide and aerosolized prostacyclin in acute respiratory distress syndrome. Am J Respir Crit Care Med 153(3):991–996

Ware LB (2005) Prognostic determinants of acute respiratory distress syndrome in adults: impact on clinical trial design. Crit Care Med 33(3 Suppl):S217–S222

Webb HH, Tierney DF (1974) Experimental pulmonary edema due to intermittent positive pressure ventilation with high inflation pressures. Protection by positive end-expiratory pressure. Am Rev Respir Dis 110(5):556–565

Weiss YG, Maloyan A et al (2002) Adenoviral transfer of HSP-70 into pulmonary epithelium ameliorates experimental acute respiratory distress syndrome. J Clin Invest 110(6):801–806

Wrigge H, Uhlig U et al (2004) The effects of different ventilatory settings on pulmonary and systemic inflammatory responses during major surgery. Anesth Analg 98(3):775–781

Yoo CG, Lee S et al (2000) Anti-inflammatory effect of heat shock protein induction is related to stabilization of I kappa B alpha through preventing I kappa B kinase activation in respiratory epithelial cells. J Immunol 164(10):5416–5423

Zilberberg MD, Epstein SK (1998) Acute lung injury in the medical ICU: comorbid conditions, age, etiology, and hospital outcome. Am J Respir Crit Care Med 157(4 Pt 1):1159–1164

Pathogens in Severe Sepsis: New Paradigms for Gram-Positive Treatment

10

Lee P. Skrupky, Scott T. Micek, and Marin H. Kollef

10.1 Introduction

Vancomycin has been considered the gold standard therapy for invasive methicillin-resistant *Staphylococcus aureus* (MRSA) infections as a result of a relatively clean safety profile, durability against resistance development and the lack of other approved alternatives for many years. However, the advent and testing of new compounds with anti-MRSA activity in comparison to vancomycin have rendered results that question vancomycin's efficacy in many serious infections. The reasons for vancomycin clinical failure are many, and have been hypothesized to include poor penetration to certain tissues (Albanese et al. 2000; Cruciani et al. 1996; Lamer et al. 1993), loss of accessory gene-regulator function in MRSA (Sakoulas et al. 2006) and potentially escalating minimum inhibitory concentrations of MRSA to vancomycin (Robert et al. 2006). Additionally, increasing reports of vancomycin-intermediate *S. aureus* (VISA) and vancomycin-resistant *S. aureus* (VRSA) have begun to populate the literature dating back to 1999. Several alternatives for the

L.P. Skrupky
Department of Pharmacy, Barnes-Jewish Hospital,
St. Louis, MO, USA

Surgery, Trauma & Burn ICU, Barnes-Jewish Hospital,
St. Louis, MO, USA

S.T. Micek
Department of Pharmacy, Barnes-Jewish Hospital,
St. Louis, MO, USA

Medical ICU, Barnes-Jewish Hospital,
St. Louis, MO, USA

M.H. Kollef (✉)
Division of Pulmonary and Critical Care Medicine,
Washington University School of Medicine,
St. Louis, MO, USA
e-mail: mkollef@dom.wustl.edu

J. Rello (eds.), *Sepsis Management*,
DOI 10.1007/978-3-642-03519-7_10, © Springer-Verlag Berlin Heidelberg 2012

treatment of MRSA infections are currently approved by the US Food and Drug Administration, including linezolid, daptomycin, tigecycline and quinopristin/dalfopristin. Additionally, there are several investigational compounds with demonstrated in vitro activity against MRSA.

10.1.1 Antibiotic Resistance of MRSA to Currently Approved Antibiotics

Methicillin-resistance in *Staphylococcus species* is encoded via the mecA gene, which results in production of PBP2A, a penicillin-binding protein with reduced affinity for β-lactams (Chambers 1997). Mec is part of a larger genomic element termed Staphylococcal chromosomal cassette (SCCmec) that contains genes mediating antibiotic resistance. Up to eight types of SCCmec have now been reported in the literature (Zhang et al. 2009), and the differences between these SCCmec types account for the primary differences between various MRSA clones. For example, SCCmec I, II and III are larger and more difficult to mobilize, and are most frequently present in hospital-acquired (HA-MRSA) clones (USA 100 and 200). SCCmec IV is a smaller, easier to mobilize genetic element that is frequently present in community-associated MRSA (CA-MRSA, USA 300 and 400) (McDougal et al. 2003). It has been observed that CA-MRSA is effectively integrating into the health care environment, and it is therefore increasingly less reliable to make this differentiation on the basis of acquisition location (Popovich et al. 2008; Schramm et al. 2007; Davis et al. 2006; Seybold et al. 2006). HA-MRSA and CA-MRSA clones are noted to display different resistance patterns as a result of their unique genetic elements. Compared with HA-MRSA, CA-MRSA isolates are more likely to be susceptible to non-β-lactam antibiotics, including trimethoprim-sulfamethoxazole (TMP-SMX), clindamycin, fluoroquinolones, gentamicin, erythromycin and tetracyclines with geographic variability (Seybold et al. 2006; Naimi et al. 2003; Fridkin et al. 2005).

Increasing attention is being paid to the issue of reduced susceptibility and resistance of MRSA to vancomycin. Although vancomycin has long been considered a reliable agent for the treatment of MRSA infections, isolates with intermediate (VISA) and full (VRSA) levels of resistance have been reported. The CLSI vancomycin minimum inhibitory concentration (MIC) breakpoints for MRSA were last updated in 2006 and resulted in a lowering of the breakpoints as follows: susceptible, ≤2 µg/mL; intermediate, 4–8 µg/mL; resistant, ≥16 µg/mL.

Vancomycin exerts its antibiotic activity by binding to the D-alanyl-D-alanine portion of cell wall precursors, which subsequently inhibits peptidoglycan polymerization and transpeptidation. High-level resistance is mediated via the vanA gene, which results in production of cell wall precursors (D-Ala-D-lac or D-Ala-D-Ser) with reduced affinity for vancomycin (Courvalin 2006). Intermediate level resistance (VISA) is believed to be preceded by the development of heteroresistant vancomycin intermediate *S. aureus* (hVISA) (Liu and Chambers 2003). Heteroresistance is the presence of resistant subpopulations within a population of bacteria determined to be susceptible to the antibiotic tested. It is thought that exposure of such a heteroresistant MRSA population to low concentrations of vancomycin may kill the fully suscepti- ble subpopulations and select out for the resistant subpopulations. The mechanisms of heteroresistance are not fully elucidated, but are hypothesized to be due to a thick- ened cell wall and increased production of false-binding sites (Liu and Chambers 2003). The accessory gene regulator type and functionality may also play a role in the development of this type of resistance (Sakoulas et al. 2002). Similar heteroresis- tance has now also been identified in methicillin-sensitive *Staphylococcus aureus* isolates as well (Pillai et al. 2009).

Reduced susceptibility to glycopeptides may also impact the susceptibility of MRSA to daptomycin. Several reports have found hVISA and VISA isolates to display resistance to daptomycin (Hayden et al. 2005; Vikram et al. 2005; Kirby et al. 2009). Daptomycin is a cyclic lipopeptide that works by binding to the cell membrane to subsequently cause destabilization resulting in bactericidal activity. It is hypothesized that the thickened cell wall noted to occur in MRSA isolates with intermediate-level vancomycin resistance may result in sequestration of daptomycin. Additionally, reduced susceptibility has been documented to develop while on pro- longed daptomycin therapy (Fowler et al. 2006; Sharma et al. 2008).

Linezolid is a synthetic oxazolidinone that inhibits the initiation of protein syn- thesis by binding to the 23S ribosomal RNA and thereby preventing formation of the 70S initiation complex. Although linezolid has generally remained a reliable antibiotic for MRSA infections, several occurrences of resistance have been observed (Tsiodras et al. 2001; Peeters and Sarria 2005; Steinkraus et al. 2007; Morales et al. 2010).The first report of resistance (Tsiodras et al. 2001) from a clini- cal isolate was reported in 2001, about 15 months after the drug was introduced to the market. Upon analysis, the organism was found to have mutations in the DNA encoding a portion of the 23S ribosomal RNA (rRNA). Linezolid resistance has been identified more commonly among *Staphylococcus epidermidis* and *Enterococcus species*, but the possibility of linezolid resistance among MRSA should be kept in mind (Morales et al. 2010). Similarly, there may be a drift in the minimum inhibitory concentration of MRSA to linezolid that occurs over time of use (Steinkraus et al. 2007).

In vitro studies have reported tigecycline to be highly active against the MRSA isolates that have been tested. No reports of resistance to clinical isolates have been reported to our knowledge, but the use of this agent for serious MRSA infections has been very limited. Quinupristin/dalfopristin has similarly been shown to be highly active in vitro against MRSA, but clinical isolates with resistance have been reported (Malbruny et al. 2002), and the use of this agent for serious MRSA infec- tions has also been limited.

10.1.2 Virulence Factors for MRSA

Virulence factors play an important role in determining the pathogenesis of MRSA infections (Lowy 1998). Colonization by MRSA is enhanced by biofilm formation, antiphagocytocic microcapsules and surface adhesions (DeLeo and Chambers 2009). Once an inoculum is established, *S. aureus* can produce a variety of virulence factors to mediate disease, including exoenzymes and toxins. Exoenzymes include proteases, lipases and hyaluronidases, which can cause tissue destruction and may facilitate the spread of infection. The toxins that can be produced are numerous and include hemolysins, leukocidins, exfoliative toxins, Panton-Valentine leukocidin (PVL) toxin, toxic shock syndrome toxin (TSST-1), enterotoxins and α-toxin (Lowy 1998; DeLeo and Chambers 2009). *S. aureus* also has a multitude of mechanisms to further elude and modulate the host immune response. Specific examples include inhibition of neutrophil chemotaxis via a secreted protein called chemotaxis inhibitory protein of staphylococci (CHIPS), resistance to phagocytosis via surface proteins [e.g., protein A and clumping factor A (ClfA)], inactivation of complement via Staphylococcus complement inhibitor (SCIN), and production of proteins that confer resistance to lysozyme (e.g., O-acetyltransferase) and antimicrobial peptides (e.g., modified Dlt proteins and MprF protein) (Foster 2005).

Various toxins have been associated with different clinical scenarios and clinical presentations (Lowy 1998; DeLeo and Chambers 2009). For example, α-toxin, enterotoxin and TSST-1 are believed to lead to extensive cytokine production and a resulting systemic inflammatory response. Epidermolytic toxins A and B cause the manifestations of Staphylococcal scalded skin syndrome. PVL is most frequently associated with CA-MRSA and may play an important role in cavitary pneumonia and necrotizing skin and soft tissue infections, as discussed in the following section.

Expression of virulence factors is largely controlled by the accessory gene regulator (agr) (Sakoulas 2006). Polymorphisms in agr account for the now five different types that have been identified. HA-MRSA is most frequently agr group II, whereas CA-MRSA is most frequently agr group I and III. Another difference is that agr is functional in a majority of CA-MRSA isolates, whereas agr may be dysfunctional in about half of the HA-MRSA isolates (Tsuji et al. 2007). When agr is active it generally results in upregulation of secreted factors and downregulation of cell surface virulence factors. This pattern of expression has been noted to occur during the stationary growth phase when studied in vitro and in animal models. During an exponential growth phase, upregulation of cell surface factors is increased and production of secreted factors is decreased. A recent study (Loughman et al. 2009) sought to examine virulence gene expression in humans by measuring transcript levels of virulence genes in samples taken directly from children with active CA-MRSA skin and soft tissue infections (superficial and invasive abscesses). This analysis showed that genes encoding secretory toxins, including PVL, were highly expressed during both superficial and invasive CA-MRSA infections, whereas surface-associated protein A (encoded by *spa*) was only associated with invasive disease. It was also demonstrated that the virulence gene expression profiles measured from in vivo samples differed from those observed when the clinical isolates were exposed to purified neutrophils in vitro. This study therefore found some differences between in vitro and animal models when compared to this in vivo assessment and supports the hypothesis that the course of an MRSA infection can be altered by recognition of host-specific signals.

10.1.3 Epidemiology and Outcomes of MRSA Infections

The era of MRSA being exclusively a nosocomial pathogen is quickly fading. An epidemiologic study conducted in metropolitan areas throughout the US found only 27% of MRSA sterile-site infections are of nosocomial origin (Klevens et al. 2007). Taking a closer look, of the 63% of patients presenting from the "community," the majority had recent healthcare exposures, including hospitalization in the previous 12 months, residence in a nursing care facility, chronic dialysis and presence of an invasive device at the time of admission. This group of patients deemed to have "healthcare-associated, community-onset" infection most often harbor strains of MRSA associated with the hospital setting; however, crossover of the CA-MRSA clone into these patients is occurring in many healthcare centers (Popovich et al. 2008; Schramm et al. 2007; Davis et al. 2006; Seybold et al. 2006).

Numerous studies have evaluated the impact methicillin resistance has on the outcome of patients with *S. aureus* infection. A meta-analysis of 31 *S. aureus* bacteremia studies found a significant increase in mortality associated with MRSA bacteremia compared to MSSA bacteremia (pooled odds ratio 1.93, 95% confidence interval 1.54–2.42; $p < 0.001$) (Cosgrove and Carmeli 2003). This finding remained evident when the analysis was limited to studies that were adjusted for potential confounding factors, most notably severity of illness. Since this publication, several other investigations comparing MRSA and MSSA bacteremia have yielded similar results (Shurland et al. 2007). The higher attributable mortality associated with MRSA could in part be explained by significant delays in the administration of an antibiotic with anti-MRSA activity, particularly in patients presenting from the community. A single-center cohort study found only 22% of MRSA sterile-site infections cultured within the first 48 h of hospital admission received an anti-MRSA antibiotic within the first 24 h of culture collection, a factor that was independently associated with hospital mortality (Schramm et al. 2006) and a significant contributor to hospital length of stay and costs (Shorr et al. 2008).

In the majority of hospitals throughout the world, the antibiotic of choice for empiric therapy of suspected MRSA infection is vancomycin. However, just as the era of MRSA occurring only in the hospital setting has ended, so too might the automatic, empiric use of vancomycin in these situations. Increasingly it is being reported that MRSA infections with vancomycin MICs in the higher end of the "susceptible" range (1.5–2 mcg/mL) may be associated with higher rates of treatment failure compared to isolates with an MIC of 1 mcg/mL or less (Lodise et al. 2008a). Additionally, a cohort analysis of MRSA bacteremia found vancomycin therapy in isolates with an MIC of 2 mcg/mL was associated with a 6.39-fold increase in the odds of hospital mortality (Soriano et al. 2008).

As the predominant genetic background of MRSA is transitioning from that of the hospital to community architecture (e.g., USA 100 to USA 300) in hospitalized patients, so too might the severity of infection. Because of its epidemiologic association with CA-MRSA and severe, necrotizing pneumonia, Panton-Valentine leukocidin (PVL) has gained much attention as an important virulence factor. However, the extent of its role in pathogenesis is a matter of significant debate, and it is likely that other factors including the expression of adhesion proteins, such as staphylococcal protein A, as well as α-toxin and phenol-soluble modulins are also responsible for the increased infection severity (DeLeo and Chambers 2009; Labandeira-Rey et al. 2007; Li et al. 2009). Regardless, the selection of antibiotics in the treatment of MRSA pneumonia characterized by hemoptysis, leukopenia, high fever and a cavitary picture on chest radiographs (Gillet et al. 2008) as well as other necrotizing infections may be of clinical significance. Secretory toxin production is likely enhanced by beta-lactams such as nafcillin or oxacillin, maintained by vancomycin and inhibited, even at sub-inhibitory concentrations, by protein-synthesis inhibitors, including clindamycin, rifampin and linezolid (Stevens et al. 2007; Dumitrescu et al. 2008). As such, it may be reasonable to combine these toxin-suppressing agents with beta-lactams or vancomycin in severe MRSA infections.

10.2   Antimicrobial Agents for MRSA

Timely provision of appropriate antimicrobial coverage in an initial anti-infective treatment regimen results in optimal outcomes for bacterial and fungal infections (Schramm et al. 2006; Kollef et al. 1999; Morrell et al. 2005). This is also true for MRSA infections where it has been shown that antimicrobial regimens not targeting MRSA when it is the cause of serious infection (e.g., pneumonia, bacteremia) results in greater mortality and longer lengths of hospitalization (Schramm et al. 2006; Shorr et al. 2008). The following represents the antimicrobial agents currently available for serious MRSA infections and those in development (Tables 10.1 and 10.2).

10.2.1 Vancomycin

Vancomycin has been considered a first-line therapy for invasive MRSA infections as a result of a relatively clean safety profile, durability against resistance development and the lack of other approved alternatives for many years. However, increasing concerns about resistance as well as the availability of alternative agents have led to questioning of vancomycin's efficacy in many serious infections. The possible reasons for vancomycin clinical failure are many and include poor penetration into certain tissues (Cruciani et al. 1996), loss of accessory gene-regulator function in MRSA (Sakoulas et al. 2002), and potentially escalating minimum inhibitory concentrations of MRSA to vancomycin (Robert et al. 2006). To circumvent the possibility of poor outcomes with vancomycin therapy in MRSA infections with MICs ≥ 1.5 mcg/mL, consensus guidelines recommend a strategy of optimizing the vancomycin pharmacokinetic-pharmacodynamic profile such that trough concentrations of 15–20 mcg/mL are achieved (American Thoracic Society 2005; Rybak et al. 2009). Unfortunately, in MRSA infections where vancomycin distribution to the site of infection is limited (e.g., lung) it is unlikely that targeted concentrations will be reached (Mohr and Murray 2007; Jeffres et al. 2006). Furthermore, when higher trough concentrations are achieved this may not improve outcome (Jeffres

Table 10.1 Antibiotics currently available for the treatment of serious MRSA infections

Antibiotic	Primary indications	Daily dose[a]	Volume of distribution (L/kg)	Elimination half-life (h)	Protein binding (%)	Main toxicity
Vancomycin	Pneumonia Skin/soft tissues Bacteremia	30 mg/kg/day	0.2–1.25	4–6	30–55	Nephrotoxicity (higher doses) Thrombocytopenia
Linezolid	Pneumonia Skin/soft tissues	600 mg q 12 h	0.5–0.6	5	31	Myelosuppression (prolonged duration generally >2 week) Lactic acidosis Peripheral & optic neuropathy Serotonin syndrome
Tigecycline	Skin/soft tissues Intra-abdominal	100 mg load 50 mg q 12 h	7–10	37–66	71–89	Nausea Vomiting Photosensitivity
Daptomycin	Bacteremia Skin/soft tissues	Bacteremia: 6 mg/kg q 24 h Skin/soft tissues: 4 mg/kg q 24 h	0.09	8–9	92	Muscle toxicity CPK elevation
Quinupristin/dalfopristin	Skin/soft tissues	7.5 mg/kg q 8 h (via central vein)	0.56–0.98	.54–1.14	11–78	Phlebitis Arthralgias & myalgias
Ceftobiprole[b]	Skin/soft tissues	500 mg q 8 h	0.25–0.30	3–4	16	Allergic reactions

(continued)

Table 10.1 (continued)

Antibiotic	Primary indications	Daily dose[a]	Volume of distribution (L/kg)	Elimination half-life (h)	Protein binding (%)	Main toxicity
Ceftaroline[c]	Skin/soft tissues Pneumonia	600 mg q 12 h	0.22–0.25	2.5–3	18	Allergic reactions
Dalbavancin[c]	Skin/soft tissues	1,000 mg day 1 500 mg weekly	0.011	147–258	93	Nausea Vomiting
Oritavancin[c]	Skin/soft tissues	1.5–3 mg/kg q 24 h	0.65–1.92	195	90	Nausea Vomiting
Telavancin[c]	Skin/soft tissues Pneumonia	7.5–10 mg/kg d	0.1	7–9	93	Renal
Iclaprim[d]	Skin/soft tissues	0.8 mg/kg q 12 h	1.15	2.5–4.1	93	Thrombocytopenia

[a]Daily dose listed assumes normal kidney and liver function
[b]Not approved for clinical use in US. Greater risk of clinical failure in ventilator-associated pneumonia compared to vancomycin plus ceftazadine
[c]Not approved for clinical use in US at the time of this writing
[d]Not approved for clinical use in US. Failed to demonstrated non-inferiority against linezolid for treatment of complicated skin and skin structure infection

et al. 2007; Hidayat et al. 2006) and could in fact increase the likelihood of nephrotoxicity (Hidayat et al. 2006; Jeffres et al. 2007; Lodise et al. 2008). The key to successful outcomes then falls to identifying patients at risk for having an MRSA infection with a vancomycin MIC that is 1.5 mcg/mL or greater and using an alternative agent. Not surprisingly, recent vancomycin exposure prior to a suspected or proven MRSA infection, even in a single dose, is a strong predictor of higher vancomycin MICs (Moise et al. 2008).

10.2.2 Linezolid

Linezolid is currently approved by the US Food and Drug Administration for the treatment of complicated skin and skin structure infections and nosocomial pneumonia caused by susceptible pathogens including MRSA. Much debate exists concerning whether linezolid should be considered the drug of choice for MRSA pneumonia on the basis of two retrospective analyses of pooled data from randomized trials comparing linezolid and vancomycin for nosocomial pneumonia (Wunderink et al. 2003; Kollef et al. 2004). In these retrospective analyses, linezolid therapy was associated with increased survival, but one limitation is that vancomycin may have been dosed inadequately, leading to suboptimal concentrations. A randomized, double-blind trial is underway in an effort to either confirm or refute these findings in hospitalized patients with nosocomial pneumonia due to MRSA. Linezolid should also be considered for necrotizing infections, including skin lesions, fasciitis and pneumonia, caused by community-associated MRSA as it has been hypothesized that antibiotics with the ability to inhibit protein synthesis may demonstrate efficacy against susceptible toxin-producing strains (Stevens et al. 2007). Recent guidelines (Mermel et al. 2009) recommend against the use of linezolid as empiric therapy for catheter-related blood stream (CRBSI) infections as one study (Wilcox et al. 2009) comparing vancomycin and linezolid for empiric therapy of complicated skin and soft tissue infections and CRBSI found a trend toward increased mortality in the linezolid group. Safety concerns that sometimes limit the use of this agent include the association of serotonin toxicity and thrombocytopenia (Taylor et al. 2006).

10.2.3 Tigecycline

Telavancin is a glycopeptide derivative of vancomycin that was recently FDA-approved for the treatment of skin and soft tissue infections due to gram-positive bacteria. Tigecycline is the first drug approved in the class of glycylcyclines, a derivative of minocycline. A modified side chain on tigecycline enhances binding to the 30S ribosomal subunit, inhibiting protein synthesis and bacterial growth against a broad spectrum of pathogens including MRSA (Rose and Rybak 2006). Tigecycline is approved in the US for the treatment of complicated MRSA skin and skin structure infections. The drug is also approved for the treatment of complicated intra-abdominal infections, but for methicillin-sensitive *Staphylococcus aureus* only. Tigecycline has a large volume of distribution producing high concentrations in tissues outside of the bloodstream, including bile, colon, and the lung (Rodvold et al. 2006). As a result of serum concentrations that rapidly decline after infusion, caution should be used in patients with proven or suspected bacteremia. Additionally, the drug may be inadequate for the treatment of hospital-acquired pneumonia, possibly due to underdosing (Chemaly et al. 2009; Anthony et al. 2008). Possible toxicities of telavancin include taste disturbance, nausea, vomiting, foamy urine, nephrotoxicity and QTc prolongation. Due to the observance of teratogenicity in animals, this agent should only be considered in women of childbearing potential when the potential benefit outweighs the risk.

10.2.4 Daptomycin

Daptomycin is indicated for MRSA-associated complicated skin and soft-tissue infections (SSTI), and bloodstream infections, including right-sided endocarditis. Of note, daptomycin should not be used in the treatment of MRSA pneumonia as the drug's activity is inhibited by pulmonary surfactant. As previously mentioned, vancomycin resistance may impact daptomycin susceptibility, and the development of reduced daptomycin susceptibility during prolonged treatment of MRSA infections has been reported (Fowler et al. 2006). These observations should be considered while assessing response to treatment of MRSA infections. As a result of dapytomycin's potential to cause myopathy, creatine phosphokinase (CPK) should be measured at baseline and weekly thereafter.

10.2.5 Quinupristin/Dalfopristin

Quinupristin/dalfopristin is a combination of two streptogramins, quinupristin and dalfopristin (in a ratio of 30:70 w/w), that inhibit different sites in protein synthesis. Each individual component demonstrates bacteriostatic activity; however, the combination is bactericidal against most gram-positive organisms. Importantly, while quinupristin/dalfopristin offers activity against MRSA and vancomycin-resistant *Enterococcus faecium*, it lacks activity against *Enterococcus faecalis*. Quinoprisitn/dalfoprisitin has FDA approval for serious infections due to VRE, and for complicated skin and skin-structure infections. Severe arthralgias and myalgias occur in up to half of patients, and as a result patient tolerability can limit this agent's utility.

10.2.6 Ceftobiprole

Ceftobiprole medocaril is a fifth-generation cephalosporin prodrug with a broad spectrum of activity. This agent was designed to maximize binding to PBP2a and yield potent anti-MRSA activity (Vidaillac and Rybak 2009). Ceftobiprole is also active against cephalosporin-resistant *Streptococcus pneumonia* and ampicillin-sensitive

Enterococus faecalis, and has a gram-negative spectrum of activity intermediate between ceftriaxone and cefepime inclusive of *Pseudomonas aeruginosa*. Two phase III clinical trials have been completed with ceftobiprole for cSSSIs (Noel et al. 2008a, b). Ceftobiprole was also compared to a combination of ceftazidime plus linezolid for treatment of nosocomial pneumonia. Ceftobiprole was unexpectedly associated with lower cure rates in patients with ventilator-associated pneumonia, particularly in those under age 45 and with high creatinine clearance (Noel et al. 2008c). This may represent a dosing issue as the same 500 mg dose was used in the nosocomial pneumonia study that was evaluated for skin infections.

10.2.7 Ceftaroline

Ceftaroline fosamil is also a fifth-generation cephalosporin prodrug, so named because of its spectrum of activity against a broad range of gram-positive and gram-negative bacteria. Ceftaroline is active against methicillin-resistant *Staphylococcus aureus* (MRSA) because of its enhanced binding to penicillin-binding protein 2a (PBP2a) as compared to other β-lactam antibiotics (Ge et al. 2008). The drug is also active against penicillin- and cephalosporin-resistant *Streptococcus pneumoniae*, β-hemolytic streptococci and *Enterococcus faecalis* (variable activity), but has little to no activity against vancomycin-resistant *Enterococcus faecium*. Against relevant gram-negative pathogens, ceftaroline has broad-spectrum activity similar to that of ceftriaxone, and the drug is expected to be inactive against *Pseudomonas* and *Acinetobacter spp.* (Ge et al. 2008). Phase III studies have been conducted for complicated skin and skin structure infections, and community-acquired pneumonia, the results of which are pending. Adverse effects in all ceftaroline studies to date have been minor and include headache, nausea, insomnia and abnormal body odor (Talbot et al. 2007).

10.2.8 Dalbavancin

Dalbavancin is an investigational lipoglycopeptide with a bactericidal mechanism of action similar to other glycopeptides in that it complexes with the D-alanyl-D-alanine (D-Ala-D-Ala) terminal of peptidoglycan, and inhibits transglycosylation and transpeptidation. Like teicoplanin, dalbavancin possesses a lipophilic side chain that leads to both high protein binding and an extended half-life, which allows for a unique once-weekly dosing of the drug (Zhanel et al. 2008). Dalbavancin is more potent than vancomycin against staphylococci, and is highly active against both methicillin-susceptible *Staphylococcus aureus* (MSSA) and MRSA. Dalbavancin is also active against vancomycin-intermediate *Staphylococcus aureus* (VISA), although MIC_{90} ranges are higher at 1–2 mcg/mL. However, dalbavancin is not active against enterococci with the VanA phenotype (Goldstein et al. 2007). Clinical data for dalbavancin include phase II and III trials in both uncomplicated and cSSSI, and catheter-related bloodstream infections. Dalbavancin has been well-tolerated throughout clinical trials, with the most commonly seen adverse effects being fever, headache and nausea.

10.2.9 Oritavancin

Oritavancin, another investigational glycopeptide, contains novel structural modifications that allow it to dimerize and anchor itself in the bacterial membrane. These
modifications also confer an enhanced spectrum of activity over traditional glycopeptide antibiotics (Mercier and Hrebickova 2005). Ortivancin has similar in vitro activity
as vancomycin against staphylococci and is equipotent against both MSSA and
MRSA. Oritavancin also has activity against VISA and VRSA, but MICs are increased
to 1 mg/L and 0.5 mg/L, respectively (Tenover et al. 1998). Oritivancin is active
against enterococci, including vancomycin-resistant enterococci (VRE); however,
MICs are significantly higher for VRE versus vancomycin-sensitive strains.

10.2.10 Telavancin

Telavancin is a glycopeptide derivative of vancomycin that was recently FDA-approved
for the treatment of skin and soft tissue infections due to gram-positive bacteria. Like
oritavancin, telavancin has the ability to anchor itself in the bacterial membrane, which
disrupts polymerization and cross-linking of peptidoglycan. Telavancin also interferes
with the normal function of the bacterial membrane, leading to a decrease in the barrier
function of the membrane. This dual mechanism helps to explain its high potency and
rapid bactericidal activity. Telavancin is bactericidal against staphylococci, including
MRSA, VISA and VRSA with MIC_{90} ranges of 0.25–1, 0.5–2, and 2–4 mg/L, respectively (Leuthner et al. 2006). Telavancin, like oritavancin, is potent against both penicillin-
susceptible and -resistant strains of *Streptococcus pneumoniae*. Telavancin is also active
against vancomycin-susceptible *Enterococcus faecium* and *Enterococcus faecalis*.
Two identical skin and skin structure trials, ATLAS I and II, compared telavancin
10 mg/kg/day to vancomycin 1 g every 12 h and found telavancin to be noninferior to
vancomycin (Zhanel et al. 2008). Telavancin has also been studied in hospital-acquired
pneumonia (HAP), but the FDA issued a complete response letter to the manufacturers
of telavancin indicating that two nosocomial pneumonia trials were inadequate to gain
approval for this indication (Theravance 2010). Possible toxicities of telavancin include
taste disturbance, nausea, vomiting, foamy urine, nephrotoxicity and QTc prolongation.
Due to the observance of teratogenicity in animals, this agent should only be considered
in women of childbearing potential when the potential benefit outweighs the risk.

10.2.11 Iclaprim

Iclaprim (formerly AR-100 and Ro 48–2622) is an investigational intravenous
diaminopyrimidine antibacterial agent that, like trimethoprim, selectively inhibits
dihydrofolate reductase of both gram-positive and gram-negative bacteria, and
exerts bactericidal effects (Schneider et al. 2003). Iclaprim is active against
MSSA, community- and nosocomial-MRSA, VISA, VRSA, groups A and B
streptococci, and pneumococci, and is variably active against enterococci (Laue
et al. 2007; Bozdogan et al. 2003). Iclaprim appears to have similar gram-negative
activity to that of trimethoprim, including activity against *E. coli*, *K. pneumoniae*,

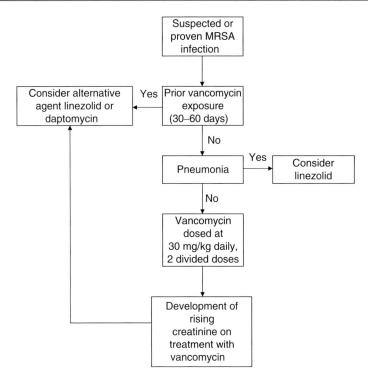

Fig. 10.1 Algorithm for the treatment of suspected or proven MRSA infections

Enterobacter, C. freundii and *P. vulgaris*. Iclaprim also appears to have activity against the atypical respiratory pathogens *Legionella* and *Chlamydia pneumoniae*, but is not active against *Pseudomonas aeruginosa* or anaerobes (Laue et al. 2007). Unfortunately, the FDA gave a negative recommendation for approval of iclaprim for skin infections since the available studies could not demonstrate noninferiority to the comparators (FDA 2009).

10.3   Conclusions

Several antibiotics with anti-MRSA activity, including linezolid, tigecycline and daptomycin, have been approved by the FDA. Additionally, there are a number of compounds in development that will likely provide a broader armamentarium for clinicians in the management of infections due to MRSA. The emergence of vanco-mycin-intermediate and vancomycin-resistant strains of *Staphylococcus aureus*, and reports of resistance to linezolid have also created a need for agents with expanded coverage. The challenge for clinicians will be to match the optimal MRSA agent, using adequate dosing and pharmacokinetic principles, to the patient's infection in order to insure the best possible outcomes (Fig. 10.1).

Acknowledgements Dr. Kollef's effort was supported by the Barnes-Jewish Hospital Foundation.

Table 10.2 Dosages, toxicities and spectrum of activity for Gram-positive antibiotics

Antibiotic	Primary indications	Daily dose[a]	Gram-positive spectrum of activity						Main toxicities
			MSSA	MRSA	VISA/VRSA	E.faecalis	E.faecium	S.pneumoniae	
Vancomycin	Pneumonia Skin/soft tissues Bacteremia	30 mg/kg/day	+	+	–	+	–	+	Nephrotoxicity (higher doses) Thrombocytopenia
Linezolid	Pneumonia Skin/soft tissues	600 mg q 12 h	+	+	+	+	+	+	Myelosuppression (prolonged duration generally >2 week) Lactic acidosis Peripheral & optic neuropathy Serotonin syndrome
Tigecycline	Skin/soft tissues Intra-abdominal	100 mg load 50 mg q 12 h	+	+	+	+	+	+	Nausea, Vomiting Photosensitivity
Daptomycin	Bacteremia Skin/soft tissues	Bacteremia: 6 mg/kg q 24 h Skin/soft tissues: 4 mg/kg q 24 h	+	+	+/–	+	+	+	Muscle toxicity CPK elevation
Quinupristin/ dalfopristin	Skin/soft tissues	7.5 mg/kg q 8 h (via central vein)	+	+	+	–	+	+	Phlebitis Arthralgias & Myalgias

Drug	Indication	Dose								Adverse effects
Telavancin	Skin/soft tissues, Pneumonia[c]	7.5–10 mg/kg d	+	+	+	+	+	+	+	Nephrotoxicity, QTc interval prolongation, Nausea, vomiting, taste disturbance
Ceftobiprole[b]	Skin/soft tissues	500 mg q 8 h	+	+	+	+	+/–	–	+	Allergic reactions
Ceftaroline[c]	Skin/soft tissues, Pneumonia	600 mg q 12 h	+	+	+	+	–	–	+	Allergic reactions
Dalbavancin[c]	Skin/soft tissues	1,000 mg day 1, 500 mg weekly	+	+	+	+	+	+/–	+	Nausea, Vomiting
Oritavancin[c]	Skin/soft tissues	1.5–3 mg/kg q 24 h	+	+	+	+	+	+	+	Nausea, Vomiting
Iclaprim[d]	Skin/soft tissues	0.8 mg/kg q 12 h	+	+	+	+	+/–	+/–	+	

[a]Daily dose listed assumes normal kidney and liver function
[b]Not approved for clinical use in US. Greater risk of clinical failure in ventilator-associated pneumonia compared to vancomycin plus ceftazadine
[c]Not approved for clinical use in US at the time of this writing
[d]Not approved for clinical use in US. Failed to demonstrated non-inferiority against linezolid for treatment of complicated skin and skin structure infection

References

Albanese J, Leone M, Bruguerolle B et al (2000) Cerebrospinal fluid penetration and pharmacokinetics of vancomycin administered by continuous infusion to mechanically ventilated patients in an intensive care unit. Antimicrob Agents Chemother 44:1356–1358

American Thoracic Society (2005) Guidelines for the management of adults with hospital-acquired, ventilator-associated, and healthcare-associated pneumonia. Am J Respir Crit Care Med 171:388–416

Anthony KB, Fishman NO, Linkin DR et al (2008) Clinical and microbiological outcomes of serious infections with multidrug-resistant gram-negative organisms treated with tigecycline. Clin Infect Dis 46:567–570

Bozdogan B, Esel D, Whitener C et al (2003) Antibacterial susceptibility of a vancomycin-resistant *Staphylococcus aureus* strain isolated at the Hershey Medical Center. J Antimicrob Chemother 52:864–868

Chambers HF (1997) Methicillin resistance in staphylococci: molecular and biochemical basis and clinical implications. Clin Microbiol Rev 10:781–791

Chemaly RF, Hanmod SS, Jiang Y et al (2009) Tigecycline use in cancer patients with serious infections: a report on 110 cases from a single institution. Medicine 88:211–220

Cosgrove SE, Carmeli Y (2003) The impact of antimicrobial resistance on health and economic outcomes. Clin Infect Dis 36:1433–1437

Courvalin P (2006) Vancomycin resistance in gram-positive cocci. Clin Infect Dis 42(Suppl 1):S25–S34

Cruciani M, Gatti G, Lazzarini L et al (1996) Penetration of vancomycin into human lung tissue. J Antimicrob Chemother 38:865–869

Davis SL, Rybak MJ, Amjad M et al (2006) Characteristics of patients with healthcare-associated infection due to SCCmec type IV methicillin-resistant *Staphylococcus aureus*. Infect Control Hosp Epidemiol 27:1025–1031

DeLeo FR, Chambers HF (2009) Reemergence of antibiotic-resistant *Staphylococcus aureus* in the genomics era. J Clin Invest 119:2464–2474

Dumitrescu O, Badiou C, Bes M et al (2008) Effect of antibiotics, alone and in combination, on Panton–Valentine leukocidin production by a *Staphylococcus aureus* reference strain. Clin Microbiol Infect 14:384–388

FDA Issues Complete Response Letter For Iclaprim (2009) Med News Today. http://www.medicalnewstoday.com/articles/135981.php. Accessed 21 Mar 2010

Foster TJ (2005) Immune evasion by staphylococci. Nat Rev Microbiol 3:948–958

Fowler VG Jr, Boucher HW, Corey GR et al (2006) Daptomycin versus standard therapy for bacteremia and endocarditis caused by *Staphylococcus aureus*. N Engl J Med 355:653–665

Fridkin SK, Hageman JC, Morrison M et al (2005) Methicillin-resistant *Staphylococcus aureus* disease in three communities. N Engl J Med 352:1436–1444

Ge Y, Biek D, Talbot GH et al (2008) In vitro profiling of ceftaroline against a collection of recent bacterial clinical isolates from across the United States. Antimicrob Agents Chemother 52:3398–3407

Gillet Y, Etienne J, Lina G et al (2008) Association of necrotizing pneumonia with Panton-Valentine leukocidin-producing *Staphylococcus aureus*, regardless of methicillin resistance. Clin Infect Dis 47:985–986

Goldstein BP, Draghi DC, Sheehan DJ et al (2007) Bactericidal activity and resistance development profiling of dalbavancin. Antimicrob Agents Chemother 51:1150–1154

Hayden MK, Rezai K, Hayes RA et al (2005) Development of daptomycin resistance in vivo in methicillin resistant *Staphylococcus aureus*. J Clin Microbiol 43:5285–5287

Hidayat LK, Hsu DI, Quist R et al (2006) High-dose vancomycin therapy for methicillin-resistant *Staphylococcus aureus* infections: efficacy and toxicity. Arch Intern Med 166:2138–2144

Jeffres MN, Isakow W, Doherty JA et al (2006) Predictors of mortality for methicillin-resistant *Staphylococcus aureus* health-care-associated pneumonia: specific evaluation of vancomycin pharmacokinetic indices. Chest 130:947–955

Jeffres MN, Isakow W, Doherty JA et al (2007) A retrospective analysis of possible renal toxicity associated with vancomycin in patients with health care-associated methicillin-resistant *Staphylococcus aureus* pneumonia. Clin Ther 29:1107–1115

Kirby A, Mohandas K, Broughton C et al (2009) In vivo development of heterogeneous glycopeptide-intermediate *Staphylococcus aureus* (hGISA), GISA and daptomycin resistance in a patient with methicillin-resistant S. aureus endocarditis. J Med Microbiol 58:376–380

Klevens RM, Morrison MA, Nadle J et al (2007) Invasive methicillin-resistant *Staphylococcus aureus* infections in the United States. JAMA 298:1763–1771

Kollef MH, Sherman G, Ward S et al (1999) Inadequate antimicrobial treatment of infections: a risk factor for hospital mortality among critically ill patients. Chest 115:462–474

Kollef MH, Rello J, Cammarata SK et al (2004) Clinical cure and survival in gram-positive ventilator-associated pneumonia: retrospective analysis of two double-blind studies comparing linezolid with vancomycin. Intensive Care Med 30:388–394

Labandeira-Rey M, Couzon F, Boisset S et al (2007) *Staphylococcus aureus* Panton-Valentine leukocidin causes necrotizing pneumonia. Science 315:1130–1133

Lamer C, de Beco V, Soler P et al (1993) Analysis of vancomycin entry into pulmonary lining fluid by bronchoalveolar lavage in critically ill patients. Antimicrob Agents Chemother 37:281–286

Laue H, Weiss L, Bernardi A et al (2007) In vitro activity of the novel diaminopyrimidine, iclaprim, in combination with folate inhibitors and other antimicrobials with different mechanisms of action. J Antimicrob Chemother 60:1391–1394

Leuthner KD, Cheung CM, Rybak MJ (2006) Comparative activity of the new lipoglycopeptide telavancin in the presence and absence of serum against 50 glycopeptide non-susceptible staphylococci and three vancomycin-resistant *Staphylococcus aureus*. J Antimicrob Chemother 58:338–343

Li M, Diep BA, Villaruz AE et al (2009) Evolution of virulence in epidemic community-associated methicillin-resistant *Staphylococcus aureus*. Proc Natl Acad Sci U S A 103:5883–5888

Liu C, Chambers HFL (2003) *Staphylococcus aureus* with heterogeneous resistance to vancomycin: epidemiology, clinical significance, and critical assessment of diagnostic methods. Antimicrob Agents Chemother 47:3040–3045

Lodise TP, Graves J, Evans A et al (2008a) Relationship between vancomycin MIC and failure among patients with methicillin-resistant *Staphylococcus aureus* bacteremia treated with vancomycin. Antimicrob Agents Chemother 52:3315–3320

Lodise TP, Lomaestro B, Graves J et al (2008b) Larger vancomycin doses (at least four grams per day) are associated with an increased incidence of nephrotoxicity. Antimicrob Agents Chemother 52:1330–1336

Loughman JA, Fritz SA, Storch GA et al (2009) Virulence gene expression in human community-acquired *Staphylococcus aureus* infection. J Infect Dis 199:294–301

Lowy FD (1998) *Staphylococcus aureus* infections. N Engl J Med 339:520–532

Malbruny B, Canu A, Bozdogan B et al (2002) Resistance to quinupristin-dalfopristin due to mutation of L22 ribisomal protein in *Staphylococcus aureus*. Antimicrob Agents Chemother 46: 2200–2207

McDougal LK, Steward CD, Killgore GE et al (2003) Pulsed-field gel electrophoresis typing of oxacillin-resistant *Staphylococcus aureus* isolates from the United States: establishing a national database. J Clin Microbiol 41:5113–5120

Mercier RC, Hrebickova L (2005) Oritavancin: a new avenue for resistant gram-positive bacteria. Expert Rev Anti Infect Ther 3:325–332

Mermel LA, Allon M, Bouza E et al (2009) Clinical Practice Guidelines for the Diagnosis and Management of Intravascular Catheter-Related Infection: 2009 Update by the Infectious Diseases Society of America. Clin Infect Dis 49:1–45

Mohr JF, Murray BE (2007) Point: Vancomycin is not obsolete for the treatment of infection caused by methicillin-resistant *Staphylococcus aureus*. Clin Infect Dis 44:1536–1542

Moise PA, Smyth DS, El-Fawal N et al (2008) Microbiological effects of prior vancomycin use in patients with methicillin-resistant *Staphylococcus aureus* bacteraemia. J Antimicrob Chemother 61:85–90

Morales G, Picazo JJ, Baos E et al (2010) Resistance to linezolid is mediated by the cfr gene in the first report of an outbreak of linezolid-resistant *Staphylococcus aureus*. Clin Infect Dis 50: 821–825

Morrell M, Fraser VJ, Kollef MH (2005) Delaying the empiric treatment of Candida bloodstream infection until positive blood culture results are obtained: a potential risk factor for hospital mortality. Antimicrob Agents Chemother 49:3640–3665

Naimi TS, LeDell KH, Como-Sabetti K et al (2003) Comparison of community- and health care-associated methicillin-resistant *Staphylococcus aureus* infection. JAMA 290:2976–2984

Noel GJ, Bush K, Bagchi P et al (2008a) A randomized, double-blind trial comparing ceftobiprole medocaril with vancomycin plus ceftazidime for the treatment of patients with complicated skin and skin structure infections. Clin Infect Dis 46:647–655

Noel GJ, Strauss RS, Amsler K et al (2008b) Results of a double-blind, randomized trial of cefto-biprole treatment of complicated skin and skin structure infections caused by gram-positive bacteria. Antimicrob Agents Chemother 52:37–44

Noel GJ, Strauss RS, Shah A et al (2008) Ceftobiprole versus ceftazidime combined with linezolid for treatment of patients with nosocomial pneumonia (abstract). In: Proceedings of the 48th Annual Interscience Conference on Antimicrobial Agents and Chemotherapy K:486

Peeters MJ, Sarria JC (2005) Clinical characteristics of linezolid-resistant *Staphylococcus aureus* infections. Am J Med Sci 330:102–104

Pillai SK, Wennersten C, Venkataraman L et al (2009) Development of reduced vancomycin susceptibility in methicillin-susceptible *Staphylococcus aureus*. Clin Infect Dis 49:1169–1174

Popovich KJ, Weinstein RA, Hota B (2008) Are community-associated methicillin-resistant *Staphylococcus aureus* (MRSA) strains replacing traditional nosocomial MRSA strains? Clin Infect Dis 46:787–794

Robert J, Bismuth R, Jarlier V (2006) Decreased susceptibility to glycopeptides in methicillin-resistant *Staphylococcus aureus*: a 20 year study in a large French teaching hospital, 1983–2002. J Antimicrob Chemother 57:506–510

Rodvold KA, Gotfried MH, Cwik M et al (2006) Serum, tissue and body fluid concentrations of tigecycline after a single 100 mg dose. J Antimicrob Chemother 58:1221–1229

Rose WE, Rybak MJ (2006) Tigecycline: first of a new class of antimicrobial agents. Pharmacotherapy 26:1099–1110

Rybak M, Lomaestro B, Rotschafer JC et al (2009) Therapeutic monitoring of vancomycin in adult patients: a consensus review of the American Society of Health-System Pharmacists, the Infectious Diseases Society of America, and the Society of Infectious Diseases Pharmacists. Am J Health Syst Pharm 66:82–98

Sakoulas G (2006) The accessory gene regulator (agr) in methicillin-resistant *Staphylococcus aureus*: role in virulence and reduced susceptibility to glycopeptide antibiotics. Drug Discov Today Dis Mech 3:287–294

Sakoulas G, Eliopoulos GM, Moellering RC Jr et al (2002) Accessory gene regulator (agr) locus in geographically diverse *Staphylococcus aureus* isolates with reduced susceptibility to vanco-mycin. Antimicrob Agents Chemother 46:1492–1502

Sakoulas G, Moellering RC Jr, Eliopoulos GM (2006) Adaptation of methicillin-resistant *Staphylococcus aureus* in the face of vancomycin therapy. Clin Infect Dis 42(Suppl 1): S40–S50

Schneider P, Hawser S, Islam K (2003) Iclaprim, a novel diaminopyrimidine with potent activity on trimethoprim sensitive and resistant bacteria. Bioorg Med Chem Lett 13:4217–4721

Schramm GE, Johnson JA, Doherty JA et al (2006) Methicillin-resistant *Staphylococcus aureus* sterile-site infection: the importance of appropriate initial antimicrobial treatment. Crit Care Med 34:2069–2074

Schramm GE, Johnson JA, Doherty JA et al (2007) Increasing incidence of sterile-site infections due to non-multidrug-resistant, oxacillin-resistant *Staphylococcus aureus* among hospitalized patients. Infect Control Hosp Epidemiol 28:95–97

Seybold U, Kourbatova EV, Johnson JG et al (2006) Emergence of community-associated methicillin-resistant *Staphylococcus aureus* USA300 genotype as a major cause of health care-associated blood stream infections. Clin Infect Dis 42:647–656

Sharma M, Riederer K, Chase P et al (2008) High rate of decreasing daptomycin susceptibility during the treatment of persistent *Staphylococcus aureus* bacteremia. Eur J Clin Microbiol Infect Dis 27:433–437

Shorr AF, Micek ST, Kollef MH (2008) Inappropriate therapy for methicillin-resistant *Staphylococcus aureus*: resource utilization and cost implications. Crit Care Med 36: 2335–2340

Shurland S, Zhan M, Bradham DD et al (2007) Comparison of mortality risk associated with bacteremia due to methicillin-resistant and methicillin-susceptible *Staphylococcus aureus*. Infect Control Hosp Epidemiol 28:273–279

Soriano A, Marco F, Martinez JA et al (2008) Influence of vancomycin minimum inhibitory concentration on the treatment of methicillin-resistant *Staphylococcus aureus* bacteremia. Clin Infect Dis 46:193–200

Steinkraus G, White R, Friedrich L (2007) Vancomycin MIC creep in non-vancomycin-intermediate *Staphylococcus aureus* (VISA), vancomycin-susceptible clinical methicillin-resistant *S. aureus* (MRSA) blood isolates from 2001 to 05. J Antimicrob Chemother 60:788–794

Stevens DL, Ma Y, Salmi DB et al (2007) Impact of antibiotics on expression of virulence-associated exotoxin genes in methicillin-sensitive and methicillin-resistant *Staphylococcus aureus*. J Infect Dis 195:202–211

Talbot GH, Thye D, Das A et al (2007) Phase 2 study of ceftaroline versus standard therapy in the treatment of complicated skin and skin structure infections. Antimicrob Agents Chemother 51:3612–3616

Taylor JJ, Wilson JW, Estes LL et al (2006) Linezolid and serotonergic drug interactions: a retrospective survey. Clin Infect Dis 43:80–87

Tenover FC, Lancaster MV, Hill BC et al (1998) Characterization of staphylococci with reduced susceptibilities to vancomycin and other glycopeptides. J Clin Microbiol 36:1020–1027

Theravance Announces Receipt of Additional FDA Communication Regarding Telavancin NDA for the Treatment of Nosocomial Pneumonia (2010) http://www.fiercebiotech.com/press-releases/-Theravance-Announces-Receipt-of-Additional-FDA-Communication-Regarding-Telavancin-NDA-tr. Accessed 21 Mar 2010

Tsiodras S, Gold HS, Sakoulas G et al (2001) Linezolid resistance in a clinical isolate of *Staphylococcus aureus* (Letter). Lancet 358:207–208

Tsuji BT, Rybak MJ, Cheung CM et al (2007) Community- and health care-associated methicillin-resistant *Staphylococcus aureus*: a comparison of molecular epidemiology and antimicrobial activities of various agents. Diagn Microbiol Infect Dis 58:41–47

Vidaillac C, Rybak MJ (2009) Ceftobiprole: first cephalosporin with activity against methicillin-resistant *Staphylococcus aureus*. Pharmacotherapy 29:511–525

Vikram HR, Havill NL, Koeth LM et al (2005) Clinical progression of methicillin-resistant *Staphylococcus aureus* vertebral osteomyelitis with reduced susceptibility to daptomycin. J Clin Microbiol 43:5384–5387

Wilcox MH, Tack KJ, Bouza E et al (2009) Complicated skin and skin-structure infections and catheter-related blood stream infections: noninferiority of linezolid in a phase 3 study. Clin Infect Dis 48:203–212

Wunderink RG, Rello J, Cammarata SK et al (2003) Linezolid vs. vancomycin: analysis of two double-blind studies of patients with methicillin-resistant *Staphylococcus aureus* nosocomial pneumonia. Chest 124:1789–1797

Zhanel GG, Trapp S, Gin AS et al (2008) Dalbavancin and telavancin: novel lipoglycopeptides for the treatment of gram-positive infections. Expert Rev Anti Infect Ther 6:67–81

Zhang K, McClure J, Elsayed S et al (2009) Novel staphylococcal cassette chromosome mec type, tentatively designated type VIII, harboring class A mec and type 4 ccr gene complexes in a Canadian epidemic strain of methicillin-resistant *Staphylococcus aureus*. Antimicrob Agents Chemother 53:531–540

Pathogens in Severe Sepsis: New Paradigms for Fungi Treatment

11

Matteo Bassetti and Malgorzata Mikulska

11.1 Introduction

Fungal infections are being increasingly diagnosed in patients admitted to the ICU. Advances in medical science allow patients with severe and complicated diseases to survive, and thus a population of subjects vulnerable to a range of infections is created. From this point of view, infections in the ICU, particularly fungal ones, are a price to pay for medical progress that allows patients to survive who in previous decades would have died.

Candida and *Aspergillus* are the main fungal pathogens affecting ICU patients, and while Aspergillus causes mainly pulmonary infections, Candida is responsible for bloodstream infections. Moreover, candidemia is by far more frequent than aspergillosis in this type of population. Therefore, this chapter will focus on candidemia, even though there are other rare fungi, both moulds and yeasts, such as *Fusarium* and *Cryptococcus*, respectively, that can cause bloodstream infections.

Candidemia is a life-threatening infection with high morbidity and mortality, especially in immunocompromised and critically ill patients (Blumberg et al. 2001; Jarvis 1995; Richards et al. 2000; Wey et al. 1989). In the ICU, it may represent up to 15% of nosocomial infections, and the crude mortality rate has been found to be

M. Bassetti (✉)
Infectious Diseases Division,
Santa Maria Della Misericordia University Hospital,
Udine, Italy

Clinica Malattie Infettive, A.O.U. Santa Maria Della Misericordia,
Udine, Italy
e-mail: mattba@tin.it

M. Mikulska
Infectious Diseases Division,
San Martino Hospital and University of Genoa School of Medicine,
Genoa, Italy

J. Rello (eds.), *Sepsis Management*,
DOI 10.1007/978-3-642-03519-7_11, © Springer-Verlag Berlin Heidelberg 2012

as high as 25%–60%, varying according to the study design and the population, with the estimated attributable mortality as high as 47% (Gudlaugsson et al. 2003; Macphail et al. 2002; Morgan et al. 2005; Zaoutis et al. 2005). Additionally, the estimated costs of each episode of invasive candidiasis in hospitalised adults are tremendous (Fridkin 2005; Morgan et al. 2005). Finally, nosocomial fungal infections have one of the highest rates of inappropriate therapy, consisting mostly of omission of initial empirical therapy and inadequate doses of fluconazole, which has been associated with increased mortality (Garey et al. 2006; Horn et al. 2009; Morrell et al. 2005; Parkins et al. 2007).

Moreover, during the last decade several new antifungal drugs have been developed and obtained approval for treatment of Candida infections. Among them, echinocandins are the most important from the point of view of treating candidemia in critically ill patients. Thus, the epidemiology, risk factors, diagnosis, and in particular treatment strategies and guidelines will be discussed further.

11.2 Epidemiology

11.2.1 Incidence

Candidemia is one of the most frequent and most serious infections in patients admitted to the intensive care unit (ICU). Indeed, in a large multicenter study that included more than 24,000 cases of bloodstream infection in North America, Candida was reported to be the fourth most frequent pathogen (Wisplinghoff et al. 2004). In Europe, where few population-based studies of Candida bloodstream infections have been conducted, the incidence of this infection was reported to be lower, remaining however one of the first ten most common pathogens (Almirante et al. 2005; Alonso-Valle et al. 2003; Bouza et al. 1999; Vincent et al. 1995).

Not only is the overall incidence of all nosocomial bloodstream infections several fold higher in patients in the ICU than in those in other hospital units (Suljagic et al. 2005), but it is also evident that in the ICU, candidemia is by far more common than in most of other wards and can affect up to about 10% of all the admitted patients (Eggimann et al. 2003; Magnason et al. 2008). Recently, the high incidence of infections due to Candida, although not all of them were bloodstream infections, was reported in a large multicenter study conducted in 13,796 patients admitted to ICUs worldwide, where 6% of all subjects experienced an infection due to Candida (Vincent et al. 2009).

The epidemiology of Candida infections, both on the worldwide scale and more importantly on the local level, has significant implications for the management of this infection. Given the well-known, albeit not universal, differences in antifungal susceptibility among different Candida species, the choice of the most appropriate empirical treatment frequently can be successfully based on epidemiological data.

11.2.2 Candida Species

11.2.2.1 Shift Versus Non-albicans Species

During the past two decades, most hospitals have reported a progressive shift in the species of Candida that causes candidemia. In the past, almost all the isolates responsible for bloodstream infections were *C. albicans*, whereas in recent years a growing proportion of episodes of candidemia have been caused by Candida species other than albicans (Bassetti et al. 2006; Chow et al. 2008a; Diekema et al. 2002; Passos et al. 2007; Shorr et al. 2007). The recently published results of a prospective surveillance study of candidemia in US hospitals demonstrated that in 2,019 patients *C. albicans* was the most frequently isolated species; however, 54% of candidemias were due to non-albicans species (Horn et al. 2009). Even though, *C. albicans* remains the predominant strain in most countries (Klingspor et al. 2004), also among critically ill patients (Diekema et al. 2002; Nolla-Salas et al. 1997; Richards et al. 2000; Voss et al. 1997), non-albicans species are increasingly common. Traditionally, isolation of non-albicans species occurred more frequently in patients with haematological malignancies and bone marrow transplant, who routinely receive fluconazole prophylaxis, and was reported to be less common among ICU patients (35–55%) (Viscoli et al. 1999). Nevertheless, recently some ICUs have reported that non-albicans species are responsible for even more than 50% of candidemia episodes in adult critically ill patients (Bassetti et al. 2006), and some alarming reports of an incidence as high as 82% of non-albicans species have been published (Pereira et al. 2010).

A review from 2002 reported that the most common non-albicans species is *C. parapsilosis*, which accounts for about one third of Candida infections, followed by *C. glabrata*, *C. tropicalis* and *C. krusei* (which is less frequently isolated from patients who are critically ill than from patients with cancer) (Krcmery and Barnes 2002). On the contrary, other more recent studies have reported *C. glabrata* to be the main non-albicans isolate, particularly in the ICU (Bassetti et al. 2006; Ruan et al. 2008; Trick et al. 2002). In 2002, Trick and colleagues reported that in the US, among all Candida species, only *C. glabrata* has increased as a cause of bloodstream infection in the ICU (Trick et al. 2002). In a study carried out in Taiwan, *C. glabrata* was the second most common species and accounted for 45 of the 147 (30%) episodes of candidemia. The incidence of *C. glabrata* fungemia was 1.3/1,000 ICU admissions, and fluconazole resistance was found in 11% of *C. glabrata* (Ruan et al. 2008). Also in a multicenter North American study, the most commonly isolated Candida species were *C. albicans* (45.6%), *C. glabrata* (26%), *C. parapsilosis* (15.7%) and *C. tropicalis* (8.1%) (Horn et al. 2009). When confronted with the study from 1999 by Ranger-Fausto and colleagues, the per cent importance of *C. albicans* and *C. glabrata* remained similar, while that of *C. parapsilosis* increased from 7% to 15.7% and that of *C. tropicalis* decreased from 19% to 8.1% (Rangel-Frausto et al. 1999). Similarly, in the ICU at our centre, the incidence of *C. glabrata* has increased significantly in the last years, and this species is now the predominant non-albicans strain in ICUs (Bassetti et al. 2006). Rare Candida species reported to cause candidemia include *C. lusitaniae*, *C. guilliermondii* and *C. rugosa* (Horn et al. 2009; Krcmery and Barnes 2002), and considering the ever more accurate laboratory systems for determining Candida species, the number of reports of infrequent strains will probably rise.

11.2.2.2 Variables Associated with Non-albicans Species

Numerous studies have tried to find reasons for this shift, and several risk factors have been associated with candidemia due to different species. In a single-centre study performed in an ICU in Greece, 56 episodes of candidemia were analysed (*C. albicans* 36 episodes and other species, 20). The following factors were associated with non-albicans candidemia: administration of corticosteroids, central venous catheter placement and pre-existing candiduria (Dimopoulos et al. 2008). Similarly, when compared with *C. albicans* infection, the receipt of fluconazole total parenteral nutrition and gastrointestinal procedures were associated with an increased risk of non-albicans candidemia (Chow et al. 2008a). However, multiple common risk factors for both non-albicans and *C. albicans* bloodstream infections can be found, and several studies failed to identify the risk factors predisposing patients to non-albicans candidemia (Chow et al. 2008b).

It is understandable that the widespread use of fluconazole can predispose patients to the development of infections due to species that are resistant to azoles, either intrinsically fully resistant, such as *C. krusei*, or in a dose-dependent fashion, such as *C. glabrata*. Indeed, the previous use of fluconazole has been found to be a risk factor for the presence of non-albicans fungemia (Bassetti et al. 2006; Chow et al. 2008a; Viscoli et al. 1999), even though some studies did not find this association (Shorr et al. 2007). Naturally, the association of fluconazole with the incidence of non-albicans candidemia should be considered only for infection due to *C. krusei* and *C. glabrata*, because other non-albicans species remain susceptible to fluconazole. Thus, the differences between the studies, as far as the role of fluconazole is concerned, might depend on the prevalence of candidemia due to these two species.

Specific risk factors for candidemia due to other non-albicans strains also have been reported, such as, for example, the presence of in-dwelling devices, hyperalimentation and being a neonate for *C. parapsilosis* (Krcmery and Barnes 2002). However, it should be highlighted that this species remains fully susceptible to azoles, while MIC for echinocandins is higher than for other species. A single US study found that *C. parapsilosis* was significantly more frequent in burn units (Davis et al. 2007). The specific risk factors associated with different Candida species are outlined in Table 11.1.

Even though the overall rise in incidence of non-albicans strains is alarming, from the clinical point of view there are important differences among the species. Specifically, the main difference between *C. albicans* and *C. kusei* or *C. glabrata* is the resistance of the latter, intrinsic or inducible, respectively, to the most frequently used antifungal agent, i.e., fluconazole. The other non-albicans species have their own particularities; however, they remain susceptible to fluconazole. The differences in susceptibility to various antifungals are partially predictable and are reported in Table 11.2. Therefore, species identification and the knowledge of local epidemiology of Candida strains causing candidemia are of utmost importance for guiding appropriate empirical therapy. On the contrary, in vitro susceptibility testing of clinical isolates of Candida proves extremely valuable for guiding therapy in patients who have received prior antifungal treatment or who are not responding to empirical therapy.

Table 11.1 Particular risk factors associated with candidemia due to different Candida species

Candida species	Risk factor
C. tropicalis	• Neutropenia and bone marrow transplantation
C. krusei	• Fluconazole use
	• Neutropenia and bone marrow transplantation
C. glabrata	• Fluconazole use
	• Surgery
	• Vascular catheters
	• Cancer
	• Diabetes
C. parapsilosis	• Parenteral nutrition
	• Vascular catheters
	• Hyperalimentation
	• Being neonate
C. lusitaniae and *C. guilliermondii*	• Previous polyene
C. rugosa	• Burns

Adapted from the following references: (Hachem et al. 2008; Krcmery and Barnes 2002)

Table 11.2 Common susceptibility of various Candida species

Species	Amphotericin B	Echinocandins[a]	Fluconazole	Itraconazole	Voriconazole[b]
C. albicans	S	S	S to R[c]	S	S
C. glabrata	S	S	S-DD to R	S-DD to R	S to R[f]
C. krusei	S	S	R	S-DD to R	S
C. lusitaniae	S to R[d]	S	S	S	S
C. parapsilosis	S	S to R[e]	S	S	S
C. tropicalis	S	S	S	S	S

Adapted from references: (Choi et al. 2007; Leroy et al. 2009; Ostrosky-Zeichner et al. 2003; Pappas et al. 2009; Pfaller and Diekema 2010)

[a]Susceptibility pattern is similar for all the echinocandins

[b]Posaconazole has the same susceptibility pattern as voriconazole, but lacking intravenous formulation has little place in treatment of candidemia in ICU

[c]Resistant in approximately 5%

[d]Resistance uncommon but can develop in initially susceptible species

[e]Higher MIC values and poor activity against *C. parapsilosis* biofilm

[f]Cross-resistance to azoles in more than 5%.

11.3 Variables Associated with Candidemia in the ICU

11.3.1 Pathogenesis of Candidemia in the ICU

Although invasive Candida infections can affect any hospitalised patient, they are more common and have unique attributes in certain populations, including patients with cancer, haematological malignancy or other immunosuppression. The predominant source of invasive Candida infection is endogenous, from superficial mucosal and cutaneous proliferation to haematogenous dissemination

(Pfaller 1996). Normal flora, which include Candida, overgrow in their habitat, and when a disruption of mucosal or skin barriers occurs, yeasts enters the bloodstream (Agvald-Ohman et al. 2008; Pappas 2006). Nevertheless, exogenous transmission of Candida has also been described and includes both contaminated solutions and materials, as happens with bacterial contamination. Especially in the ICU environment, exogenous transmissions from healthcare workers to patients and from patients to patients have been documented (Asmundsdottir et al. 2008; Bliss et al. 2008).

Indeed, numerous risk factors for candidemia have been reported, and the pathogenesis of this infection in the ICU setting is complex. Since alterations in the host defence can lead to overgrowth of *C. albicans*, which is frequently present as part of the microflora of the gastrointestinal tract or the oropharynx in the normal human host, factors such as hospitalisation, diabetes, thermal trauma and disease resulting in a compromised immune response are all associated with such colonisation. The suppression of the normal bacterial flora in the gastrointestinal tract by broad-spectrum antibiotic therapy also allows the yeast to proliferate. Both in neutropenic patients with haematological malignancies (Richet et al. 1991) and in non-neutropenic patients (Pittet et al. 1994), long-term and high-density colonisation has been shown to lead to candidemia. Many factors common to ICU patients, such as poor nutrition, trauma, hypotension, therapy with steroids or cyclosporine, and ischemia and reperfusion, may damage the integrity of the gastrointestinal mucosa with penetration by the yeast, potentially leading to systemic infection. Although it appears that most systemic infections with *C. albicans* are caused by endogenous organisms via translocation from the gastrointestinal tract or by sequential spread from other body sites, apparent outbreaks of infection have been reported in association with the use of parenteral nutrition in ICU patients (Vaudry et al. 1988). The presence of Candida on the hands of healthcare workers has been demonstrated, suggesting that infection-control measures may be valuable (Rangel-Frausto et al. 1999). Both endogenous and exogenous colonisation can, however, coexist in the clinical setting. Furthermore, ICU patients are subjected to a number of therapeutic and supportive interventions (e.g., mechanical ventilation and intravascular catheters) that interfere with natural barriers to microorganisms' entry or with mechanisms for clearing them.

11.3.2 Risk Factors for Candidemia in the ICU

Indeed, both ICU and non-ICU patients share well-recognised risks for invasive candidiasis, such as the use of broad-spectrum antibacterial agents, vascular access and total parenteral nutrition; however, the former group of patients is more likely to have had recent surgery, but less likely to have malignancy, neutropenia or immunosuppression (DiNubile et al. 2007). Moreover, a variety of recognised high-risk groups, such as neutropenic cancer patients and recipients of bone marrow or solid organ transplants, are increasingly found in the ICU. However,

Table 11.3 Factors predisposing ICU patients to candidemia

Risk factors	
In all the patients	• Prior abdominal surgery
	• Intravascular catheters
	• Parenteral nutrition
	• Use of broad-spectrum antibiotics
	• Immunosuppression, including corticosteroid therapy
	• Acute renal failure
	• Diabetes
	• Transplantation
	• Haemodialysis
	• Pancreatitis
Specific for ICU patients	• Prolonged stay in the ICU
	• *Candida* colonization, particularly if multifocal
	• High Acute Physiology and Chronic Health Evaluation (APACHE) II score
	• Low birth weight for neonatal ICU

Adapted from the following references: (Blumberg et al. 2001; De Waele et al. 2003; Wey et al. 1989)

outside these very high-risk groups, it is possible to identify specific risk factors that predispose ICU patients to systemic Candida infection. The factors predisposing critically ill patients to candidemia are shown in Table 11.3, and the presence of vascular catheters or disruption of gut or skin barrier are among the most important ones.

Multiple logistic regression analysis has identified the use of Hickman catheters as an independent predictor of Candida infection (Wey et al. 1989), and univariate analysis showed that the use of Swan-Ganz catheters, parenteral nutrition, multiple blood transfusions and artificial ventilator support were also significant risk factors. In fact, up to 80% of cases of candidemia arise from or evolve in the presence of a vascular access, including access related to central venous catheters, haemodialysis catheters, peripherally inserted central catheters and implanted ports (Ben-Ami et al. 2008).

Another risk factor to be mentioned, which appears to have a major influence on the probability of developing systemic Candida infection in the ICU, is the severity of the patient's underlying condition, often represented by APACHE II score. Its significance has a mainly descriptive, but not predictive, value in showing infection (Fraser et al. 1992). Specific therapeutic interventions may actually reflect the severity of the patient's underlying condition and therefore serve only as secondary, dependent risk factors. Also the dynamic progression of risk factors in critical patients is reported to be significant: a rapid increase should prompt clinicians to obtain surveillance fungal cultures and consider empirical antifungal therapy (McKinnon et al. 2001).

11.3.3 Predictive Value of Candida Colonisation in ICU Patients

Candida is present in small numbers in the physiological flora of the mucosal surfaces and skin of many healthy hosts. However, in the last decade, several studies have shown that ICU patients with mucosal Candida colonisation, particularly if multifocal, are at a higher risk for candidemia. Thus, patients with such a colonisation may benefit from antifungal prophylaxis or pre-emptive strategies (Leon et al. 2006; Ostrosky-Zeichner et al. 2007; Saiman et al. 2001; Singhi et al. 2008).

Important efforts have focused on identifying critically ill patients that are at high risk of developing candidemia in order to apply the most efficacious management strategy and avoid mortality. Several risk prediction scores have been developed, and simple parameters were combined to predict which patients would develop candidemia. In 2006, Leon and colleagues published the results of a retrospective analysis of prospectively collected data on 1,699 ICU patients (Leon et al. 2006). Four parameters, parenteral nutrition, surgery, multifocal colonisation and severe sepsis, were considered in order to define patients at high risk of candidemia (sensitivity 81%, specificity 74%). Similarly, in 2007 Ostrosky-Zeichner and colleagues published the results of a retrospective analysis identifying patients at high risk for invasive candidiasis among 2,890 subjects admitted to the ICU (Ostrosky-Zeichner et al. 2007). Namely, the presence of systemic antibiotic treatment or the presence of a central venous catheter plus two of the following—parenteral nutrition, dialysis, major surgery, pancreatitis, steroids or other immunosuppressive agents—identified the patients with 10% risk of developing invasive candidiasis (sensitivity 34%, specificity 90%).

11.4 Diagnosis of Candidemia

Blood cultures remain the mainstay for diagnosing candidemia; however, the sensitivity reported frequently is not optimal. Moreover, the time from the blood sample collection and the microbiological response of growing yeast is often lengthy. Furthermore, several more days are required for species identification and susceptibility testing. Therefore, new methods of diagnosing invasive Candida infection have been investigated, and they include serological markers (mannan and beta-D-glucan) and real-time polymerase chain reaction. Even though the results of testing for the presence of mannan antigen and antimannan antibody have been promising in ICU patients (Sendid et al. 1999), the test is not routinely used in clinical practice. On the contrary, a new assay searching for another structural protein of many fungi, including Candida, is beta-D-glucan. Its use has been included in the 2008 IDSA guidelines for diagnosing invasive fungal disease: in fact, in severely immunocompromised patients with positive serum beta-D-glucan results, a diagnosis of probable fungal infection can be made (Pappas et al. 2009).

11.5 Management of Candidemia in the ICU

As far as the management of candidemia in the ICU is concerned, there is no single strategy that can be considered the most appropriate. In fact, different approaches can be chosen and can be judged as the best for a given clinical situation. In particular, three management options are available: prophylaxis, empirical therapy and treatment of a culture-proven infection. So how the best strategy is chosen? Knowledge of epidemiological data, the above-mentioned risk factors and primarily the analysis of the local epidemiology of candidemia in a singular ICU allow determining if a patient is at low, moderate or high risk of developing this infection. Consequently, the choice of the most appropriate management strategies, which include prophylaxis, pre-emptive strategy and evidence-based therapy, can be made. Moreover, knowing the most frequent species and susceptibility patterns of Candida isolated in a single ICU is a basis for choosing the adequate prophylaxis or empirical treatment.

11.5.1 Prophylaxis in the ICU

Prophylaxis, defined as the administration of an antifungal agents to a patient with no evidence of infection, has been evaluated in several studies and meta-analyses (Calandra and Marchetti 2004; Cruciani et al. 2005; Lipsett 2004; Shorr et al. 2005), and its main advantage is a possible reduction in the rate of candidemia. Since morbidity and mortality rates in patients with systemic fungal infections are exceedingly high, the use of an effective antifungal prophylaxis in selected high-risk patients is very attractive and might be an option in selected populations. The strategy of antifungal prophylaxis is now well established in patients with persistent neutropenia after treatment for haematological malignancies or after bone marrow transplantation (Bow et al. 2002; Hughes et al. 2002). On the contrary, routine use of antifungal prophylaxis in the general ICU setting is discouraged (Rex and Sobel 2001). Nonetheless, the implementation of targeted antifungal prophylaxis has been shown to be effective in certain ICU settings (Calandra and Marchetti 2004; Lipsett 2004), and three randomised placebo-controlled trails reported a decrease in the incidence of Candida infection with fluconazole prophylaxis (Eggimann et al. 1999; Garbino et al. 2002; Pelz et al. 2001). Moreover, two meta-analyses confirmed that prophylactic fluconazole administration in ICU patients reduced the rate of Candida infection, but no clear survival advantage was observed (Playford et al. 2006; Shorr et al. 2005). Only the meta-analysis by Cruciani and colleagues reported, along with a relative risk reduction in candidemia, a decrease in overall mortality; however, the benefit on mortality was mainly driven by a study by Savino and colleagues from 1994 that used clotrimazole, ketoconazole and nystatin as prophylaxis (Cruciani et al. 2005; Savino et al. 1994).

On the other hand, the disadvantages of fluconazole prophylaxis include possible toxicity and a profound influence on the local epidemiology with the emergence of fluconazole-resistant isolates (Bassetti et al. 2009). Therefore, in expert opinion expressed in reviews and guidelines (Ostrosky-Zeichner 2004; Pappas et al. 2009), antifungal prophylaxis might be warranted only for ICUs with high rates of invasive candidiasis, as compared to the normal rates of 1–2%, particularly for selected patients who are at the highest risk (>10%) (Ostrosky-Zeichner et al. 2007). The approach of limiting prophylaxis to a subgroup of patients with the highest risk of candidemia may help to limit the quantity of antifungals used and delay the emergence of infections due to fluconazole-resistant Candida strains seen in immunocompromised patients. In fact, this approach is supported by the recent IDSA guidelines that recommend fluconazole prophylaxis at a dose of 400 mg (6 mg/kg) daily for high-risk adult patients hospitalised in ICUs that have a high incidence of invasive candidiasis (Pappas et al. 2009).

11.5.2 Empirical Therapy

Empirical treatment is defined as administration of antifungals in the presence of persistent and refractory fever in patients who are at high risk for fungal infection. This strategy was developed almost 3 decades ago for neutropenic patients when it became evident that the lack of sensitivity of microbiological and clinical findings resulted in delayed diagnosis and increased morbidity and mortality. Even though the first studies on empirical therapy have been underpowered, they are being used in different clinical settings, and numerous antifungals are being registered and recommended for empirical treatment of invasive candidiasis, both in neutropenic and non-neutropenic patients (Pappas et al. 2009). All these efforts are aimed at reducing morbidity and mortality by starting treatment as early as possible, given the evidence that a delay in antifungal prescribing significantly increases mortality rates in candidemia (Garey et al. 2006; Morrell et al. 2005). However, in the ICU, where numerous patients have different risk factors for fungal infections, the routine use of empirical therapy in case of persistent fever may result in significant overtreatment. Therefore, a new spre-emptive approach strategy, which originates from the idea of empirical therapy and is frequently described together with it, appears very promising. In fact, the US guidelines recommend that such an approach (although they continue to call it empirical treatment) should be considered for critically ill patients with risk factors for invasive candidiasis and no other known cause of fever, based on clinical assessment of risk factors, serologic markers for invasive candidiasis and/or culture data from non-sterile sites (Pappas et al. 2009).

11.5.3 Pre-emptive Therapy

The main concept of a pre-emptive strategy is to better identify patients at high risk for developing candidemia. Therefore, the overall use of antifungals in the ICU can be reduced, without delaying therapy in patients who mostly need it.

Table 11.4 Choice of antifungals for treatment of candidemia in critically ill patients

Treatment	First choice	Alternative
Pre-emptive or empirical	Echinocandin	L-AmB
Culture-proven candidemia		
C. albicans	Echinocandin	Fluconazole or L-AmB
C. glabrata	Echinocandin	L-AmB
C. krusei	Echinocandin	L-AmB
C. parapsilosis	L-AmB	Echinocandin or fluconazole

Adapted from IDSA guidelines (Pappas et al. 2009)
L-AmB lipid formulation of Amphotericin B

The recent availability of more sensitive and specific clinical and laboratory tools allows for better identification of high-risk patients, and this approach has been used successfully (Maertens et al. 2005). However, the question arises how to define which patients are at high risk for developing candidemia. No clear predictive rule exists, but the two above-described score systems for ICU patients can be of some help. In brief, multifocal colonisation by Candida and/ or the presence of the well-described factors outlined in Table 11.4 make a patient a suitable candidate for empirical therapy if any signs or symptoms of infection compare. In particular, the efficacy of a pre-emptive strategy in ICU patients has been recently established in a single-institution study where the use of fluconazole in patients with a corrected colonisation index (CCI) ≥0.5, described previously by Pittet and colleagues (Pittet et al. 1994), significantly decreased the incidence of invasive candidiasis (Piarroux et al. 2004). Moreover, surrogate markers of invasive fungal infections have been extensively studied. In particular, beta-D-glucan is a component of the cell wall of Candida and other fungi, and has been investigated as a serological marker for fungal infections, including candidemia (Ostrosky-Zeichner et al. 2005). Even though false-positive results have been reported and its routine use in the ICU requires further validation, persistently high serum levels of beta-D-glucan in ICU patients were found indicative of fungal disease (Presterl et al. 2009).

Therefore, a pre-emptive approach in critically ill patients might be defined as starting antifungals when the following conditions are satisfied: the presence of a long ICU stay (<96 h) and broad-spectrum antibiotic therapy; any of the other risk factors such as severe sepsis, gastrointestinal surgery and parenteral nutrition; plus microbiological evidence of Candida infection, including multifocal colonisation or a positive result of serum beta-D-glucan. The proposed approach is shown in Fig. 11.1, and as for any new strategy, it will warrant validation in prospective trails. One of the main advantages of such an approach is limiting the use of antifungal agents in low-risk patients, while starting treatment for candidemia without delay when symptoms appear in patients at high risk for this infection. Thus, the benefit of early therapy, in terms of morbidity and mortality, can be obtained, while overtreatment can be avoided (Fig. 11.2).

Fig. 11.1 Different
approaches for management
of candidemia in critically ill
patients

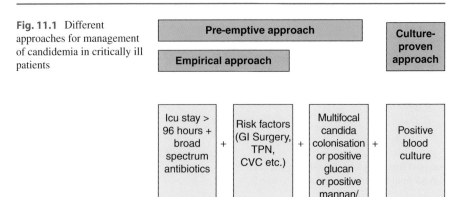

Fig. 11.2 Number of ICU
patients who are exposed to
antifungals according to
various management
strategies applied

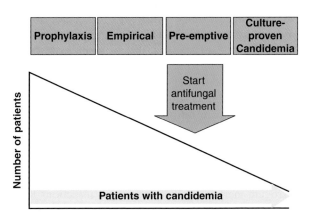

11.5.4 Treatment of a Culture-Documented Candidemia

For ICU patients with low/medium risk of developing candidemia, blood cultures should be performed if a clinical suspicion of systemic infection is present, even in the absence of fever. Numerous blood cultures, both from CVC and peripheral line, remain the cornerstone of the diagnosis of candidemia. As any delay before administering primary therapy can lead to a noticeable increase in mortality, antifungal agents should be prescribed as soon as there is a growth of yeast in blood samples. The choice of antifungal for an unknown Candida species should be based on the knowledge of the local epidemiology. In the ICU, where most infections are due to *C. albicans* and where fluconazole-resistance is low, the latter is the drug of choice. On the other hand, in an ICU where fluconazole-resistant species are common (for example, *C. glabrata*), or in patients colonised with fluconazole-resistant strains, echinocandins are the drugs of choice. Moreover, for patients in severe or moderately severe clinical conditions, echinocandins are recommended because of their cidal activity against Candida. Moreover, their side effects are less common that those reported for the other fungicidal agent, liposomal amphotericin B.

11.5.5 Other Aspects of Treating Candidemia in the ICU

Once the initial therapy for candidemia has been started, several clinical issues remain open. Firstly, the efficacy of the treatment should be assessed by the documentation of blood cultures returning sterile. Moreover, the date of the first negative blood culture is important, because the recommended length of treatment is 14 days after the documented clearance of Candida from the bloodstream and resolution of symptoms attributable to candidemia.

Secondly, the antifungal chosen empirically can be changed based on the results of species determination or susceptibility testing. Thus, for stable patients with *C. albicans* or other fluconazole-susceptible strains, fluconazole is the drug of choice. Importantly, fluconazole is the preferred treatment for *C. parapsilosis*, as resistance to echinocandins has been reported (Forrest et al. 2008).

Thirdly, patients who improve clinically and clear Candida from the bloodstream may be suitable for step-down oral therapy to complete the course of 14 days. The available oral antifungals are fluconazole, itraconazole, voriconazole and posaconazole. Fluconazole is an obvious choice for susceptible species, while voriconazole can be indicated as step-down therapy for *C. krusei* or voriconazole-susceptible *C. glabrata*.

Last but not least, ophthalmologic fundus examination is warranted in all the patients to exclude disseminated endovascular infection, and intravenous catheter removal is strongly recommended for non-neutropenic patients with candidemia. Also in neutropenic patients, catheter removal should be considered, but the benefit should be weighted against other clinical problems.

Biofilm production is a well-documented phenomenon for Candida species that significantly contributes to Candida pathogenicity in catheter-related bloodstream infections, resulting in recurrent or persistent infections, and biofilm-mediated antifungal resistance leading to treatment failure (Lewis et al. 2002). Moreover, the mortality in patients with invasive infections due to biofilm-producing Candida species has been reported to be significantly higher (Tumbarello et al. 2007). Therefore, the activity of antifungals against biofilm has important clinical implications and is known to vary among different agents. In particular, fluconazole and azoles, which are static against Candida, are also not active against sessile forms, while echinocandins and amphotericin B offer both bactericidal activity and good penetration into biofilms formed on vascular devices. However, a study performed on 43 Candida species, including 12 *C. albicans*, 12 *C. parapsilosis*, 10 *C. tropicalis* and 9 *C. glabrata* isolates, found that the activity of caspofungin and micafungin against biofilm of *C. parapsilosis* and *C. tropicalis* was significantly lower than that of amphotericin B (Choi et al. 2007). Table 11.5 outlines the susceptibility of different Candida species to two antifungals that are active against biofilm-producing strains.

11.6 Antifungal Agents

In recent years, numerous new antifungal drugs have been developed, studied and approved for various indications, and almost all of these new drugs are licensed to treat candidemia in different patient populations. Other compounds are being

Table 11.5 Activity against different Candida species of two antifungals that are active against Candida biofilm-producing stains

Species	Amphotericin B	Echinocandins
C. albicans	S	S
C. glabrata	S	S
C. krusei	S	S
C. lusitaniae	S to R[a]	S
C. parapsilosis	S	S to R[b]
C. tropicalis	S	S to R[b]

[a]Resistance uncommon but can develop in initially susceptible species
[b]Higher MIC values and poor activity against biofilm for caspofungin and micafungin (Choi et al. 2007)

Table 11.6 Currently available antifungals for treating candidemia

Drug	Dose	
	Loading dose (first 24 h)	Daily dose
Fluconazole	800 mg (12 mg/kg)	400 mg (6 mg/kg)
Itraconazole	–	200 mg/day
Voriconazole	6 mg/kg every 12 h for the first two doses	3 mg/kg every 12 h
Posaconazole	–	200 mg × 3/day
AmB deoxycholate	–	0.5–1 mg/kg
Liposomal AmB	–	3 mg/kg
Lipid complex AmB	–	5 mg/kg
Anidulafungin	200 mg	100 mg
Caspofungin	70 mg	50 mg
Micafungin	–	100 mg

AmB Amphotericin B

developed and tested in clinical trials. The most appropriate antifungal drug can be chosen from the three main groups: (1) the polyenes (amphotericin B deoxycholate, lipid complex, liposomal); (2) the azoles (fluconazole, voriconazole, posaconazole, itraconazole, ravuconazole); and (3) the echinocandins (caspofungin, micafungin, anidulafungin). Of note, most of the studies on efficacy in candidemia have not shown significant differences between various agents. However, the differences in drug-related toxicity are significant, and the possibility of drug-drug interactions, so important in critically ill patients who receive numerous medications, varies significantly among the single agents. Therefore, the choice of the best antifungal agent still poses a challenge for the clinician. The detailed description of various agents used for treating candidemia is beyond the scope of this chapter; however, the dosages of the main antifungals are reported in Table 11.6. Moreover, given that echinocandins are the most recently introduced class of antifungals and general recommendations do not usually specify which of them should be used, Table 11.7 outlines the differences in indication, dosing, etc., of three echinocandin compounds. All the echinocandins are approved for treatment of candidemia, other forms of Candida infections (intraabdominal abscess, peritonitis) and oesophageal

Table 11.7 Main differences between the three echinocandins available

Variable	Anidulafungin	Caspofungin	Micafungin
Loading dose	–200 mg –100 mg for oesophageal candidiasis	–70 mg – No loading dose for oesophageal candidiasis	None
Daily dose for different indications	–100 mg/day –50 mg/day for oesophageal candidiasis	– 50 mg/day	–100 mg/day for candidemia –150 mg/day for oesophageal candidiasis –50 mg/day in prophylaxis
Age of patients	Adults	>3 months	Adults
Metabolism	Slow chemical degradation at physiologic temperature and pH	Hepatic metabolism+spontaneous chemical degradation	Hepatic metabolism+enzymatic biotransformation
Indication for *Aspergillus* infection	None	Yes, in patients who are refractory to or intolerant of other therapies	None
Indications in neutropenic patients	None	Empirical therapy for presumed fungal infections in febrile, neutropenic patients	Prophylaxis of *Candida* infections in HSCT recipients
Dose adjustment in moderate hepatic impairment	None	Dose reduced (see Table 11.9)	None
Dose adjustment in severe hepatic impairment	None	Unknown	Unknown

HSCT haematopoietic stem cell transplant recipients (Data deriving from FDA labels)

Table 11.8 Dose adjustment required in case of renal impairment

Drug	Dose adjustment	Comments
• Anidulafungin	None	–
• Caspofungin	None	–
• Micafungin	None	–
• Voriconazole, oral formulation only	None	Do not use IV formulation due to carrier accumulation (cyclodextrin) if CrCl < 50
• Itraconazole oral solution	None	Do not use IV formulation due to carrier accumulation (cyclodextrin) if CrCl < 30
• Amphotericin B deoxycholate	Do not use	Switch to less nephrotoxic formulation
• Amphotericin B lipid formulations	Unknown	–
• Fluconazole	Yes	50% of the dose if CrCl < 50
• Posaconazole	None	If CrCl < 20 monitor closely for break-through infections due to the variability in exposure

CrCl creatinine clearance, expressed in mL/min

Table 11.9 Dose adjustment required in case of hepatic impairment

Drug	Dose adjustment	Comments
• Anidulafungin	None	–
• Caspofungin	Yes	Moderate hepatic impairment (Child-Pugh score 7–9) 35 mg daily, with 70 mg loading dose
• Micafungin	None	No data in severe hepatic impairment
• Voriconazole	Yes	50% of maintenance dose in mild to moderate hepatic impairment (Child-Pugh Class A and B); no data in Child-Pugh Class C; patients with hepatic insufficiency must be carefully monitored for drug toxicity
• Itraconazole oral solution	Unknown	Patients with impaired hepatic function should be carefully monitored when taking itraconazole.
• Amphotericin B	Unknown	–
• Fluconazole	None	–
• Posaconazole	None	–

candidiasis. Considering that many ICU patients have other significant comorbidities, the data on the treatment with various antifungals in case of renal or hepatic insufficiency are reported in Tables 11.8 and 11.9, respectively.

11.7 Management of Candidemia in the Neonatal ICU

The incidence of candidemia in the neonatal ICU has been increasing, mostly due to the fact that more low birth weight and very low birth weight newborns survive longer thanks to advances in medical technology. Therefore, they are more likely to

Table 11.10 Dosing of antifungals in paediatric patients (in order of strength in recommendation for invasive candidiasis)

Drug	Dose
Amphotericin B deoxycholate	1 mg/kg daily
Liposomal amphotericin B	3 mg/kg daily
Lipid complex amphotericin B	5 mg/kg daily
Fluconazole	12 mg/kg daily
Caspofungin	50 mg/m², with a single 70 mg/m² loading dose
Micafungin	2–4 mg/kg daily in children
	10–12 mg/kg daily in neonates
Anidulafungin	1.5 mg/kg/day in children 2–17 years old
Voriconazole	7 mg/kg every 12 h, up to the age of 12 years

develop infectious complications, and candidemia is one of the most frequent nosocomial BSIs in this population. The reported risk factors for candidemia in neonates and adults are similar, and include central venous catheters and arterial lines, parenteral nutrition, mechanical ventilation and the extended use of antibiotics. Unlike in the adult ICU, in the NICU, *C. albicans* remains the most common isolate, although non-albicans species such as *C. parapsilosis* and *C. tropicalis* are increasingly common (Filioti et al. 2007; Fridkin et al. 2006). Fortunately, these species are susceptible to fluconazole.

The recent IDSA guidelines on the management of Candida infections offer recommendations for paediatric patients. In particular, for neonatal candidiasis the following treatments are regarded as first line: amphotericin B deoxycholate or liposomal amphotericin B if urinary tract involvement is excluded, and fluconazole. The guidelines also state that echinocandins should be used with caution and are generally limited to situations in which resistance or toxicity precludes the use of fluconazole or amphotericin B. Dosing of antifungals in paediatric patients is outlined in Table 11.10.

Additionally, a lumbar puncture and a dilated retinal examination, preferably by an ophthalmologist, are recommended in neonates with sterile body fluid and/or urine cultures positive for Candida, and removing an intravascular catheter is strongly recommended. Finally, in nurseries with high rates of invasive candidiasis, fluconazole prophylaxis can be considered in neonates with birth weight is below 1,000 g.

11.8 Conclusions

Candida is one of the most common causes of nosocomial bloodstream infections. Morbidity and mortality associated with candidemia are significant, and the epidemiology of the species have been changing, both on the local and worldwide levels. Even though numerous risk factors for invasive Candida infection have been reported and several antifungals are widely available, the optimal management of candidemia remains a challenge. The agents recommended for initial treatment of candidemia in critically ill patients include echinocandins and lipid formulation of amphotericin B, but the choice among prophylactic, empirical and pre-emptive therapy is crucial.

Compared to prophylaxis, empirical and pre-emptive approaches allow reducing the exposure to antifungals by targeting only the patients at high risk of candidemia, without delaying therapy until yeast is identified in blood cultures. Pre-emptive strategy is based on the presence of numerous risk factors, together with microbiological documentation of the presence of Candida, such as multifocal colonisation or positive serum beta-D-glucan. Further prospective studies are warranted to confirm the benefits of routine use of pre-emptive treatment of candidemia.

References

Agvald-Ohman C, Klingspor L, Hjelmqvist H et al (2008) Invasive candidiasis in long-term patients at a multidisciplinary intensive care unit: Candida colonization index, risk factors, treatment and outcome. Scand J Infect Dis 40:145–153

Almirante B, Rodriguez D, Park BJ et al (2005) Epidemiology and predictors of mortality in cases of Candida bloodstream infection: results from population-based surveillance, Barcelona, Spain, from 2002 to 2003. J Clin Microbiol 43:1829–1835

Alonso-Valle H, Acha O, Garcia-Palomo JD et al (2003) Candidemia in a tertiary care hospital: epidemiology and factors influencing mortality. Eur J Clin Microbiol Infect Dis 22: 254–257

Asmundsdottir LR, Erlendsdottir H, Haraldsson G et al (2008) Molecular epidemiology of candidemia: evidence of clusters of smoldering nosocomial infections. Clin Infect Dis 47:e17–e24

Bassetti M, Righi E, Costa A et al (2006) Epidemiological trends in nosocomial candidemia in intensive care. BMC Infect Dis 6:21

Bassetti M, Ansaldi F, Nicolini L et al (2009) Incidence of candidaemia and relationship with fluconazole use in an intensive care unit. J Antimicrob Chemother 64:625–629

Ben-Ami R, Weinberger M, Orni-Wasserlauff R et al (2008) Time to blood culture positivity as a marker for catheter-related candidemia. J Clin Microbiol 46:2222–2226

Bliss JM, Basavegowda KP, Watson WJ et al (2008) Vertical and horizontal transmission of Candida albicans in very low birth weight infants using DNA fingerprinting techniques. Pediatr Infect Dis J 27:231–235

Blumberg HM, Jarvis WR, Soucie JM et al (2001) Risk factors for candidal bloodstream infections in surgical intensive care unit patients: the NEMIS prospective multicenter study. The National Epidemiology of Mycosis Survey. Clin Infect Dis 33:177–186

Bouza E, Perez-Molina J, Munoz P (1999) Report of ESGNI01 and ESGNI02 studies. Bloodstream infections in Europe. Clin Microbiol Infect 5(2):S1–S12

Bow EJ, Laverdiere M, Lussier N et al (2002) Antifungal prophylaxis for severely neutropenic chemotherapy recipients: a meta analysis of randomized-controlled clinical trials. Cancer 94:3230–3246

Calandra T, Marchetti O (2004) Clinical trials of antifungal prophylaxis among patients undergoing surgery. Clin Infect Dis 39(Suppl 4):S185–S192

Choi HW, Shin JH, Jung SI et al (2007) Species-specific differences in the susceptibilities of biofilms formed by Candida bloodstream isolates to echinocandin antifungals. Antimicrob Agents Chemother 51:1520–1523

Chow JK, Golan Y, Ruthazer R et al (2008a) Factors associated with candidemia caused by non-albicans Candida species versus Candida albicans in the intensive care unit. Clin Infect Dis 46:1206–1213

Chow JK, Golan Y, Ruthazer R et al (2008b) Risk factors for albicans and non-albicans candidemia in the intensive care unit. Crit Care Med 36:1993–1998

Cruciani M, de Lalla F, Mengoli C (2005) Prophylaxis of Candida infections in adult trauma and surgical intensive care patients: a systematic review and meta-analysis. Intensive Care Med 31:1479–1487

Davis SL, Vazquez JA, McKinnon PS (2007) Epidemiology, risk factors, and outcomes of Candida albicans versus non-albicans candidemia in nonneutropenic patients. Ann Pharmacother 41:568–573

De Waele JJ, Vogelaers D, Blot S et al (2003) Fungal infections in patients with severe acute pancreatitis and the use of prophylactic therapy. Clin Infect Dis 37:208–213

Diekema DJ, Messer SA, Brueggemann AB et al (2002) Epidemiology of candidemia: 3-year results from the emerging infections and the epidemiology of Iowa organisms study. J Clin Microbiol 40:1298–1302

Dimopoulos G, Ntziora F, Rachiotis G et al (2008) Candida albicans versus non-albicans intensive care unit-acquired bloodstream infections: differences in risk factors and outcome. Anesth Analg 106:523–529; table of contents

DiNubile MJ, Lupinacci RJ, Strohmaier KM et al (2007) Invasive candidiasis treated in the intensive care unit: observations from a randomized clinical trial. J Crit Care 22:237–244

Eggimann P, Francioli P, Bille J et al (1999) Fluconazole prophylaxis prevents intra-abdominal candidiasis in high-risk surgical patients. Crit Care Med 27:1066–1072

Eggimann P, Garbino J, Pittet D (2003) Epidemiology of Candida species infections in critically ill non-immunosuppressed patients. Lancet Infect Dis 3:685–702

Filioti J, Spiroglou K, Panteliadis CP et al (2007) Invasive candidiasis in pediatric intensive care patients: epidemiology, risk factors, management, and outcome. Intensive Care Med 33: 1272–1283

Forrest GN, Weekes E, Johnson JK (2008) Increasing incidence of Candida parapsilosis candidemia with caspofungin usage. J Infect 56:126–129

Fraser VJ, Jones M, Dunkel J et al (1992) Candidemia in a tertiary care hospital: epidemiology, risk factors, and predictors of mortality. Clin Infect Dis 15:414–421

Fridkin SK (2005) The changing face of fungal infections in health care settings. Clin Infect Dis 41:1455–1460

Fridkin SK, Kaufman D, Edwards JR et al (2006) Changing incidence of Candida bloodstream infections among NICU patients in the United States: 1995–2004. Pediatrics 117:1680–1687

Garbino J, Lew DP, Romand JA et al (2002) Prevention of severe Candida infections in nonneutropenic, high-risk, critically ill patients: a randomized, double-blind, placebo-controlled trial in patients treated by selective digestive decontamination. Intensive Care Med 28:1708–1717

Garey KW, Rege M, Pai MP et al (2006) Time to initiation of fluconazole therapy impacts mortality in patients with candidemia: a multi-institutional study. Clin Infect Dis 43:25–31

Gudlaugsson O, Gillespie S, Lee K et al (2003) Attributable mortality of nosocomial candidemia, revisited. Clin Infect Dis 37:1172–1177

Hachem R, Hanna H, Kontoyiannis D et al (2008) The changing epidemiology of invasive candidiasis: Candida glabrata and Candida krusei as the leading causes of candidemia in hematologic malignancy. Cancer 112:2493–2499

Horn DL, Neofytos D, Anaissie EJ et al (2009) Epidemiology and outcomes of candidemia in 2019 patients: data from the prospective antifungal therapy alliance registry. Clin Infect Dis 48:1695–1703

Hughes WT, Armstrong D, Bodey GP et al (2002) 2002 guidelines for the use of antimicrobial agents in neutropenic patients with cancer. Clin Infect Dis 34:730–751

Jarvis WR (1995) Epidemiology of nosocomial fungal infections, with emphasis on Candida species. Clin Infect Dis 20:1526–1530

Klingspor L, Tornqvist E, Johansson A et al (2004) A prospective epidemiological survey of candidaemia in Sweden. Scand J Infect Dis 36:52–55

Krcmery V, Barnes AJ (2002) Non-albicans Candida spp. causing fungaemia: pathogenicity and antifungal resistance. J Hosp Infect 50:243–260

Leon C, Ruiz-Santana S, Saavedra P et al (2006) A bedside scoring system ("Candida score") for early antifungal treatment in nonneutropenic critically ill patients with Candida colonization. Crit Care Med 34:730–737

Leroy O, Gangneux JP, Montravers P et al (2009) Epidemiology, management, and risk factors for death of invasive Candida infections in critical care: a multicenter, prospective, observational study in France (2005–2006). Crit Care Med 37:1612–1618

Lewis RE, Kontoyiannis DP, Darouiche RO et al (2002) Antifungal activity of amphotericin B, fluconazole, and voriconazole in an in vitro model of Candida catheter-related bloodstream infection. Antimicrob Agents Chemother 46:3499–3505

Lipsett PA (2004) Clinical trials of antifungal prophylaxis among patients in surgical intensive care units: concepts and considerations. Clin Infect Dis 39(Suppl 4):S193–S199

Macphail GL, Taylor GD, Buchanan-Chell M et al (2002) Epidemiology, treatment and outcome of candidemia: a five-year review at three Canadian hospitals. Mycoses 45:141–145

Maertens J, Theunissen K, Verhoef G et al (2005) Galactomannan and computed tomography-based preemptive antifungal therapy in neutropenic patients at high risk for invasive fungal infection: a prospective feasibility study. Clin Infect Dis 41:1242–1250

Magnason S, Kristinsson KG, Stefansson T et al (2008) Risk factors and outcome in ICU-acquired infections. Acta Anaesthesiol Scand 52:1238–1245

McKinnon PS, Goff DA, Kern JW et al (2001) Temporal assessment of Candida risk factors in the surgical intensive care unit. Arch Surg 136:1401–1408; discussion 1409

Morgan J, Meltzer MI, Plikaytis BD et al (2005) Excess mortality, hospital stay, and cost due to candidemia: a case-control study using data from population-based candidemia surveillance. Infect Control Hosp Epidemiol 26:540–547

Morrell M, Fraser VJ, Kollef MH (2005) Delaying the empiric treatment of candida bloodstream infection until positive blood culture results are obtained: a potential risk factor for hospital mortality. Antimicrob Agents Chemother 49:3640–3645

Nolla-Salas J, Sitges-Serra A, Leon-Gil C et al (1997) Candidemia in non-neutropenic critically ill patients: analysis of prognostic factors and assessment of systemic antifungal therapy. Study Group of Fungal Infection in the ICU. Intensive Care Med 23:23–30

Ostrosky-Zeichner L (2004) Prophylaxis and treatment of invasive candidiasis in the intensive care setting. Eur J Clin Microbiol Infect Dis 23:739–744

Ostrosky-Zeichner L, Rex JH, Pappas PG et al (2003) Antifungal susceptibility survey of 2,000 bloodstream Candida isolates in the United States. Antimicrob Agents Chemother 47:3149–3154

Ostrosky-Zeichner L, Alexander BD, Kett DH et al (2005) Multicenter clinical evaluation of the (1–>3) beta-D-glucan assay as an aid to diagnosis of fungal infections in humans. Clin Infect Dis 41:654–659

Ostrosky-Zeichner L, Sable C, Sobel J et al (2007) Multicenter retrospective development and validation of a clinical prediction rule for nosocomial invasive candidiasis in the intensive care setting. Eur J Clin Microbiol Infect Dis 26:271–276

Pappas PG (2006) Invasive candidiasis. Infect Dis Clin North Am 20:485–506

Pappas PG, Kauffman CA, Andes D et al (2009) Clinical practice guidelines for the management of candidiasis: 2009 update by the Infectious Diseases Society of America. Clin Infect Dis 48:503–535

Parkins MD, Sabuda DM, Elsayed S et al (2007) Adequacy of empirical antifungal therapy and effect on outcome among patients with invasive Candida species infections. J Antimicrob Chemother 60:613–618

Passos XS, Costa CR, Araujo CR et al (2007) Species distribution and antifungal susceptibility patterns of Candida spp. bloodstream isolates from a Brazilian tertiary care hospital. Mycopathologia 163:145–151

Pelz RK, Hendrix CW, Swoboda SM et al (2001) Double-blind placebo-controlled trial of fluconazole to prevent candidal infections in critically ill surgical patients. Ann Surg 233:542–548

Pereira GH, Muller PR, Szeszs MW et al (2010) Five-year evaluation of bloodstream yeast infections in a tertiary hospital: the predominance of non-C albicans Candida species. Med Mycol 48(6):839–842

Pfaller MA (1996) Nosocomial candidiasis: emerging species, reservoirs, and modes of transmission. Clin Infect Dis 22(Suppl 2):S89–S94

Pfaller MA, Diekema DJ (2010) Epidemiology of invasive mycoses in North America. Crit Rev Microbiol 36:1–53

Piarroux R, Grenouillet F, Balvay P et al (2004) Assessment of preemptive treatment to prevent severe candidiasis in critically ill surgical patients. Crit Care Med 32:2443–2449

Pittet D, Monod M, Suter PM et al (1994) Candida colonization and subsequent infections in critically ill surgical patients. Ann Surg 220:751–758

Playford EG, Webster AC, Sorrell TC et al (2006) Antifungal agents for preventing fungal infections in non-neutropenic critically ill and surgical patients: systematic review and meta-analysis of randomized clinical trials. J Antimicrob Chemother 57:628–638

Presterl E, Parschalk B, Bauer E et al (2009) Invasive fungal infections and (1,3)-beta-D-glucan serum concentrations in long-term intensive care patients. Int J Infect Dis 13:707–712

Rangel-Frausto MS, Wiblin T, Blumberg HM et al (1999) National epidemiology of mycoses survey (NEMIS): variations in rates of bloodstream infections due to Candida species in seven surgical intensive care units and six neonatal intensive care units. Clin Infect Dis 29:253–258

Rex JH, Sobel JD (2001) Prophylactic antifungal therapy in the intensive care unit. Clin Infect Dis 32:1191–1200

Richards MJ, Edwards JR, Culver DH et al (2000) Nosocomial infections in combined medical-surgical intensive care units in the United States. Infect Control Hosp Epidemiol 21:510–515

Richet HM, Andremont A, Tancrede C et al (1991) Risk factors for candidemia in patients with acute lymphocytic leukemia. Rev Infect Dis 13:211–215

Ruan SY, Lee LN, Jerng JS et al (2008) Candida glabrata fungaemia in intensive care units. Clin Microbiol Infect 14:136–140

Saiman L, Ludington E, Dawson JD et al (2001) Risk factors for Candida species colonization of neonatal intensive care unit patients. Pediatr Infect Dis J 20:1119–1124

Savino JA, Agarwal N, Wry P et al (1994) Routine prophylactic antifungal agents (clotrimazole, ketoconazole, and nystatin) in nontransplant/nonburned critically ill surgical and trauma patients. J Trauma 36:20–25; discussion 25–26

Sendid B, Tabouret M, Poirot JL et al (1999) New enzyme immunoassays for sensitive detection of circulating Candida albicans mannan and antimannan antibodies: useful combined test for diagnosis of systemic candidiasis. J Clin Microbiol 37:1510–1517

Shorr AF, Chung K, Jackson WL et al (2005) Fluconazole prophylaxis in critically ill surgical patients: a meta-analysis. Crit Care Med 33:1928–1935; quiz 1936

Shorr AF, Lazarus DR, Sherner JH et al (2007) Do clinical features allow for accurate prediction of fungal pathogenesis in bloodstream infections? Potential implications of the increasing prevalence of non-albicans candidemia. Crit Care Med 35:1077–1083

Singhi S, Rao DS, Chakrabarti A (2008) Candida colonization and candidemia in a pediatric intensive care unit. Pediatr Crit Care Med 9:91–95

Suljagic V, Cobeljic M, Jankovic S et al (2005) Nosocomial bloodstream infections in ICU and non-ICU patients. Am J Infect Control 33:333–340

Trick WE, Fridkin SK, Edwards JR et al (2002) Secular trend of hospital-acquired candidemia among intensive care unit patients in the United States during 1989–1999. Clin Infect Dis 35:627–630

Tumbarello M, Posteraro B, Trecarichi EM et al (2007) Biofilm production by Candida species and inadequate antifungal therapy as predictors of mortality for patients with candidemia. J Clin Microbiol 45:1843–1850

Vaudry WL, Tierney AJ, Wenman WM (1988) Investigation of a cluster of systemic Candida albicans infections in a neonatal intensive care unit. J Infect Dis 158:1375–1379

Vincent JL, Bihari DJ, Suter PM et al (1995) The prevalence of nosocomial infection in intensive care units in Europe. Results of the European Prevalence of Infection in Intensive Care (EPIC). Study EPIC International Advisory Committee. JAMA 274:639–644

Vincent JL, Rello J, Marshall J et al (2009) International study of the prevalence and outcomes of infection in intensive care units. JAMA 302:2323–2329

Viscoli C, Girmenia C, Marinus A et al (1999) Candidemia in cancer patients: a prospective, multicenter surveillance study by the Invasive Fungal Infection Group (IFIG) of the European Organization for Research and Treatment of Cancer (EORTC). Clin Infect Dis 28:1071–1079

Voss A, le Noble JL, Verduyn Lunel FM et al (1997) Candidemia in intensive care unit patients: risk factors for mortality. Infection 25:8–11

Wey SB, Mori M, Pfaller MA et al (1989) Risk factors for hospital-acquired candidemia. A matched case-control study. Arch Intern Med 149:2349–2353

Wisplinghoff H, Bischoff T, Tallent SM et al (2004) Nosocomial bloodstream infections in US hospitals: analysis of 24,179 cases from a prospective nationwide surveillance study. Clin Infect Dis 39:309–317

Zaoutis TE, Argon J, Chu J et al (2005) The epidemiology and attributable outcomes of candidemia in adults and children hospitalized in the United States: a propensity analysis. Clin Infect Dis 41:1232–1239

Importance of High Creatinine Clearance for Antibacterial Treatment in Sepsis

12

Jeffrey Lipman and Andrew Udy

12.1 Introduction

In-hospital and intensive care unit (ICU) mortality rates for sepsis remain unacceptably high (Finfer et al. 2004), and while there have been major developments in such areas as cardiology and oncology, the development of new antibacterial agents has largely stopped. This is in the context of an ever-increasing incidence of multiresistant organisms, resulting in the previously unimaginable scenario of "un-treatable" infection. As such, the timely and effective application of existing antibacterial therapies must be optimised, not only to increase the chance of therapeutic success, but also to reduce the risk of selecting multiresistant strains (Roberts et al. 2008). In particular, this process must consider the inherent virulence of the infecting pathogen, the host's immune/inflammatory response, the nature of additional "non-infectious" therapies provided, and the relevant interplay with the pharmacokinetic-pharmacodynamic properties of the antibacterial agent (Fig. 12.1). Importantly, this process is dynamic and requires constant re-evaluation to ensure optimal antibacterial application.

This chapter will review the key pharmacological properties relevant to dosing antibacterials in the intensive care unit, with specific emphasis on the interaction among the host's response, therapeutic interventions and changes in antibacterial

J. Lipman (✉)
Critical Care and Anaesthesiology, The University of Queensland,
Brisbane, QLD, Australia

Department of Intensive Care Medicine, Royal Brisbane and Women's Hospital,
Herston Road, 4029 Herston, Brisbane, QLD, Australia
e-mail: j.lipman@uq.edu.au

A. Udy
Department of Intensive Care Medicine, Royal Brisbane and Women's Hospital,
Herston, Brisbane, QLD, Australia

Burns, Trauma and Critical Care Research Center, The University of Queensland,
Brisbane, QLD, Australia

J. Rello (eds.), *Sepsis Management*,
DOI 10.1007/978-3-642-03519-7_12, © Springer-Verlag Berlin Heidelberg 2012

Fig. 12.1 Important factors in optimising bacterial eradication

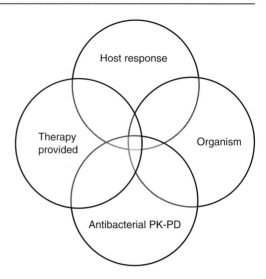

pharmacokinetics. The focus will be on the potential for augmented renal clearance of these agents, predisposing to sub-therapeutic drug concentrations, treatment failure or the selection of resistant organisms. The likely pathophysiology driving this phenomenon will be reviewed, in addition to consideration of subgroups of critically ill patients "at risk". Dosing strategies to improve drug exposure in such a setting will be identified, as will the role for routine application of therapeutic drug monitoring (TDM).

12.2 Basic Pharmacological Principles

The aim of clinical pharmacology is to optimise the effects of pharmaceuticals on the body such that an optimum response is achieved while avoiding toxicity and side effects. Two major disciplines key to the application of this process are that of pharmacokinetics and pharmacodynamics. Pharmacokinetics (PK) is primarily interested in the changes in drug concentration (ideally at the effect site) over time and is graphically represented by a concentration time curve (Fig. 12.2). Typically this involves considering the absorption, distribution, metabolism and elimination of pharmaceuticals from the body. A variety of PK parameters can be employed to define this process for different agents, examples of which are defined below:

- *Volume of distribution (Vd)* = Hypothetical volume of fluid that the total amount of administered drug distributes into, generating a concentration equal to that measured in plasma.
- *Clearance (CL)* = Volume of plasma effectively cleared of the drug per unit time. Total drug clearance is the combination of the clearances for each eliminating organ or tissue.
- *Plasma half-life (T1/2)* = Time required for the plasma concentration to fall by one half.
- C_{max} = The maximum concentration measured after one dose. Ideally at the effect site, although commonly measured in plasma.

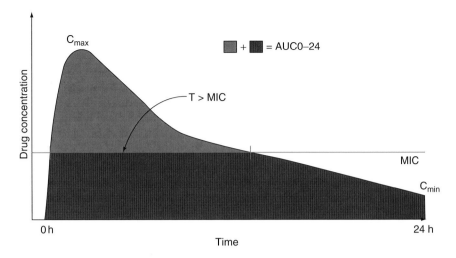

Fig. 12.2 Concentration versus time curve. *Cmax* maximum drug concentration, *Cmin* minimum drug concentration, *MIC* minimum inhibitory concentration, *AUC0-24* area under the concentration time curve from 0 to 24 h

- C_{min} = The minimum concentration during a dosing period. Commonly determined in plasma prior to the next dose.
- *Area under the curve (AUC)* = The area under the concentration–time curve. Typically estimated from time zero to infinity using plasma concentrations.

    The distribution of any given antibacterial agent will vary significantly depending upon its inherent pharmacochemical properties (such as molecular weight and electrochemical charge) and its degree of plasma protein binding. Those agents with a higher affinity for lipids (lipophilic) will tend towards a higher Vd and longer elimination times, with extensive distribution into tissues and the intracellular space. In contrast, hydrophilic agents will primarily be limited to the extracellular space, favouring a lower Vd and more rapid elimination. Those agents that are highly bound (to albumin or alpha-1 acid glycoprotein) may have very limited distribution (primarily in plasma) and a longer duration of action. Importantly, it is the free (or unbound) fraction that is pharmacologically active, and this will be influenced by plasma protein concentrations and binding competition from other agents.

    Pharmacodynamics (PD) in contrast involves the study of the effects of the drug and is typically represented by a dose response curve. In terms of antibacterials, this refers to the ability of the agent to kill or inhibit the growth of an infecting organism following a given dose. Significantly, there is an important interplay between the PK properties of these agents and their efficacy, which is referred to as the pharmacokinetic-pharmacodynamic (PK-PD) characteristics. The PK-PD parameters of note for antibacterial agents are summarised below:

- $T > MIC$ = The time for which the concentration of the antibacterial agent remains above the minimum inhibitory concentration (MIC) for bacterial growth during a given dosing period

- C_{max}/MIC = The ratio of the maximum antibacterial concentration (C_{max}) to the MIC of the infecting organism
- AUC_{0-24}/MIC = The ratio of the area under the concentration time curve during a 24 h time period to the MIC of the infecting organism.

12.3   Antibacterial Pharmacokinetics-Pharmacodynamics

Using this established framework, different antibacterial agents can be broadly classified on the basis of their kill characteristics into time-dependant, concentration-dependant or concentration-time-dependant killers (Table 12.1). These kill characteristics describe the PK-PD parameters that represent optimal bactericidal activity (Nicolau 2003). Of note, any significant change in antibacterial PK (as might be expected in the critically ill) will largely alter the efficacy of these agents on the basis of this classification.

12.3.1 Concentration-Dependant Killing

The aminoglycosides (gentamicin, tobramycin, amikacin) represent the most extensively studied group of antibacterials in this category, and the PK-PD factor most

Table 12.1 Categories of antibacterials based on PK-PD "kill" characteristic

Category	Concentration dependant	Time dependant	Concentration-time dependant
PK-PD factor	C_{max}/MIC	T > MIC	AUC_{0-24}/MIC
Examples	Aminoglycosides	β-lactams	Glycopeptides
	Daptomycin	Linezolid	Fluoroquinolones
	Fluoroquinolones	Lincosamides	Tigecycline
			Azithromycin
PK-PD aim	Aminoglycosides:	β-lactams and linezolid:	Glycopeptides:
	– $C_{max}/MIC > 10$	– 100% T > MIC	– $AUC_{0-24}/MIC > 400$
	– Low C_{min}	Lincosamides:	Fluoroquinolones:
	Fluoroquinolones:	– 50% T > MIC	– $AUC_{0-24}/MIC > 125$
	– $C_{max}/MIC > 10$		Azithromycin:
			– $AUC_{0-24}/MIC > 25$
Implications of ARC	Increased CL/Low C_{min}	Less T > MIC	Lower AUC_{0-24}/MIC
Dosing strategies	Weight based	Increased frequency	Increased frequency
	Increased frequency	Extended or continuous infusion	Continuous infusion
	Use of TDM	Use of TDM	Use of TDM

PK-PD pharmacokinetics-pharmacodynamics, C_{max} maximum drug concentration, *MIC* minimum inhibitory concentration, AUC_{0-24} area under the concentration-time curve, *CL* drug clearance, C_{min} minimum drug concentration closely linked with therapeutic success is the C_{max}/MIC ratio (Moore et al. 1987; Mouton and Vinks 2005; Vogelman and Craig 1985, 1986). In contrast, C_{min} levels and the total dose administered are more closely associated with toxicity (Craig 1998). This group also displays a significant post-antibacterial effect (PAE) (Vogelman and Craig 1985), and as such, recommended dosing strategies aim to achieve a high peak concentration, ensuring a C_{max}/MIC ratio of at least 10 (Buijk et al. 2002; Kashuba et al. 1999), with preferably undetectable trough levels. The aminoglycosides are largely hydrophilic, distributing primarily into the extracellular space, and making the Vd the most relevant PK parameter for effective initial dosing (Beckhouse et al. 1988). As these agents are excreted almost entirely unchanged by glomerular filtration (Chambers and Sande 1996), drug elimination will be significantly altered with changes in renal function.

Daptomycin is a novel lipopolypeptide antibacterial agent that demonstrates concentration-dependant killing against most gram-positive pathogens (Safdar et al. 2004). The C_{max}/MIC ratio is the PK-PD parameter most closely associated with clinical efficacy (Safdar et al. 2004), while this agent also demonstrates a moderate PAE (Pankuch et al. 2003). Similarly to aminoglycosides, distribution is limited to extracellular fluid, such that increases in the Vd will result in a sub-optimal peak concentration. In addition, daptomycin is highly protein bound, and the primary route of elimination is via the kidneys (Schriever et al. 2005).

12.3.2 Time-Dependant Killing

The most widely used group of agents in this category is the β-lactams (penicillins, cephalosporins, carbapenems and monobactams), and the PK-PD target for optimal bacterial killing is the T>MIC (Craig 1984; Vogelman and Craig 1986). In this respect, dosing strategies employing agents without any significant post-antibacterial effect, should ideally achieve drug concentrations a factor of 4–5 times above the MIC (Angus et al. 2000; Mouton and den Hollander 1994), for 90–100% of the dosing interval (McKinnon et al. 2008; Turnidge 1998). Because of their inherent PAE (Bustamante et al. 1984), the carbepenems have been considered to require less T>MIC for both bacteriostatic (20%) and bacteriocidal (40%) activity (Drusano 2003). The majority of these agents are excreted via glomerular filtration and tubular secretion, leading to potentially significant changes in drug CL with altered renal function. Ceftriaxone (Joynt et al. 2001), and ertapenem (Brink et al. 2009) are agents within this class that are highly protein bound, and as such, their PK can be significantly altered in the setting of hypoalbuminaemia (Goldstein 1949).

Linezolid is an example of an oxazolidinone antibacterial that also displays time-dependant killing (Andes et al. 2002; Gentry-Nielsen et al. 2002). Previous animal research has suggested that a T>MIC of 40–80% of the dosing interval is required for a successful outcome (Gentry-Nielsen et al. 2002), although recently, longer durations (approaching of 100% of the dosing interval) have been advocated for maximal bacterial eradication, particularly with *Staphylococcus aureus* (Craig 2003). Although hydrophilic in nature, linezolid is widely distributed in the body, and undergoes hepatic metabolism before the parent drug and metabolites are excreted in the urine (MacGowan 2003). The lincosamides (lincomycin, clindamycin) are also time-dependant killers, with previous authors suggesting that free drug levels be maintained above the MIC for 40–50% of the dosing interval (Craig 2001). These lipophilic agents distribute widely in the body (Gwilt and Smith 1986; Mueller et al. 1999) and undergo extensive hepatic metabolism (Avant et al. 1975; Bellamy et al. 1966).

12.3.3 Concentration-Time-Dependant Killing

Agents within this group often display both time- and concentration-dependant features, and include a number of commonly prescribed agents. For example, despite an increased understanding of vancomycin pharmacokinetics in the critically ill, the optimal PK-PD parameter predictive of clinical success is not entirely certain. In particular, some data suggest that the bactericidal activity of vancomycin is time dependent (Larsson et al. 1996; Lowdin et al. 1998), while separate research proposes the C_{max}/MIC ratio as more important for efficacy against some organisms (Knudsen et al. 2000). Others advocate the AUC_{0-24}/MIC ratio as the most important PK-PD parameter correlating with efficacy (Craig 2003; Rybak 2006), and a clinical advantage to AUC_{0-24}/MIC vales ≥ 400 in the treatment of methicillin-resistant *Staphylococcus aureus* (MRSA) lower respiratory tract infections has been demonstrated (Moise-Broder et al. 2004). A predominantly hydrophilic drug, vancomycin has a limited volume of distribution and poor penetration into tissues (Cruciani et al. 1996). The primary route of elimination is renal (Pea et al. 2000), via a combination of glomerular filtration and tubular secretion. Teicoplanin shares a number of features with vancomycin, although its high degree of protein binding leads to a prolonged elimination half-life (Del Favero et al. 1991) and facilitates once a day dosing.

The fluoroquinolones, including ciprofloxacin, levofloxacin, moxifloxacin and gatifloxacin, also display both concentration- and time-dependant effects in terms of their optimal PK-PD parameter. Specifically, while a C_{max}/MIC ratio > 10 has been considered necessary to ensure adequate bacterial kill (Blaser et al. 1987; Preston et al. 1998), others have proposed an AUC_{0-24}/MIC value > 125 as essential when treating gram-negative infections in the critically ill (Forrest et al. 1993). Lower values appear to be more acceptable when targeting gram-positive infections (>30) (Nix et al. 1992), although ratios < 100 may promote the emergence of bacterial resistance (Schentag 1999; Thomas et al. 1998). These agents are particularly lipophilic and distribute widely in tissues (Gous et al. 2005). Ciprofloxacin is hepatically metabolized, although dose adjustment is recommended in renal dysfunction (Hoffken et al. 1985). In comparison, both gatifloxacin and levofloxacin are renally eliminated (Nakashima et al. 1995; Rebuck et al. 2002), and drug CL can be expected be significantly altered with changes in renal function.

Other agents that demonstrate concentration-time-dependant killing include tigecycline and azithromycin. Tigecycline is a member of the glycylcyclines, a novel group of tetracyclines with enhanced gram-positive and gram-negative activity.

Tigecycline demonstrates rapid and extensive penetration into body tissues (Meagher et al. 2005a), along with time-dependent killing against *Streptococcus pneumoniae*, *Haemophilus influenzae* and *Neisseria gonorrhoea* (Petersen et al. 1999). Despite this, the AUC_{0-24}/MIC ratio is considered to more closely correlate with efficacy (Meagher et al. 2005b), largely due to the agent's long elimination half-life (via biliary excretion) and prolonged PAE (Muralidharan et al. 2005). Azithromycin is an "azalide" antibiotic, with improved tissue penetration, a longer plasma half-life and increased activity against gram-negative organisms compared with the macrolides (Piscitelli et al. 1992). AUC_{0-24}/MIC appears to be the PK-PD parameter most closely associated with clinical efficacy, with work suggesting that values ≥ 25 are needed to achieve and maintain bactericidal activity against *S. pneumoniae* (Sevillano et al. 2006). Azithromycin is primarily eliminated via biliary excretion.

12.4 Physiological Changes in the Critically Ill Affecting Renal Function

Critical illness represents a state of significant homeostatic disruption, causing marked alteration in organ function from baseline. Such changes are often similar regardless of the insult and at least initially are characterised by a systemic inflammatory response (SIRS). This syndrome has been well described in the literature (Bone et al. 1992), and can be identified with both infectious and non-infectious aetiologies (Ishikawa et al. 2006; Kohl and Deutschman 2006). The presence of a proven or suspected infection in combination with this inflammatory state is then termed sepsis, while the developments of organ dysfunction and hypotension refractory to fluid resuscitation are termed severe sepsis and septic shock respectively (Calandra and Cohen 2005; Levy et al. 2003). Consideration of the underlying cellular and humoral cascades that drive this phenomenon are beyond the scope of this chapter, although macrovascular, microvascular and cellular dysfunction can be identified in a number of organs (Parrillo 1993; Rice and Bernard 2005). Importantly, a key cardiovascular component of this inflammatory response is that of a "hyperdynamic" circulation, characterised by an increase in cardiac output (CO), systemic vasodilation and increased blood flow to major organs (Di Giantomasso et al. 2003b; Parrillo et al. 1990).

Separate to the underlying disease phenomenon, admission to the ICU is associated with the application of aggressive haemodynamic therapies in an attempt to restore cardiovascular homeostasis. In this manner, current international guidelines recommend the administration of intravenous resuscitation fluids and/or the application of vasoactive agents (such as norepinephrine or dobutamine) to achieve a set of pre-defined haemodynamic targets (Dellinger et al. 2008). With the limited evidence available, such a strategy favours a survival advantage (Rivers et al. 2001), although recent research has raised concerns over the validity of such arbitrary endpoints, particularly when associated with the need for a high vasopressor load (Dunser et al. 2009).

How such changes influence renal function is the subject of ongoing research. A subgroup of patients in this setting will go on to manifest acute kidney injury (AKI) (Bagshaw et al. 2007), potentially requiring the application of renal replacement therapy, and the rationalisation of renally excreted drugs. The nature of this insult is not entirely clear and may be multifactorial in many circumstances. However, septic AKI per se appears to be distinct from other causes, in that renal blood flow (RBF) is maintained or even enhanced in concert with an increase in CO (Langenberg et al. 2006). An important additional consideration is that RBF is the most important determinant of glomerular filtration (GFR) and is usually autoregulated over a range of perfusion pressures (Shipley and Study 1951).

The influence of resuscitative strategies on RBF and GFR are also of interest. In particular, Wan and colleagues have previously shown a positive effect of crystalloid administration on creatinine clearance (CL_{CR}), despite no significant change in RBF (Wan et al. 2007). The likely mechanism underlying this phenomenon involves haemodilution of circulating plasma proteins, resulting in a fall in plasma oncotic pressure. The role of vasopressor infusion (particularly norepinephrine) in this setting has recently been reviewed, and in general, the application of such therapies appears safe, if not beneficial from a renal point of view (Bellomo et al. 2008). Specifically, large animal research has confirmed a positive effect of norepinephrine infusion on CO, RBF and CL_{CR} (Di Giantomasso et al. 2002, 2003a), and studies in human sepsis and septic shock have demonstrated similar results (Desjars et al. 1989; Marin et al. 1990; Redl-Wenzl et al. 1993). Low-dose vasopressin infusion is also associated with an increase in CL_{CR} (Di Giantomasso et al. 2006; Holmes et al. 2001), while adrenaline appears to have less of an effect (Day et al. 2000; Di Giantomasso et al. 2005).

Previous work examining the renal response to moderate protein ingestion (Bosch et al. 1983) or intravenous administration of amino acids (Castellino et al. 1988) has led investigators to propose the concept of a "renal reserve" (Thomas et al. 1994). Although controversial, one potential model encompasses a population of dormant nephrons that are recruitable in the face of a large nitrogenous load, the implication being that the kidneys are not working at maximal capacity under basal conditions and at times of biological stress can respond with an increase in filtration. The role of this "renal reserve" in critical illness is still uncertain, but as the clinical state is often characterised by increased catabolism and inflammation, a potential role in maintaining renal function in this setting is not implausible. Significantly, the capacity of this "reserve" appears to decline with age.

In summary, critical illness is defined by significant alterations in organ function, often exacerbated by therapeutic interventions. In this setting, renal function can significantly deteriorate, often as a part of multiple organ dysfunction (MODS) (Bagshaw et al. 2007), whereby consideration of dose reduction of antibacterials may be necessary (see Chap. 13). However, in a significant subset, renal function can be enhanced, leading to supra-normal clearance of circulating solute, including renally eliminated antibacterial agents. We term this phenomenon augmented renal clearance (ARC), the mechanisms of which are graphically illustrated in Fig. 12.3.

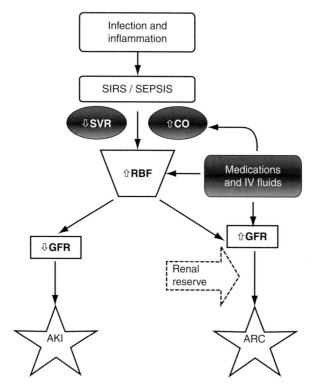

Fig. 12.3 Mechanisms underlying augmented renal clearance in the critically ill. *SIRS* systemic inflammatory response syndrome *CO* cardiac output, *SVRI* systemic vascular resistance index, *RBF* renal blood flow, *GFR* glomerular filtration rate, *IV* intra-venous, *AKI* acute kidney injury, *ARC* augmented renal clearance

12.5   Augmented Renal Clearance

The most widely accepted index of renal *function* in health and disease is the glomerular filtration rate (Stevens et al. 2006), as opposed to biomarkers of kidney *injury*, such as neutrophil gelatinase-associated lipoprotein (NGAL), which are continuing to be evaluated in clinical practice (Parikh and Devarajan 2008). The accepted norms for GFR are 120–130 mL/min/1.73 m^2 in healthy young adults, although these values do decline with age (Stevens et al. 2006). ARC refers to the enhanced renal elimination of circulating solute (such as waste products or pharmaceuticals) and may manifest as a consequence of enhanced glomerular filtration, tubular secretion or both (Udy et al. 2010c). As "baseline" values are available for comparison and laboratory assessment is relatively straightforward, measuring GFR is the most convenient method of monitoring changes in renal function and, in particular, identifying the presence of ARC. However, important pitfalls in this approach are numerous, including a lack of consensus on the upper limit of normal filtration, and the most reliable and accurate method of measuring GFR in clinical practice.

Furthermore, focusing solely on filtration provides no information on tubular function, which can be particularly important for some antibacterial agents.

What constitutes *hyperfiltration* is largely uncertain, particularly as there are no robust data to link any specific GFR value with adverse outcomes. Previously authors have attempted to apply categorisation systems based on arbitrary cutoffs, such as that proposed by Sunder-Plassmann and Horl, where GFRs ≥ 120 mL/min/1.73 m^2 (> 149 mL/min/1.73 m^2 in the young adult) were considered "glomerular hyperfiltration" (Sunder-Plassmann and Horl 2004). To date, this definition has not gained widespread acceptance, and the term "glomerular hyperfiltration" is perhaps more suited to subsets of chronic kidney disease (CKD) and is not representative of the mechanisms involved in critical illness. Recently, we have employed significantly higher definitions of ARC (> 160 mL/min/1.73 m^2 and > 150 mL/min/1.73 m^2 in men and women, respectively) (Udy et al. 2010a), although more work is needed in this area to better refine these values and correlate them with drug exposure.

How to measure GFR in clinical practice is equally as controversial. The traditional biomarker of renal function has been the plasma creatinine concentration, although it lacks sensitivity in identifying those patients with augmented clearances (Hoste et al. 2005). As such, some form of assessment of GFR is necessary to optimise drug exposure, and although ideal filtration markers [such as inulin (Orlando et al. 1998)] or radionucleotide imaging are available, neither is particularly feasible in the critically ill population. As most patients in the ICU are immobile and require a urinary catheter, it is our opinion that the most reliable and feasible estimate of GFR is a measured CL$_{CR}$. By measuring the concentration of creatinine in plasma and urine, and noting the volume of urine produced over the given time period, an accurate and repeatable estimate of GFR can be calculated.

Previously, 2- (Herrera-Gutierrez et al. 2007; Sladen et al. 1987), 6- (Cherry et al. 2002), 4- (Fuster-Lluch et al. 2008), 8- (Lipman et al. 2003) and 24-h (Conil et al. 2006a) time intervals have been used, with acceptable precision and bias between results (Herrera-Gutierrez et al. 2007). We favour 8-h collections, as these provide the best balance between accuracy and feasibility (Baumann et al. 1987; Cherry et al. 2002), and can usually be reported daily, allowing the clinician to monitor trends and tailor therapy accordingly. An important consideration is that creatinine is both freely filtered by the glomerulus and secreted by the proximal tubule, meaning that at lower filtration rates, a measured CL$_{CR}$ will tend to overestimate the true GFR (Kim et al. 1969, 1972). However, as sub-therapeutic dosing is only a realistic concern at higher filtration rates, and measured CL$_{CR}$ has been correlated with drug elimination in the ICU (Lipman et al. 1999b, 2001), such values are an important guide to those patients with potential inadequate drug exposure.

12.5.1 Prevalence in the ICU

Although there are few robust data, there are an emerging number of studies that are documenting ARC in the critically ill (Udy et al. 2010c). In a prospective single-centre study using 4-h CL$_{CR}$ measures, Fuster-Lluch et al. documented an incidence of "glomerular hyperfiltration" of 17.9% on the first day of ICU admission using 4-h CL_{CR} measures (Fuster-Lluch et al. 2008). Of those patients remaining in the ICU, the percentage manifesting hyperfiltration peaked on day 5, as did the absolute mean CL_{CR} value (> 165 mL/min/1.73 m²). Elevated filtration rates were associated with younger age, lower APACHE II scores, higher urine outputs and a higher diastolic blood pressure (Fuster-Lluch et al. 2008).

More recently, Claus and colleagues have examined the incidence of ARC (CL_{CR} > 120 mL/min) in patients receiving anti-infective therapy in the ICU. Daily 24-h CL_{CR} measurements were performed in 141 patients, of whom 53.9% demonstrated ARC at some point during their treatment (Claus et al. 2010). In addition, age, surgical admission and administration of anti-infective therapy were identified as independent predictors of augmented glomerular filtration (Claus et al. 2010). Further evidence supporting ARC as a potentially common, albeit under-recognised phenomenon in the critically ill is a number of PK studies in general ICU patients demonstrating elevated clearances of β-lactams (Boselli et al. 2006; Brink et al. 2009; Burkhardt et al. 2007; Gomez et al. 1999; Joynt et al. 2001; Lipman et al. 1999b, 2001; Roberts et al. 2009b), glycopeptides (Barbot et al. 2003; Pea et al. 2000), fluoroquinolones (Pea et al. 2003a), linezolid (Adembri et al. 2008) and aminoglycosides (Beckhouse et al. 1988).

12.5.2 Trauma and Surgery

Multitrauma and postoperative patients represent important subgroups of the critically ill at risk of ARC (Udy et al. 2010b). In the work by Fuster-LLuch et al. those with higher filtration rates were predominantly multitrauma or postoperative admissions (Fuster-Lluch et al. 2008), while similar results were documented by Brown and colleagues in 50 critically ill post-surgical patients (Brown et al. 1980). In this study, CL_{CR} reached a peak of 190 mL/min/1.73 m² on the 4th postoperative day in the trauma cohort ($n = 17$), and CO demonstrated a modest correlation with CL_{CR} in both trauma and non-trauma patients, although those receiving vasoactive medications or displaying sepsis were excluded (Brown et al. 1980). In addition, Cherry and colleagues, in their work investigating the accuracy of shorter duration CL_{CR} collections, demonstrated significantly elevated clearances across all time points in the trauma versus non-trauma patients (Cherry et al. 2002).

Further qualifying these data are a number of PK studies demonstrating augmented drug clearances in this population. For example, Hanes et al. demonstrated increased clearance of ceftazidime in trauma patients (Hanes et al. 2000), while Toschlog and colleagues reported rapid elimination of gentamicin in over 50% of their trauma cohort (Toschlog et al. 2003). Similarly, in the surgical ICU, significantly elevated clearances of piperacillin have been demonstrated in a young septic cohort (Shikuma et al. 1990a), while in a multicentre randomised clinical trial, investigators demonstrated augmented piperacillin CL as compared with healthy volunteers when it was used in the treatment of complicated intra-abdominal infection (Li et al. 2005).

12.5.3 Neurosurgery

Neurosurgical patients are another population where ARC may manifest frequently and is a reflection of the disease process, patient demographic and the treatment provided (Udy et al. 2010b). Isolated traumatic brain injury is associated with the release of cytokines and inflammatory mediators (Ott et al. 1994) or may occur in the setting of multitrauma, with associated global tissue injury and inflammation (Nuytinck et al. 1988). Younger patients, often without significant comorbidity, tend to be over-represented in this group, and ICU management focuses on aggressively restoring blood flow to the injured brain. Routinely this involves the administration of resuscitation fluids and vasoactive medications, particularly in the defence of an adequate cerebral perfusion pressure (CPP) (Bratton et al. 2007a, b). In addition, refractory intracranial hypertension often prompts the use of concentrated saline solutions or osmotic diuretics in an attempt to reduce cerebral free water (Bratton et al. 2007c). In this respect, ARC has been demonstrated in traumatically brain injured patients receiving vasopressor therapy (Albanese et al. 2004; Benmalek et al. 1999) and mannitol (Valdes et al. 1979), while in an animal model, hypertonic saline solutions promote an increase in CL_{CR} (Wan et al. 2007). The use of induced hypertension and hypervolaemia in subarachnoid haemorrhage complicated by delayed cerebral ischaemia is likely to produce a similar phenomenon, although there are no data in this area currently.

12.5.4 Burn Injury

The initial phase of burn injury lasts approximately 48–72 h and is characterised by an inflammatory response and marked protein capillary leak syndrome. Largely determined by the extent of the injury, significant volumes of fluid can translocate into the interstitial space, leading to relative hypovolaemia and haemoconcentration. Initial treatment is therefore focused on the restoration of an adequate circulating blood volume and organ perfusion (Latenser 2009). Current data also favour early debridement of the burn tissue (Latenser 2009), often meaning return visits to the operating theatre, bleeding and administration of blood products. Once complete, the burnt patient enters a hypermetabolic phase associated with wound healing, typically lasting several weeks and often complicated by nosocomial infection. During this phase cardiac output tends to be elevated, leading to increased RBF and GFR (Loirat et al. 1978; Udy et al. 2010b).

In this setting a significant percentage to patients will manifest ARC ($CL_{CR} > 120$ mL/min/1.73 m^2), and the most accurate method of estimating GFR is a measured CL_{CR} (Conil et al. 2007c). As such, the elimination of renally cleared antibacterials would be expected to be increased, and this has been demonstrated for β-lactams (Adam et al. 1989; Bonapace et al. 1999; Conil et al. 2007a, b, d; Dailly et al. 2003; Shikuma et al. 1990b), glycopeptides (Dailly et al. 2008; Dolton et al. 2010), aminoglycosides (Conil et al. 2006b; Loirat et al. 1978), daptomycin (Mohr et al. 2008) and fluoroquinolones (Garrelts et al. 1996) with burn injury.

12.5.5 Other "At Risk" Groups

Low plasma albumin concentrations can be frequently recognised in the critically ill (Finfer et al. 2006), the cause of which is often multifactorial, and can involve a poor pre-morbid nutritional status, large volume crystalloid resuscitation, hepatic dysfunction or an inability to establish adequate nutrition in the ICU. In addition, critical illness significantly increases energy expenditure, leading to exaggerated catabolism and protein degradation. The relevance to antibacterial PK primarily concerns those agents that are highly protein bound and renally eliminated, such that a higher free (or unbound) fraction is associated with an increase in drug clearance. Examples include ceftriaxone (Joynt et al. 2001), teicoplanin (Barbot et al. 2003) and ertapenem (Brink et al. 2009; Burkhardt et al. 2007), where clearances have been demonstrated to be elevated with hypoalbuminaemia.

Patients presenting with haematological malignancy, and perhaps more specifically febrile neutropaenia, can also manifest ARC. Broad-spectrum antibacterial therapy is often warranted in this group without prior isolates, and it is in this setting that significant changes in drug CL have been noted (Lortholary et al. 2008). In particular, Pea et al. have demonstrated that significantly higher empirical doses of teicoplanin were needed to achieve adequate trough concentrations in patients with acute leukaemia, as well as a moderate inverse linear correlation between levels and estimated CL_{CR} (Pea et al. 2004). Similarly, augmented clearances and/or higher dosing requirements have been demonstrated with β-lactams (Lamoth et al. 2009; Nyhlen et al. 2001), aminoglycosides (Higa and Murray 1987; Romano et al. 1999), daptomycin (Bubalo et al. 2009) and vancomycin (Fernandez de Gatta et al. 1993) in this setting. Although we are not aware of any descriptive studies of CL_{CR} in this population, the recruitment of a "renal reserve" (particularly in younger patients) may help to explain this phenomenon.

12.6   Relevance to Antibacterial Pharmacokinetics and Implications for Dosing

With an established framework for understanding the relevant "kill characteristics" of any given antibacterial agent, the implications of ARC on dosing strategies in the critically ill can be more fully considered. Furthermore, while the following discussion primarily considers those agents that are renally eliminated, it is possible to hypothesise that a similar mechanism may alter the elimination of hepatically cleared agents through an increase in liver blood flow and upregulation of metabolic pathways. Further work in this area is needed.

12.6.1 Concentration-Dependant Agents

As the aminoglycosides are primarily eliminated by glomerular filtration (Chambers and Sande 1996), ARC will significantly increase drug clearance (Beckhouse et al.

1988; Toschlog et al. 2003). In addition, ICU interventions have been shown to have a significant impact on aminoglycoside PK (Lugo and Castaneda-Hernandez 1997), meaning that traditional dosing regimens are routinely unlikely to meet the required PK-PD targets in this population (Rea et al. 2008). An altered Vd will be a key component (Marik et al. 1991b), stressing the importance of a weight-based dosing strategy. However, doses of 7 mg/kg generally confer a C_{max}/MIC ratio of at least 10 [maximising bacterial killing (Kashuba et al. 1999)], and multiple studies have confirmed comparable if not superior clinical outcomes with extended interval dosing (Marik et al. 1991a; Olsen et al. 2004; Prins et al. 1993). Reducing the frequency to 18 hourly can be considered and has the added advantage of continuing to utilise these agents PAE. Importantly, trough level monitoring will be essential in avoiding toxicity.

Daptomycin is also primarily eliminated by the kidneys, and while dose reduction has been recommended with renal impairment (Schriever et al. 2005), there are only limited data examining the impact of ARC on its prescription in the critically ill. Of note, augmented total body CL of daptomycin has been demonstrated in neutropaenic patients, although there was no correlation with estimated CL_{CR} (Bubalo et al. 2009). This may suggest a possible non-renal mechanism, although no *measured* values of GFR were obtained (Bubalo et al. 2009).

12.6.2 Time-Dependant Agents

In respect to the β-lactams, drug elimination has been correlated with CL_{CR} in a number of studies (Angus et al. 2000; Conil et al. 2007b; Ikawa et al. 2008; Joukhadar et al. 2002; Joynt et al. 2001; Kitzes-Cohen et al. 2002; Li et al. 2005; Lipman et al. 1999b, 2001; Lovering et al. 1995; Roos et al. 2007; Tam et al. 2003; Van Dalen et al. 1987; Young et al. 1997), and given the time-dependant nature of their bactericidal action, ARC must be considered when determining the optimum dosing regimen. For example, recent work in the critically ill has revealed a robust inverse linear relationship between CL_{CR} and trough piperacillin levels (Conil et al. 2006a), reinforcing this parameter as a key covariate in predicting drug exposure. Furthermore, while no PK or outcome studies have been performed with β-lactams and ARC per se, a recent non-inferiority study of ceftobiprole versus linezolid and ceftazidime in nosocomial pneumonia has raised some important clinical concerns. Specifically, although there was no difference in the overall cure rate in the 781 enrolled patients, inferior outcomes were noted with ceftobiprole in the subgroup with ventilator-associated pneumonia (VAP), who were either young (< 45 years) or had an elevated CL_{CR} at baseline (≥ 150 mL/min) (Noel et al. 2008). Of note, a higher frequency of male patients with brain injury was assigned to the ceftobiprole arm (Noel et al. 2008), introducing ARC as a potential confounder, although no PK data were supplied.

As such, strategies that maintain sufficient drug concentrations throughout the dosing interval, typically by means of more frequent administration, and extended or continuous infusions, would seem the most sensible in the setting of ARC.

However, while relevant PK-PD data support this approach in the critically ill (Angus et al. 2000; Georges et al. 2005; Hanes et al. 2000; Lipman et al. 1999a; McNabb et al. 2001; Mouton et al. 1997; Nicolau et al. 2001; Roberts et al. 2007a, b, 2009a, b; Roberts and Lipman 2007), and superior clinical outcomes have been reported by some investigators (Lodise et al. 2007; Lorente et al. 2006, 2007, 2009; Roberts et al. 2007b), a recent systematic review of continuous infusion of β-lactams did not demonstrate any clinical advantage in this setting (Roberts et al. 2009c). Importantly, this analysis included a heterogeneous group of critically ill patients, and as yet there are no data to define any particular role of such strategies in patients manifesting ARC.

Although dose modification is currently not recommended for linezolid in renal dysfunction (Brier et al. 2003), the fact that it undergoes at least partial renal elimination and demonstrates time-dependant characteristics suggests ARC could significantly impact upon the optimal dosing regimen. In this respect, an alternate dosing strategy has been trialled in the critically ill, with a reported PK advantage to continuous infusion (Adembri et al. 2008). However, no specific dose modification can be recommended at this time, as conflicting data have been presented, suggesting no difference in key PK parameters between healthy volunteers and those manifesting severe sepsis and septic shock (Thallinger et al. 2008).

12.6.3 Concentration-Time-Dependant Agents

The glycopeptides undergo primarily renal elimination (Pea et al. 2000), and as such, a significant correlation with CL_{CR} has been demonstrated with both vancomycin (Dailly et al. 2008; Llopis-Salvia and Jimenez-Torres 2006; Pea et al. 2009) and teicoplanin CL (Barbot et al. 2003; Lortholary et al. 1996; Pea et al. 2003b) in the critically ill. ARC is therefore a significant consideration when dosing these agents, and the importance of reviewing glycopeptide schedules regularly is reinforced by the need to administer higher doses in the ICU in order to meet the desired PK-PD targets, particularly with intermediate or drug-resistant pathogens (del Mar Fernandez de Gatta Garcia et al. 2007). While there are no specific studies examining dosing in ARC, current guidelines recommend dosing using total body weight (~30 mg/kg) with the aim of achieving trough concentrations between 15 and 20 mg/L (MacGowan 1998) (vancomycin) in order to ensure an adequate AUC_{0-24}:MIC ratio. As such, an increased frequency of dosing or continuous infusion would appear to be an attractive solution, although current data are conflicted on this point. Specifically, while investigators have demonstrated a clinical benefit with continuous infusions in ventilator-associated pneumonia (Rello et al. 2005), a large prospective multicentre study failed to reveal any significant difference in microbiological or clinical outcomes with continuous versus intermittent dosing (Wysocki et al. 2001). As such, a specific dosing strategy cannot be recommended at this time.

An added complexity when using teicoplanin is this drug's high degree of protein binding, leading to potentially elevated drug CL in the setting of hypoalbuminaemia and ARC. As such, while standard dosing regimens routinely use a loading dose of 6 mg/kg 12-hourly for three doses (Pea et al. 2003b), followed by 6 mg/kg 24-hourly thereafter, more frequent administration may be advocated in the future. In addition, current data also favour higher loading doses in septic patients (Brink et al. 2008), and at least 12 mg/kg in endocarditis, bone and joint infections (Wilson 2000), and ventilator-associated pneumonia (Mimoz et al. 2006).

The prescription of fluoroquinolones is also particularly challenging in this setting, as currently there are only limited data examining the impact of ARC (Udy et al. 2010c). This is coupled with a large Vd and variable renal elimination for some agents. Specifically, although reported PK data for ciprofloxacin reveal a close correlation between total drug CL and estimated CL_{CR} (Conil et al. 2008), and elevated renal clearances of levofloxacin have been reported in early onset VAP (Pea et al. 2003a), specific dose recommendations are hard to determine. While 8-hourly dosing of ciprofloxacin in severe sepsis and normal renal function has been demonstrated to be both safe and effective (Lipman et al. 1998), this may still not produce the desired PK-PD targets for optimum bacterial killing (Sun et al. 2005). Of the agents in this class, levofloxacin is perhaps the most "susceptible" to ARC, as it is renally eliminated, and of note, higher doses are currently being advocated in the critically ill (Graninger and Zeitlinger 2004). Additional research concerning these agents is urgently needed, particularly with the recognition that inappropriate dosing may not only lead to therapeutic failure, but also stimulate the development of drug resistant strains (Drusano 2003).

12.7 You Only Find What You Look For – The Importance of Measuring Creatinine Clearance

Most dosing strategies for antibacterial agents are derived from studies in healthy volunteers and fail to consider the unique setting of the critical care environment. As such, the empirical application of these regimes, without considering the underlying pathophysiology of the patient, is likely to result in sub-optimal drug exposure, promoting either treatment failure or toxicity. It is therefore essential that the clinician assess the need for revision of dosing schedules as early as possible. In those patients manifesting AKI, the plasma creatinine concentration tends to rise, alerting the clinician to the potential need for dose modification. In this respect, the use of these values almost entirely focuses on identifying renal impairment, triggering dose reduction for those agents that are renally eliminated. However, the converse, increasing doses in those patients with normal or low plasma creatinine concentrations, is seldom considered in clinical practice.

In order to improve sensitivity, particularly in identifying early stages of CKD, formulae have been developed to mathematically estimate GFR using plasma creatinine concentrations and simple demographic measures. The modification of diet in the renal disease (MDRD) formula (Levey et al. 1999) in particular has gained worldwide acceptance in this respect, although recent concerns have been raised about its validity in optimising drug prescription (Martin et al. 2009), particularly in the critical care environment. The Cockcroft-Gault equation, an equally popular estimate of CL_{CR} (Cockcroft and Gault 1976), has traditionally been used extensively in pharmaceutical research. However, while these estimates may provide more useful information than plasma creatinine concentrations alone (Herrera-Gutierrez et al. 2007), neither equation was designed for use in the critically ill, and ongoing research confirms that they are less accurate in this setting (Cherry et al. 2002; Conil et al. 2007c; Martin et al. 2010; Poggio et al. 2005a; Snider et al. 1995), as well as in those manifesting higher filtration rates (Lin et al. 2003; Poggio et al. 2005b; Rule et al. 2004). It is therefore our view that the most robust and feasible manner of measuring GFR in the critically ill, is the collection of a timed urinary creatinine clearance. Furthermore, this should be applied regularly to patients in the ICU, particularly in settings where therapeutic drug monitoring is not available, as a means to identifying those patients "at risk" of sub-therapeutic drug exposure.

12.7.1 Therapeutic Drug Monitoring

TDM has an established role in improving efficacy and limiting toxicity in the prescription of aminoglycosides, as well as optimising the dosing of glycopeptides in the critically ill (Roberts and Lipman 2006). However, outside of these examples, TDM has been infrequently available to the clinician. Nevertheless, our increasing knowledge of the relevant PK-PD properties of many agents, coupled with an improved capability to measure plasma and even tissue concentrations with increasing accuracy, means that TDM is likely to have a central role in improving antibacterial dosing schedules in the future. This must also be considered in the context of an increasing prevalence of antibacterial drug resistance, whereby optimisation of drug levels is paramount to achieving clinical success (Roberts et al. 2008). As such, TDM should be considered as an absolutely necessary component to antibacterial prescription in the critically ill and ideally should be available for a wide variety of agents.

12.8   Conclusion

Early, appropriate application of antibacterial therapy has been demonstrated to significantly improve survival in critically ill septic patients (Ibrahim et al. 2000; Kollef et al. 1999; Kumar et al. 2006), and as such, it is mandatory for the prescriber to consider any intervention that will improve drug exposure in this setting. The host response, additional non-antibacterial therapy, the organism and antibacterial PK-PD have an important interplay in determining optimal dosing in such patients and, as a consequence, the chances of therapeutic success. To date, assessment of renal function in the critically ill has largely focused on identifying renal dysfunction, often triggering appropriate modification of drug dosing. However, a new and significantly under-recognised paradigm is that of augmented renal clearance, whereby increasing the dose and/or frequency of administration may be appropriate. Important subgroups at risk include young postoperative, trauma, burn and head-injured patients.

A key component in effectively modifying dosing regimens is the recognition of suboptimal drug concentrations. While titration of drug therapy to readily available clinical endpoints is common in the ICU, such as adjusting vasopressor infusions to a desired mean arterial pressure, this task is more challenging with agents that manifest silent pharmacodynamic indices, such as antibacterial agents. In this respect, therapeutic drug monitoring, as part of an active clinical pharmacology programme, is a key component of this process, such that inadequate drug concentrations can lead to appropriate dose modification. In situations where TDM is not available, a measured CL_{CR} can act as a useful surrogate of drug elimination, prompting the clinician to consider alternative dosing regimens. In particular, *you only find what you look for*, suggesting that clinicians must regularly consider this phenomenon in daily practice in order to improve the delivery of antibacterial therapy in this setting.

References

Adam D, Zellner PR, Koeppe P et al (1989) Pharmacokinetics of ticarcillin/clavulanate in severely burned patients. J Antimicrob Chemother 24(Suppl B):121–129

Adembri C, Fallani S, Cassetta MI et al (2008) Linezolid pharmacokinetic/pharmacodynamic profile in critically ill septic patients: intermittent versus continuous infusion. Int J Antimicrob Agents 31:122–129

Albanese J, Leone M, Garnier F et al (2004) Renal effects of norepinephrine in septic and nonseptic patients. Chest 126:534–539

Andes D, van Ogtrop ML, Peng J et al (2002) In vivo pharmacodynamics of a new oxazolidinone (linezolid). Antimicrob Agents Chemother 46:3484–3489

Angus BJ, Smith MD, Suputtamongkol Y et al (2000) Pharmacokinetic-pharmacodynamic evaluation of ceftazidime continuous infusion vs. intermittent bolus injection in septicaemic melioidosis. Br J Clin Pharmacol 50:184–191

Avant GR, Schenker S, Alford RH (1975) The effect of cirrhosis on the disposition and elimination of clindamycin. Am J Dig Dis 20:223–230

Bagshaw SM, Uchino S, Bellomo R et al (2007) Septic acute kidney injury in critically ill patients: clinical characteristics and outcomes. Clin J Am Soc Nephrol 2:431–439

Barbot A, Venisse N, Rayeh F et al (2003) Pharmacokinetics and pharmacodynamics of sequential intravenous and subcutaneous teicoplanin in critically ill patients without vasopressors. Intensive Care Med 29:1528–1534

Baumann TJ, Staddon JE, Horst HM et al (1987) Minimum urine collection periods for accurate determination of creatinine clearance in critically ill patients. Clin Pharm 6:393–398

Beckhouse MJ, Whyte IM, Byth PL et al (1988) Altered aminoglycoside pharmacokinetics in the critically ill. Anaesth Intensive Care 16:418–422

Bellamy HM Jr, Bates BB, Reinarz JA (1966) Lincomycin metabolism in patients with hepatic insufficiency: effect of liver disease on lincomycin serum concentrations. Antimicrob Agents Chemother (Bethesda) 6:36–41

Bellomo R, Wan L, May C (2008) Vasoactive drugs and acute kidney injury. Crit Care Med 36:S179–S186

Benmalek F, Behforouz N, Benoist JF et al (1999) Renal effects of low-dose dopamine during vasopressor therapy for posttraumatic intracranial hypertension. Intensive Care Med 25:399–405

Blaser J, Stone BB, Groner MC et al (1987) Comparative study with enoxacin and netilmicin in a pharmacodynamic model to determine importance of ratio of antibiotic peak concentration to MIC for bactericidal activity and emergence of resistance. Antimicrob Agents Chemother 31:1054–1060

Bonapace CR, White RL, Friedrich LV et al (1999) Pharmacokinetics of cefepime in patients with thermal burn injury. Antimicrob Agents Chemother 43:2848–2854

Bone RC, Balk RA, Cerra FB et al (1992) Definitions for sepsis and organ failure and guidelines for the use of innovative therapies in sepsis. The ACCP/SCCM Consensus Conference Committee. American College of Chest Physicians/Society of Critical Care Medicine. Chest 101:1644–1655

Bosch JP, Saccaggi A, Lauer A et al (1983) Renal functional reserve in humans. Effect of protein intake on glomerular filtration rate. Am J Med 75:943–950

Boselli E, Breilh D, Saux MC et al (2006) Pharmacokinetics and lung concentrations of ertapenem in patients with ventilator-associated pneumonia. Intensive Care Med 32:2059–2062

Bratton SL, Chestnut RM, Ghajar J et al (2007a) Guidelines for the management of severe traumatic brain injury. I. Blood pressure and oxygenation. J Neurotrauma 24(Suppl 1):S7–S13

Bratton SL, Chestnut RM, Ghajar J et al (2007b) Guidelines for the management of severe traumatic brain injury. IX. Cerebral perfusion thresholds. J Neurotrauma 24(Suppl 1):S59–S64

Bratton SL, Chestnut RM, Ghajar J et al (2007c) Guidelines for the management of severe traumatic brain injury. II. Hyperosmolar therapy. J Neurotrauma 24(Suppl 1):S14–S20

Brier ME, Stalker DJ, Aronoff GR et al (2003) Pharmacokinetics of linezolid in subjects with renal dysfunction. Antimicrob Agents Chemother 47:2775–2780

Brink AJ, Richards GA, Cummins RR et al (2008) Recommendations to achieve rapid therapeutic teicoplanin plasma concentrations in adult hospitalised patients treated for sepsis. Int J Antimicrob Agents 32:455–458

Brink AJ, Richards GA, Schillack V et al (2009) Pharmacokinetics of once-daily dosing of ertapenem in critically ill patients with severe sepsis. Int J Antimicrob Agents 33:432–436

Brown R, Babcock R, Talbert J et al (1980) Renal function in critically ill postoperative patients: sequential assessment of creatinine osmolar and free water clearance. Crit Care Med 8:68–72

Bubalo JS, Munar MY, Cherala G et al (2009) Daptomycin pharmacokinetics in adult oncology patients with neutropenic fever. Antimicrob Agents Chemother 53:428–434

Buijk SE, Mouton JW, Gyssens IC et al (2002) Experience with a once-daily dosing program of aminoglycosides in critically ill patients. Intensive Care Med 28:936–942

Burkhardt O, Kumar V, Katterwe D et al (2007) Ertapenem in critically ill patients with early-onset ventilator-associated pneumonia: pharmacokinetics with special consideration of free-drug concentration. J Antimicrob Chemother 59:277–284

Bustamante CI, Drusano GL, Tatem BA et al (1984) Postantibiotic effect of imipenem on Pseudomonas aeruginosa. Antimicrob Agents Chemother 26:678–682

Calandra T, Cohen J (2005) The International Sepsis Forum consensus conference on definitions of infection in the intensive care unit. Crit Care Med 33:1538–1548

Castellino P, Giordano C, Perna A et al (1988) Effects of plasma amino acid and hormone levels on renal hemodynamics in humans. Am J Physiol 255:F444–F449

Chambers HE, Sande MA (1996) Goodman and Gillman's The pharmacological basis of therapeutics. McGraw Hill, New York

Cherry RA, Eachempati SR, Hydo L et al (2002) Accuracy of short-duration creatinine clearance determinations in predicting 24-hour creatinine clearance in critically ill and injured patients. J Trauma 53:267–271

Claus B, Colpaert K, Hoste EA et al (2010) Increased glomerular filtration in the critically ill patient receiving anti-infective treatment. Crit Care 14(Suppl 1):P509

Cockcroft DW, Gault MH (1976) Prediction of creatinine clearance from serum creatinine. Nephron 16:31–41

Conil JM, Georges B, Mimoz O et al (2006a) Influence of renal function on trough serum concentrations of piperacillin in intensive care unit patients. Intensive Care Med 32:2063–2066

Conil JM, Georges B, Breden A et al (2006b) Increased amikacin dosage requirements in burn patients receiving a once-daily regimen. Int J Antimicrob Agents 28:226–230

Conil JM, Georges B, Lavit M et al (2007a) A population pharmacokinetic approach to ceftazidime use in burn patients: influence of glomerular filtration, gender and mechanical ventilation. Br J Clin Pharmacol 64:27–35

Conil JM, Georges B, Fourcade O et al (2007b) Intermittent administration of ceftazidime to burns patients: influence of glomerular filtration. Int J Clin Pharmacol Ther 45:133–142

Conil JM, Georges B, Fourcade O et al (2007c) Assessment of renal function in clinical practice at the bedside of burn patients. Br J Clin Pharmacol 63:583–594

Conil JM, Georges B, Lavit M et al (2007d) Pharmacokinetics of ceftazidime and cefepime in burn patients: the importance of age and creatinine clearance. Int J Clin Pharmacol Ther 45: 529–538

Conil JM, Georges B, de Lussy A et al (2008) Ciprofloxacin use in critically ill patients: pharmacokinetic and pharmacodynamic approaches. Int J Antimicrob Agents 32:505–510

Craig W (1984) Pharmacokinetic and experimental data on beta-lactam antibiotics in the treatment of patients. Eur J Clin Microbiol 3:575–578

Craig WA (1998) Pharmacokinetic/pharmacodynamic parameters: rationale for antibacterial dosing of mice and men. Clin Infect Dis 26:1–10; quiz 11–12

Craig WA (2001) Does the dose matter? Clin Infect Dis 33(Suppl 3):S233–S237

Craig WA (2003) Basic pharmacodynamics of antibacterials with clinical applications to the use of beta-lactams, glycopeptides, and linezolid. Infect Dis Clin North Am 17:479–501

Cruciani M, Gatti G, Lazzarini L et al (1996) Penetration of vancomycin into human lung tissue. J Antimicrob Chemother 38:865–869

Dailly E, Kergueris MF, Pannier M et al (2003) Population pharmacokinetics of imipenem in burn patients. Fundam Clin Pharmacol 17:645–650

Dailly E, Le Floch R, Deslandes G et al (2008) Influence of glomerular filtration rate on the clearance of vancomycin administered by continuous infusion in burn patients. Int J Antimicrob Agents 31:537–539

Day NP, Phu NH, Mai NT et al (2000) Effects of dopamine and epinephrine infusions on renal hemodynamics in severe malaria and severe sepsis. Crit Care Med 28:1353–1362

Del Favero A, Patoia L, Rosina R et al (1991) Pharmacokinetics and tolerability of teicoplanin in healthy volunteers after single increasing doses. Antimicrob Agents Chemother 35: 2551–2557

del Mar Fernandez de Gatta Garcia M, Revilla N, Calvo MV et al (2007) Pharmacokinetic/pharmacodynamic analysis of vancomycin in ICU patients. Intensive Care Med 33:279–285

Dellinger RP, Levy MM, Carlet JM et al (2008) Surviving Sepsis Campaign: international guidelines for management of severe sepsis and septic shock: 2008. Crit Care Med 36:296–327

Desjars P, Pinaud M, Bugnon D et al (1989) Norepinephrine therapy has no deleterious renal effects in human septic shock. Crit Care Med 17:426–429

Di Giantomasso D, May CN, Bellomo R (2002) Norepinephrine and vital organ blood flow. Intensive Care Med 28:1804–1809

Di Giantomasso D, May CN, Bellomo R (2003a) Norepinephrine and vital organ blood flow during experimental hyperdynamic sepsis. Intensive Care Med 29:1774–1781

Di Giantomasso D, May CN, Bellomo R (2003b) Vital organ blood flow during hyperdynamic sepsis. Chest 124:1053–1059

Di Giantomasso D, Bellomo R, May CN (2005) The haemodynamic and metabolic effects of epinephrine in experimental hyperdynamic septic shock. Intensive Care Med 31:454–462

Di Giantomasso D, Morimatsu H, Bellomo R et al (2006) Effect of low-dose vasopressin infusion on vital organ blood flow in the conscious normal and septic sheep. Anaesth Intensive Care 34:427–433

Dolton M, Xu H, Cheong E et al (2010) Vancomycin pharmacokinetics in patients with severe burn injuries. Burns 36(4):469–76, Epub 2009 Oct 28

Drusano GL (2003) Prevention of resistance: a goal for dose selection for antimicrobial agents. Clin Infect Dis 36:S42–S50

Dunser MW, Ruokonen E, Pettila V et al (2009) Association of arterial blood pressure and vaso-pressor load with septic shock mortality: a post hoc analysis of a multicenter trial. Crit Care 13:R181

Fernandez de Gatta MM, Fruns I, Hernandez JM et al (1993) Vancomycin pharmacokinetics and dosage requirements in hematologic malignancies. Clin Pharm 12:515–520

Finfer S, Bellomo R, Lipman J et al (2004) Adult-population incidence of severe sepsis in Australian and New Zealand intensive care units. Intensive Care Med 30:589–596

Finfer S, Bellomo R, McEvoy S et al (2006) Effect of baseline serum albumin concentration on outcome of resuscitation with albumin or saline in patients in intensive care units: analysis of data from the saline versus albumin fluid evaluation (SAFE) study. BMJ 333:1044

Forrest A, Nix DE, Ballow CH et al (1993) Pharmacodynamics of intravenous ciprofloxacin in seriously ill patients. Antimicrob Agents Chemother 37:1073–1081

Fuster-Lluch O, Geronimo-Pardo M, Peyro-Garcia R et al (2008) Glomerular hyperfiltration and albuminuria in critically ill patients. Anaesth Intensive Care 36:674–680

Garrelts JC, Jost G, Kowalsky SF et al (1996) Ciprofloxacin pharmacokinetics in burn patients. Antimicrob Agents Chemother 40:1153–1156

Gentry-Nielsen MJ, Olsen KM, Preheim LC (2002) Pharmacodynamic activity and efficacy of linezolid in a rat model of pneumococcal pneumonia. Antimicrob Agents Chemother 46: 1345–1351

Georges B, Conil JM, Cougot P et al (2005) Cefepime in critically ill patients: continuous infusion vs. an intermittent dosing regimen. Int J Clin Pharmacol Ther 43:360–369

Goldstein A (1949) The interactions of drugs and plasma proteins. J Pharmacol Exp Ther 95(Pt. 2):102–165

Gomez CM, Cordingly JJ, Palazzo MG (1999) Altered pharmacokinetics of ceftazidime in criti-cally ill patients. Antimicrob Agents Chemother 43:1798–1802

Gous A, Lipman J, Scribante J et al (2005) Fluid shifts have no influence on ciprofloxacin pharma-cokinetics in intensive care patients with intra-abdominal sepsis. Int J Antimicrob Agents 26: 50–55

Graninger W, Zeitlinger M (2004) Clinical applications of levofloxacin for severe infections. Chemotherapy 50(Suppl 1):16–21

Gwilt PR, Smith RB (1986) Protein binding and pharmacokinetics of lincomycin following intra-venous administration of high doses. J Clin Pharmacol 26:87–90

Hanes SD, Wood GC, Herring V et al (2000) Intermittent and continuous ceftazidime infusion for critically ill trauma patients. Am J Surg 179:436–440

Herrera-Gutierrez ME, Seller-Perez G, Banderas-Bravo E et al (2007) Replacement of 24-h creatinine clearance by 2-h creatinine clearance in intensive care unit patients: a single-center study. Intensive Care Med 33:1900–1906

Higa GM, Murray WE (1987) Alterations in aminoglycoside pharmacokinetics in patients with cancer. Clin Pharm 6:963–966

Hoffken G, Lode H, Prinzing C et al (1985) Pharmacokinetics of ciprofloxacin after oral and parenteral administration. Antimicrob Agents Chemother 27:375–379

Holmes CL, Walley KR, Chittock DR et al (2001) The effects of vasopressin on hemodynamics and renal function in severe septic shock: a case series. Intensive Care Med 27:1416–1421

Hoste EA, Damen J, Vanholder RC et al (2005) Assessment of renal function in recently admitted critically ill patients with normal serum creatinine. Nephrol Dial Transplant 20: 747–753

Ibrahim EH, Sherman G, Ward S et al (2000) The influence of inadequate antimicrobial treatment of bloodstream infections on patient outcomes in the ICU setting. Chest 118:146–155

Ikawa K, Morikawa N, Ikeda K et al (2008) Pharmacokinetic-pharmacodynamic target attainment analysis of biapenem in adult patients: a dosing strategy. Chemotherapy 54:386–394

Ishikawa M, Nishioka M, Hanaki N et al (2006) Postoperative metabolic and circulatory responses in patients that express SIRS after major digestive surgery. Hepatogastroenterology 53:228–233

Joukhadar C, Klein N, Mayer BX et al (2002) Plasma and tissue pharmacokinetics of cefpirome in patients with sepsis. Crit Care Med 30:1478–1482

Joynt GM, Lipman J, Gomersall CD et al (2001) The pharmacokinetics of once-daily dosing of ceftriaxone in critically ill patients. J Antimicrob Chemother 47:421–429

Kashuba AD, Nafziger AN, Drusano GL et al (1999) Optimizing aminoglycoside therapy for nosocomial pneumonia caused by gram-negative bacteria. Antimicrob Agents Chemother 43:623–629

Kim KE, Onesti G, Ramirez O et al (1969) Creatinine clearance in renal disease. A reappraisal. Br Med J 4:11–14

Kim KE, Onesti G, Swartz C (1972) Creatinine clearance and glomerular filtration rate. Br Med J 1:379–380

Kitzes-Cohen R, Farin D, Piva G et al (2002) Pharmacokinetics and pharmacodynamics of meropenem in critically ill patients. Int J Antimicrob Agents 19:105–110

Knudsen JD, Fuursted K, Raber S et al (2000) Pharmacodynamics of glycopeptides in the mouse peritonitis model of Streptococcus pneumoniae or Staphylococcus aureus infection. Antimicrob Agents Chemother 44:1247–1254

Kohl BA, Deutschman CS (2006) The inflammatory response to surgery and trauma. Curr Opin Crit Care 12:325–332

Kollef MH, Sherman G, Ward S et al (1999) Inadequate antimicrobial treatment of infections: a risk factor for hospital mortality among critically ill patients. Chest 115:462–474

Kumar A, Roberts D, Wood KE et al (2006) Duration of hypotension before initiation of effective antimicrobial therapy is the critical determinant of survival in human septic shock. Crit Care Med 34:1589–1596

Lamoth F, Buclin T, Csajka C et al (2009) Reassessment of recommended imipenem doses in febrile neutropenic patients with hematological malignancies. Antimicrob Agents Chemother 53:785–787

Langenberg C, Wan L, Egi M et al (2006) Renal blood flow in experimental septic acute renal failure. Kidney Int 69:1996–2002

Larsson AJ, Walker KJ, Raddatz JK et al (1996) The concentration-independent effect of monoexponential and biexponential decay in vancomycin concentrations on the killing of Staphylococcus aureus under aerobic and anaerobic conditions. J Antimicrob Chemother 38:589–597

Latenser BA (2009) Critical care of the burn patient: the first 48 hours. Crit Care Med 37:2819–2826

Levey AS, Bosch JP, Lewis JB et al (1999) A more accurate method to estimate glomerular filtration rate from serum creatinine: a new prediction equation. Modification of Diet in Renal Disease Study Group. Ann Intern Med 130:461–470

Levy MM, Fink MP, Marshall JC et al (2003) 2001 SCCM/ESICM/ACCP/ATS/SIS International Sepsis Definitions Conference. Intensive Care Med 29:530–538

Li C, Kuti JL, Nightingale CH et al (2005) Population pharmacokinetics and pharmacodynamics of piperacillin/tazobactam in patients with complicated intra-abdominal infection. J Antimicrob Chemother 56:388–395

Lin J, Knight EL, Hogan ML et al (2003) A comparison of prediction equations for estimating glomerular filtration rate in adults without kidney disease. J Am Soc Nephrol 14:2573–2580

Lipman J, Scribante J, Gous AG et al (1998) Pharmacokinetic profiles of high-dose intravenous ciprofloxacin in severe sepsis. The Baragwanath Ciprofloxacin Study Group. Antimicrob Agents Chemother 42:2235–2239

Lipman J, Gomersall CD, Gin T et al (1999a) Continuous infusion ceftazidime in intensive care: a randomized controlled trial. J Antimicrob Chemother 43:309–311

Lipman J, Wallis SC, Rickard C (1999b) Low plasma cefepime levels in critically ill septic patients: pharmacokinetic modeling indicates improved troughs with revised dosing. Antimicrob Agents Chemother 43:2559–2561

Lipman J, Wallis SC, Rickard CM et al (2001) Low cefpirome levels during twice daily dosing in critically ill septic patients: pharmacokinetic modelling calls for more frequent dosing. Intensive Care Med 27:363–370

Lipman J, Wallis SC, Boots RJ (2003) Cefepime versus cefpirome: the importance of creatinine clearance. Anesth Analg 97:1149–1154; table of contents

Llopis-Salvia P, Jimenez-Torres NV (2006) Population pharmacokinetic parameters of vancomycin in critically ill patients. J Clin Pharm Ther 31:447–454

Lodise TP Jr, Lomaestro B, Drusano GL (2007) Piperacillin-tazobactam for Pseudomonas aeruginosa infection: clinical implications of an extended-infusion dosing strategy. Clin Infect Dis 44:357–363

Loirat P, Rohan J, Baillet A et al (1978) Increased glomerular filtration rate in patients with major burns and its effect on the pharmacokinetics of tobramycin. N Engl J Med 299: 915–919

Lorente L, Lorenzo L, Martin MM et al (2006) Meropenem by continuous versus intermittent infusion in ventilator-associated pneumonia due to gram-negative bacilli. Ann Pharmacother 40:219–223

Lorente L, Jimenez A, Palmero S et al (2007) Comparison of clinical cure rates in adults with ventilator-associated pneumonia treated with intravenous ceftazidime administered by continuous or intermittent infusion: a retrospective, nonrandomized, open-label, historical chart review. Clin Ther 29:2433–2439

Lorente L, Jimenez A, Martin MM et al (2009) Clinical cure of ventilator-associated pneumonia treated with piperacillin/tazobactam administered by continuous or intermittent infusion. Int J Antimicrob Agents 33:464–468

Lortholary O, Tod M, Rizzo N et al (1996) Population pharmacokinetic study of teicoplanin in severely neutropenic patients. Antimicrob Agents Chemother 40:1242–1247

Lortholary O, Lefort A, Tod M et al (2008) Pharmacodynamics and pharmacokinetics of antibacterial drugs in the management of febrile neutropenia. Lancet Infect Dis 8:612–620

Lovering AM, Vickery CJ, Watkin DS et al (1995) The pharmacokinetics of meropenem in surgical patients with moderate or severe infections. J Antimicrob Chemother 36:165–172

Lowdin E, Odenholt I, Cars O (1998) In vitro studies of pharmacodynamic properties of vancomycin against Staphylococcus aureus and Staphylococcus epidermidis. Antimicrob Agents Chemother 42:2739–2744

Lugo G, Castaneda-Hernandez G (1997) Relationship between hemodynamic and vital support measures and pharmacokinetic variability of amikacin in critically ill patients with sepsis. Crit Care Med 25:806–811

MacGowan AP (1998) Pharmacodynamics, pharmacokinetics, and therapeutic drug monitoring of glycopeptides. Ther Drug Monit 20:473–477

MacGowan AP (2003) Pharmacokinetic and pharmacodynamic profile of linezolid in healthy volunteers and patients with Gram-positive infections. J Antimicrob Chemother 51(Suppl 2): ii17–ii25

Marik PE, Lipman J, Kobilski S et al (1991a) A prospective randomized study comparing once- versus twice-daily amikacin dosing in critically ill adult and paediatric patients. J Antimicrob Chemother 28:753–764

Marik PE, Havlik I, Monteagudo FS et al (1991b) The pharmacokinetic of amikacin in critically ill adult and paediatric patients: comparison of once- versus twice-daily dosing regimens. J Antimicrob Chemother 27(Suppl C):81–89

Marin C, Eon B, Saux P et al (1990) Renal effects of norepinephrine used to treat septic shock patients. Crit Care Med 18:282–285

Martin JH, Fay MF, Ungerer JP (2009) eGFR–use beyond the evidence. Med J Aust 190: 197–199

Martin JH, Fay MF, Udy A et al (2010) Pitfalls of using estimations of glomerular filtration in an intensive care population. Intern Med J. doi:10.1111/j.1445-5994.2010.02160.x

McKinnon PS, Paladino JA, Schentag JJ (2008) Evaluation of area under the inhibitory curve (AUIC) and time above the minimum inhibitory concentration (T>MIC) as predictors of outcome for cefepime and ceftazidime in serious bacterial infections. Int J Antimicrob Agents 31:345–351

McNabb JJ, Nightingale CH, Quintiliani R et al (2001) Cost-effectiveness of ceftazidime by continuous infusion versus intermittent infusion for nosocomial pneumonia. Pharmacotherapy 21:549–555

Meagher AK, Ambrose PG, Grasela TH et al (2005a) Pharmacokinetic/pharmacodynamic profile for tigecycline-a new glycylcycline antimicrobial agent. Diagn Microbiol Infect Dis 52: 165–171

Meagher AK, Ambrose PG, Grasela TH et al (2005b) The pharmacokinetic and pharmacodynamic profile of tigecycline. Clin Infect Dis 41(Suppl 5):S333–S340

Mimoz O, Rolland D, Adoun M et al (2006) Steady-state trough serum and epithelial lining fluid concentrations of teicoplanin 12 mg/kg per day in patients with ventilator-associated pneumonia. Intensive Care Med 32:775–779

Mohr JF 3rd, Ostrosky-Zeichner L, Wainright DJ et al (2008) Pharmacokinetic evaluation of single-dose intravenous daptomycin in patients with thermal burn injury. Antimicrob Agents Chemother 52:1891–1893

Moise-Broder PA, Forrest A, Birmingham MC et al (2004) Pharmacodynamics of vancomycin and other antimicrobials in patients with Staphylococcus aureus lower respiratory tract infections. Clin Pharmacokinet 43:925–942

Moore RD, Lietman PS, Smith CR (1987) Clinical response to aminoglycoside therapy: importance of the ratio of peak concentration to minimal inhibitory concentration. J Infect Dis 155:93–99

Mouton JW, den Hollander JG (1994) Killing of Pseudomonas aeruginosa during continuous and intermittent infusion of ceftazidime in an in vitro pharmacokinetic model. Antimicrob Agents Chemother 38:931–936

Mouton JW, Vinks AA (2005) Pharmacokinetic/pharmacodynamic modelling of antibacterials in vitro and in vivo using bacterial growth and kill kinetics: the minimum inhibitory concentration versus stationary concentration. Clin Pharmacokinet 44:201–210

Mouton JW, Vinks AA, Punt NC (1997) Pharmacokinetic-pharmacodynamic modeling of activity of ceftazidime during continuous and intermittent infusion. Antimicrob Agents Chemother 41:733–738

Mueller SC, Henkel KO, Neumann J et al (1999) Perioperative antibiotic prophylaxis in maxillo-facial surgery: penetration of clindamycin into various tissues. J Craniomaxillofac Surg 27: 172–176

Muralidharan G, Micalizzi M, Speth J et al (2005) Pharmacokinetics of tigecycline after single and multiple doses in healthy subjects. Antimicrob Agents Chemother 49:220–229

Nakashima M, Uematsu T, Kosuge K et al (1995) Single- and multiple-dose pharmacokinetics of AM-1155, a new 6-fluoro-8-methoxy quinolone, in humans. Antimicrob Agents Chemother 39:2635–2640

Nicolau DP (2003) Optimizing outcomes with antimicrobial therapy through pharmacodynamic profiling. J Infect Chemother 9:292–296

Nicolau DP, McNabb J, Lacy MK et al (2001) Continuous versus intermittent administration of ceftazidime in intensive care unit patients with nosocomial pneumonia. Int J Antimicrob Agents 17:497–504

Nix DE, Spivey JM, Norman A et al (1992) Dose-ranging pharmacokinetic study of ciprofloxacin after 200-, 300-, and 400-mg intravenous doses. Ann Pharmacother 26:8–10

Noel G, Strauss R, Shah A et al (2008) Poster K-486. Ceftobiprole versus Ceftazidime combined with Linezolid for Treatment of Patients with Noscomial Pneumonia. 48th Interscience Conference on Antimicrobial Agents and Chemotherapy & 46th Infectious Diseases Society of America Joint Scientific Meeting, October 25-28, Washington, USA

Nuytinck HK, Offermans XJ, Kubat K et al (1988) Whole-body inflammation in trauma patients. An autopsy study. Arch Surg 123:1519–1524

Nyhlen A, Ljungberg B, Nilsson-Ehle I (2001) Pharmacokinetics of ceftazidime in febrile neutropenic patients. Scand J Infect Dis 33:222–226

Olsen KM, Rudis MI, Rebuck JA et al (2004) Effect of once-daily dosing vs. multiple daily dosing of tobramycin on enzyme markers of nephrotoxicity. Crit Care Med 32:1678–1682

Orlando R, Floreani M, Padrini R et al (1998) Determination of inulin clearance by bolus intravenous injection in healthy subjects and ascitic patients: equivalence of systemic and renal clearances as glomerular filtration markers. Br J Clin Pharmacol 46:605–609

Ott L, McClain CJ, Gillespie M et al (1994) Cytokines and metabolic dysfunction after severe head injury. J Neurotrauma 11:447–472

Pankuch GA, Jacobs MR, Appelbaum PC (2003) Postantibiotic effects of daptomycin against 14 staphylococcal and pneumococcal clinical isolates. Antimicrob Agents Chemother 47: 3012–3014

Parikh CR, Devarajan P (2008) New biomarkers of acute kidney injury. Crit Care Med 36: S159–S165

Parrillo JE (1993) Pathogenetic mechanisms of septic shock. N Engl J Med 328:1471–1477

Parrillo JE, Parker MM, Natanson C et al (1990) Septic shock in humans. Advances in the understanding of pathogenesis, cardiovascular dysfunction, and therapy. Ann Intern Med 113: 227–242

Pea F, Porreca L, Baraldo M et al (2000) High vancomycin dosage regimens required by intensive care unit patients cotreated with drugs to improve haemodynamics following cardiac surgical procedures. J Antimicrob Chemother 45:329–335

Pea F, Di Qual E, Cusenza A et al (2003a) Pharmacokinetics and pharmacodynamics of intravenous levofloxacin in patients with early-onset ventilator-associated pneumonia. Clin Pharmacokinet 42:589–598

Pea F, Brollo L, Viale P et al (2003b) Teicoplanin therapeutic drug monitoring in critically ill patients: a retrospective study emphasizing the importance of a loading dose. J Antimicrob Chemother 51:971–975

Pea F, Viale P, Candoni A et al (2004) Teicoplanin in patients with acute leukaemia and febrile neutropenia: a special population benefiting from higher dosages. Clin Pharmacokinet 43: 405–415

Pea F, Furlanut M, Negri C et al (2009) Prospectively validated dosing nomograms for maximizing the pharmacodynamics of vancomycin administered by continuous infusion in the critically ill patients: the Optivanco study. Antimicrob Agents Chemother 53(5):1863–7, Epub 2009 Feb 17

Petersen PJ, Jacobus NV, Weiss WJ et al (1999) In vitro and in vivo antibacterial activities of a novel glycylcycline, the 9-t-butylglycylamido derivative of minocycline (GAR-936). Antimicrob Agents Chemother 43:738–744

Piscitelli SC, Danziger LH, Rodvold KA (1992) Clarithromycin and azithromycin: new macrolide antibiotics. Clin Pharm 11:137–152

Poggio ED, Nef PC, Wang X et al (2005a) Performance of the Cockcroft-Gault and modification of diet in renal disease equations in estimating GFR in ill hospitalized patients. Am J Kidney Dis 46:242–252

Poggio ED, Wang X, Greene T et al (2005b) Performance of the modification of diet in renal disease and Cockcroft-Gault equations in the estimation of GFR in health and in chronic kidney disease. J Am Soc Nephrol 16:459–466

Preston SL, Drusano GL, Berman AL et al (1998) Pharmacodynamics of levofloxacin: a new paradigm for early clinical trials. JAMA 279:125–129

Prins JM, Buller HR, Kuijper EJ et al (1993) Once versus thrice daily gentamicin in patients with serious infections. Lancet 341:335–339

Rea RS, Capitano B, Bies R et al (2008) Suboptimal aminoglycoside dosing in critically ill patients. Ther Drug Monit 30:674–681

Rebuck JA, Fish DN, Abraham E (2002) Pharmacokinetics of intravenous and oral levofloxacin in critically ill adults in a medical intensive care unit. Pharmacotherapy 22:1216–1225

Redl-Wenzl EM, Armbruster C, Edelmann G et al (1993) The effects of norepinephrine on hemodynamics and renal function in severe septic shock states. Intensive Care Med 19:151–154

Rello J, Sole-Violan J, Sa-Borges M et al (2005) Pneumonia caused by oxacillin-resistant Staphylococcus aureus treated with glycopeptides. Crit Care Med 33:1983–1987

Rice TW, Bernard GR (2005) Therapeutic intervention and targets for sepsis. Annu Rev Med 56:225–248

Rivers E, Nguyen B, Havstad S et al (2001) Early goal-directed therapy in the treatment of severe sepsis and septic shock. N Engl J Med 345:1368–1377

Roberts JA, Lipman J (2006) Antibacterial dosing in intensive care: pharmacokinetics, degree of disease and pharmacodynamics of sepsis. Clin Pharmacokinet 45:755–773

Roberts JA, Lipman J (2007) Optimizing use of beta-lactam antibiotics in the critically ill. Semin Respir Crit Care Med 28:579–585

Roberts JA, Paratz J, Paratz E et al (2007a) Continuous infusion of beta-lactam antibiotics in severe infections: a review of its role. Int J Antimicrob Agents 30:11–18

Roberts JA, Boots R, Rickard CM et al (2007b) Is continuous infusion ceftriaxone better than once-a-day dosing in intensive care? A randomized controlled pilot study. J Antimicrob Chemother 59:285–291

Roberts JA, Kruger P, Paterson DL et al (2008) Antibiotic resistance–what's dosing got to do with it? Crit Care Med 36:2433–2440

Roberts JA, Kirkpatrick CM, Roberts MS et al (2009a) Meropenem dosing in critically ill patients with sepsis and without renal dysfunction: intermittent bolus versus continuous administration? Monte Carlo dosing simulations and subcutaneous tissue distribution. J Antimicrob Chemother 64(1):142–150, Epub 2009 Apr 27

Roberts JA, Roberts MS, Robertson TA et al (2009b) Piperacillin penetration into tissue of critically ill patients with sepsis–bolus versus continuous administration? Crit Care Med 37:926–933

Roberts JA, Webb SA, Paterson DL et al (2009c) A systematic review on clinical benefits of continuous administration of beta-lactam antibiotics. Crit Care Med 37:2071–2078

Romano S, Fdez de Gatta MM, Calvo MV et al (1999) Population pharmacokinetics of amikacin in patients with haematological malignancies. J Antimicrob Chemother 44:235–242

Roos JF, Lipman J, Kirkpatrick CM (2007) Population pharmacokinetics and pharmacodynamics of cefpirome in critically ill patients against gram-negative bacteria. Intensive Care Med 33:781–788

Rule AD, Larson TS, Bergstralh EJ et al (2004) Using serum creatinine to estimate glomerular filtration rate: accuracy in good health and in chronic kidney disease. Ann Intern Med 141:929–937

Rybak MJ (2006) The pharmacokinetic and pharmacodynamic properties of vancomycin. Clin Infect Dis 42(Suppl 1):S35–S39

Safdar N, Andes D, Craig WA (2004) In vivo pharmacodynamic activity of daptomycin. Antimicrob Agents Chemother 48:63–68

Schentag JJ (1999) Antimicrobial action and pharmacokinetics/pharmacodynamics: the use of AUIC to improve efficacy and avoid resistance. J Chemother 11:426–439

Schriever CA, Fernandez C, Rodvold KA et al (2005) Daptomycin: a novel cyclic lipopeptide antimicrobial. Am J Health Syst Pharm 62:1145–1158

Sevillano D, Alou L, Aguilar L et al (2006) Azithromycin iv pharmacodynamic parameters predicting Streptococcus pneumoniae killing in epithelial lining fluid versus serum: an in vitro pharmacodynamic simulation. J Antimicrob Chemother 57:1128–1133

Shikuma LR, Ackerman BH, Weaver RH et al (1990a) Effects of treatment and the metabolic response to injury on drug clearance: a prospective study with piperacillin. Crit Care Med 18:37–41

Shikuma LR, Ackerman BH, Weaver RH et al (1990b) Thermal injury effects on drug disposition: a prospective study with piperacillin. J Clin Pharmacol 30:632–637

Shipley RE, Study RS (1951) Changes in renal blood flow, extraction of inulin, glomerular filtration rate, tissue pressure and urine flow with acute alterations of renal artery blood pressure. Am J Physiol 167:676–688

Sladen RN, Endo E, Harrison T (1987) Two-hour versus 22-hour creatinine clearance in critically ill patients. Anesthesiology 67:1013–1016

Snider RD, Kruse JA, Bander JJ et al (1995) Accuracy of estimated creatinine clearance in obese patients with stable renal function in the intensive care unit. Pharmacotherapy 15:747–753

Stevens LA, Coresh J, Greene T et al (2006) Assessing kidney function–measured and estimated glomerular filtration rate. N Engl J Med 354:2473–2483

Sun HK, Kuti JL, Nicolau DP (2005) Pharmacodynamics of antimicrobials for the empirical treatment of nosocomial pneumonia: a report from the OPTAMA Program. Crit Care Med 33:2222–2227

Sunder-Plassmann G, Horl WH (2004) A critical appraisal for definition of hyperfiltration. Am J Kidney Dis 43:396; author reply 396–397

Tam VH, McKinnon PS, Akins RL et al (2003) Pharmacokinetics and pharmacodynamics of cefepime in patients with various degrees of renal function. Antimicrob Agents Chemother 47:1853–1861

Thallinger C, Buerger C, Plock N et al (2008) Effect of severity of sepsis on tissue concentrations of linezolid. J Antimicrob Chemother 61:173–176

Thomas DM, Coles GA, Williams JD (1994) What does the renal reserve mean? Kidney Int 45:411–416

Thomas JK, Forrest A, Bhavnani SM et al (1998) Pharmacodynamic evaluation of factors associated with the development of bacterial resistance in acutely ill patients during therapy. Antimicrob Agents Chemother 42:521–527

Toschlog EA, Blount KP, Rotondo MF et al (2003) Clinical predictors of subtherapeutic aminoglycoside levels in trauma patients undergoing once-daily dosing. J Trauma 55:255–260; discussion 260–252

Turnidge JD (1998) The pharmacodynamics of beta-lactams. Clin Infect Dis 27:10–22

Udy A, Boots R, Senthuran S et al (2010a) Augmented creatinine clearance in traumatic brain injury. Anesth Analg 111:1505–1510

Udy AA, Putt MT, Shanmugathasan S et al (2010b) Augmented renal clearance in the Intensive Care Unit: an illustrative case series. Int J Antimicrob Agents. doi:10.1016/j.ijantimicag.2010.02.013

Udy AA, Roberts JA, Boots RJ et al (2010c) Augmented renal clearance: implications for antibacterial dosing in the critically ill. Clin Pharmacokinet 49:1–16

Valdes ME, Landau SE, Shah DM et al (1979) Increased glomerular filtration rate following mannitol administration in man. J Surg Res 26:473–477

Van Dalen R, Vree T, Baars IM (1987) Influence of protein binding and severity of illness on renal elimination of four cephalosporin drugs in intensive-care patients. Pharm Weekbl Sci 9:98–103

Vogelman BS, Craig WA (1985) Postantibiotic effects. J Antimicrob Chemother 15(Suppl A):37–46

Vogelman B, Craig WA (1986) Kinetics of antimicrobial activity. J Pediatr 108:835–840

Wan L, Bellomo R, May CN (2007) The effects of normal and hypertonic saline on regional blood flow and oxygen delivery. Anesth Analg 105:141–147

Wilson AP (2000) Clinical pharmacokinetics of teicoplanin. Clin Pharmacokinet 39:167–183

Wysocki M, Delatour F, Faurisson F et al (2001) Continuous versus intermittent infusion of vancomycin in severe Staphylococcal infections: prospective multicenter randomized study. Antimicrob Agents Chemother 45:2460–2467

Young RJ, Lipman J, Gin T et al (1997) Intermittent bolus dosing of ceftazidime in critically ill patients. J Antimicrob Chemother 40:269–273

How do I Adjust Antimicrobial Daily Dosage in Patients with MODS? A Pharmacist's Contribution

13

Marta Ulldemolins and Jason A. Roberts

13.1 Introduction

Treatment of severe infections remains a daily challenge to clinicians. Added to the reduced susceptibilities of nosocomial pathogens, the natural complexity of the critically ill patient makes antimicrobial choice and dosing particularly difficult (Roberts and Lipman 2009). In this situation, the effectiveness of the therapeutic armamentarium is frequently compromised. Recent data describe an escalation of the incidence of bacteria and fungi that are resistant to the available antimicrobials (Spellberg et al. 2008), and the dearth of antimicrobial drugs with new mechanisms of action in the pipeline (source: Pharmaceutical Research and Manufactures of America) make it vital that we use presently available antimicrobials appropriately in order to extend their life. One of the essential components for the optimization of antimicrobial use is dosing, because of the causal relationship that is thought to

M. Ulldemolins
Critical Care Department, Vall d'Hebron University Hospital;
Institut de Recerca Vall d'Hebron-Universitat Autònoma de Barcelona (UAB),
Barcelona, Spain

Centro de Investigación Biomédica En Red de Enfermedades Respiratorias (CIBERES),
Madrid, Spain

J.A. Roberts (✉)
Department of Intensive Care Medicine, Royal Brisbane and Women's Hospital,
Herston, Brisbane, QLD, Australia

Burns, Trauma and Critical Care Research Centre, The University of Queensland,
Herston, Brisbane, QLD, Australia

Pharmacy Department, Royal Brisbane and Women's Hospital,
Herston, Brisbane, QLD, Australia

Burns, Trauma and Critical Care Research Centre, Royal Brisbane and Women's Hospital,
Herston, QLD, Australia
e-mail: j.roberts2@uq.edu.au

J. Rello (eds.), *Sepsis Management*,
DOI 10.1007/978-3-642-03519-7_13, © Springer-Verlag Berlin Heidelberg 2012

exist between inappropriate dosing and the development of bacterial resistance (Roberts et al. 2008). Moreover, optimization of antimicrobial dosing in critically ill patients is very relevant in terms of clinical outcomes, as early and appropriate antimicrobial therapy has been sufficiently demonstrated to be the most effective intervention for reducing mortality (Garnacho-Montero et al. 2003; Kollef et al. 1999; Kumar et al. 2006; Rello et al. 1997). Therefore, optimization of antimicrobial dosing is a significant priority in the clinical management of severe infections in critically ill patients in the intensive care unit (ICU).

Multiple organ dysfunction syndrome (MODS) occurs as a severe worsening in the physiology of patients with severe infections and systemic inflammation response syndrome (SIRS). MODS is defined by consensus as the worsening of organ function in critically ill patients such that homeostasis cannot be maintained without clinical intervention, frequently involving two or more organ systems (American College of Chest Physicians/Society of Critical Care Medicine 1992). The impact of MODS on antimicrobial dose requirements is significant, as the syndrome itself, in concert with aggressive medical management, is likely to produce significant variations in the volume of distribution (Vd) and clearance (CL) of antimicrobials (Roberts and Lipman 2009). Therefore, a detailed understanding of the triumvirate of patient, antimicrobial and disease state are required for dose individualization. This component of an antimicrobial use optimization program could be ideally governed by an ICU pharmacist, whose function would be, among other tasks, to give support on antimicrobial dose adjustments. Such interventions would complement the other activities of the infection management working group composed of intensivists, microbiologists and infectious disease specialists.

The contribution of the ICU pharmacist in the care of critically ill patients with community-acquired infections, hospital-acquired infections and sepsis has been demonstrated to impact positively in clinical outcomes, length of hospital stay and hospital resource utilization (MacLaren et al. 2008). Hence, it is advisable to include an ICU pharmacist as a member of the clinical team. In this chapter we aim to review the contribution of ICU pharmacists to the optimization of antimicrobial use in patients with MODS. This chapter aims to emphasize the bases for dose adjustments in terms of disease-driven variations in antimicrobial pharmacokinetics and pharmacokinetics/ pharmacodynamics and in terms of the physicochemical properties of the selected antimicrobial. We will provide dose recommendations with the objective of optimizing both initial and maintenance dosing of antimicrobials in critically ill patients with MODS.

13.2 Physicochemical Properties of Antimicrobials

The concept "antimicrobial" includes a wide range of families of compounds that exhibit great differences between them in terms of their physicochemical properties. These properties can be crucial determinants of the distribution and elimination processes in a patient. The uniqueness of each class of antimicrobial makes independent study essential to provide accurate characterization of antimicrobial behavior.

Antimicrobials are usually classified, from a chemical perspective, by water affinity. The partition coefficient for octanol/water describes the degree of water

Table 13.1 Antimicrobials commonly used in the ICU classified by affinity for water

Hydrophilic antimicrobials	Lipophilic antimicrobials[a]
β-lactams (penicillins, cephalosporins, carbapenems, monobactams)	Macrolides
Glycopeptides	Fluoroquinolones
Aminoglycosides	Tetracyclines and tigecycline
Polymixins	Daptomycin (amphiphilic)
Daptomycin (amphiphilic)	Rifampicin
Linezolid	Fusidic Acid
	Pentamidine
	Metronidazole
	Lincosamides
	Triazoles
	Echinocandins
	Sulfamethoxazole-trimethoprim

[a]The level of lipophilicity and Vd of these compounds can vary significantly

affinity, or hydrophilicity, of a compound, allowing their classification as either hydrophilic or lipophilic. Table 13.1 classifies the most commonly used antimicrobial classes in the ICU according to their physicochemical properties.

The distribution of antimicrobials within and elimination from the body are affected heavily by the chemical properties of the antimicrobial. For example, hydrophilic antimicrobials have a distribution in line with extracellular water and generally penetrate into tissues with high water content, including intravascular fluid, extravascular (but not intracellular) water and muscle tissue. However, hydrophilic antimicrobials are unable to significantly cross lipid membranes and, therefore, do not distribute intracellularly or into adipose tissue. Their volume of distribution (Vd) is, hence, almost equivalent to the extracellular water (ECW), which usually corresponds to a value between 0.1 and 0.3 L/kg (Roberts and Lipman 2009).

Lipophilic drugs can dissolve across the lipid cellular membranes and therefore reach the intracellular compartment in significant concentrations. As a result, lipophilic antimicrobials distribute into the total body water (TBW) and lipid tissues, such as adipose tissue. The Vd of lipophilic drugs depends on the level of lipophilicty of the compound, with very lipophilic compounds having highly significant sequestration into lipid tissue, giving them a very high Vd. Other compounds that are not as lipophilic will have a decreased sequestration into lipid tissue, giving them a smaller Vd, but still significantly larger than that observed with hydrophilic antimicrobials. (Roberts and Lipman 2009).

13.3   Overview of Clinical Pharmacokinetics

Pharmacokinetics is the study of the dose of drug administered to its concentration in plasma and tissues (Rowland and Tozer 1995). The principal pharmacokinetic parameters are summarized below and include:

- C_{max}: peak concentration achieved after a single dose.
- t_{max}: time after administration when C_{max} is achieved.

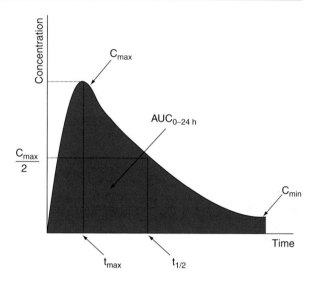

- *Volume of distribution (Vd)*: apparent volume of fluid that contains the total drug dose administered at the same concentration as in plasma.
- *Clearance (CL)*: quantifies the irreversible loss of drug from the body by metabolism and/or excretion. Is an apparent measure of the volume of plasma cleared of drug per unit time.
- *Elimination half-life ($t_{1/2}$)*: time required for the plasma concentration to fall by one-half. Half-life is a parameter derived from both clearance and volume of distribution.
- *Protein binding*: extent to which the drug binds to plasma proteins (mainly albumin and α_1- acid glycoprotein). This binding is an equilibrium that depends on the drug-protein affinity, drug concentration and protein concentration.
- AUC_{0-24h}: total Area Under the concentration-time Curve over a 24-h period. AUC_{0-24h} is calculated from the integration of the concentration/time function and provides information about drug exposure.

  Figure 13.1 represents a plasmatic concentration-time curve of a drug administered by bolus. Some of the pharmacokinetic parameters described above are marked in the graph.

13.4 Overview of Pharmacodynamics and Pharmacokinetics-Pharmacodynamics

Pharmacodynamics is the study of the relationship between drug concentration and pharmacological effect (Rowland and Tozer 1995). The study of pharmacodynamics, however, is very difficult to perform, as the determination of the drug concentration at the target site (such as the site of the infection) can be very difficult to obtain. It follows that the pharmacokinetic/pharmacodynamic approach was designed to bridge the gap between pharmacokinetics and pharmacodynamics, and seeks a relationship

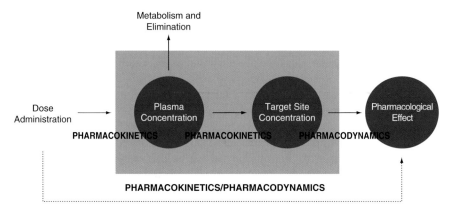

Fig. 13.2 Interrelationship among pharmacokinetics, pharmacodynamics and pharmacokinetics-pharmacodynamics

between dose and pharmacological effect (Rowland and Tozer 1995). Figure 13.2 illustrates the relationship among these three concepts.

Focusing on antimicrobials, the pharmacokinetic/pharmacodynamic indices associated with optimal activity are (Craig 1998):

$f_{T>MIC}$: time in a dosing interval that the free (unbound) concentration of the antimicrobial in plasma exceeds the minimum inhibitory concentration (MIC) of the bacteria.

C_{max}/MIC: ratio between the peak free concentration and the MIC of the bacteria.

AUC_{0-24}/MIC: ratio between the area under the concentration-time curve (free concentrations) during a 24-h period and the MIC of the bacteria.

Pharmacokinetics/pharmacodynamics classifies antimicrobials into three classes depending on the pharmacodynamic index that describes optimal bacterial killing activity (Craig 1998) for the drug class:

Time-dependent antimicrobials: the optimal killing activity is achieved when plasma concentrations are maintained above the MIC of the bacteria for a defined fraction of the dosing interval ($f_{T>MIC}$).

Concentration-dependent antimicrobials: the optimal killing activity is correlated with the magnitude of the peak achieved, quantified by the ratio between the C_{max} and the MIC (C_{max}/MIC).

Concentration-dependent antimicrobials with time-dependence: a defined AUC_{0-24}/MIC ratio is correlated with optimal killing activity.

13.5   Clinical Scenarios in MODS Likely to Affect Drug Vd and CL

MODS derived from a septic insult is dependent on alterations in hemodynamic homeostasis. Hypovolemia and cardiovascular depression leading to tissue hypoxia are the main phenomena that lead ultimately to a dysfunction of many organ systems (Jones and Puskarich 2009). Endotoxins from the lipopolysaccharide of microorganisms produce a proinflammatory effect on the vascular endothelium by inducing the production of endogenous molecules. This leads to vasodilatation and transcapillary leakage of fluid and plasma proteins (such as albumin) from the intravascular to the extravascular space (Fleck et al. 1985; van der Poll 2001). The hemodynamic insufficiency leads to tissue and organ hypoperfusion, which may result in myocardial dysfunction (Thijs et al. 1990). Altered perfusion of tissues and eliminating organs (e.g., kidney, liver) can compromise the processes of distribution and elimination of a drug and therefore impact on its pharmacological effect. As antimicrobials can be considered a group of drugs with "silent" pharmacodynamics, where it is almost impossible to identify pharmacological effect in "real time," knowledge of likely concentrations at the site of infection is essential for maximizing microbial killing. Therefore, consideration of the scenarios likely to vary antimicrobial concentrations and dosage requirements because of altered Vd and CL is necessary for optimization of antimicrobial therapy.

Below we have detailed the main scenarios likely to affect pharmacokinetics.

13.5.1 Tissue Hypoperfusion

Tissue hypoperfusion is a consequence of the sepsis-mediated maldistribution of blood flow, leading to perfusion of "vital" organs (i.e., brain or lung) to the detriment of peripheral tissues (e.g., subcutaneous or muscular tissue) (Jones and Puskarich 2009). Tissue hypoperfusion significantly compromises antimicrobial distribution, which is especially relevant as peripheral tissues are frequently the source of infection (Ryan 1993). It follows that failure to attain therapeutic antimicrobial concentrations is likely to lead to therapeutic failure and development of bacterial resistance (Joukhadar et al. 2001; Roberts et al. 2008). In this case, the results of some studies that evaluate tissue penetration of β-lactams in continuous infusion versus intermittent bolus would suggest that continuous or extended infusions would achieve more consistent antimicrobial concentrations in tissues and should be considered when treating infections by poorly susceptible bacteria (Roberts et al. 2009a, b).

13.5.2 Gastrointestinal Dysfunction

Impaired gastrointestinal (GI) absorption is a collateral effect of cardiovascular depression-related hypoperfusion that results in decreased absorption of nutrition and enterally administered drugs (Heyland et al. 1996; Singh et al. 1994). This phenomenon has been well described in critically ill patients (Heyland et al. 1996). Another group of patients that exhibits considerable degrees of GI dysfunction is post-thoracic surgery patients (Paul et al. 2009), whereby enteral administration of the antimicrobial may be ineffective because of poor absorption, in which case intravenous administration should be preferred.

13.5.3 Renal Dysfunction

Several clinical scenarios and drugs can precipitate acute kidney injury (AKI) in critically ill patients (Pannu and Nadim 2008; Wan et al. 2008). Regardless of the cause, early identification of AKI and accurate assessment of renal function are essential for dose adjustment of antimicrobials, or their metabolites, that are predominantly renally cleared.

As renal function worsens, homeostasis cannot be maintained, and waste metabolic products accumulate in the bloodstream, with subsequent toxic effects. It follows then that prescription of renal replacement therapy (RRT) should be considered. The effect of RRT on drug clearance is extremely variable and heavily dependent on many factors related to the patient, the drug and the dialysis settings prescribed (Joynt et al. 2001).

13.5.4 Hepatic Dysfunction

Hepatic dysfunction may appear in critically ill patients with severe sepsis because of tissue hypoperfusion itself or the administration of hepatotoxic drugs, such as rifampicin (Marshall 2001). Hepatic damage can impair the metabolic capacity of this organ, which can lead to the accumulation of hepatically cleared antimicrobials (Greenfield et al. 1983; Westphal and Brogard 1993). A decrease in the hepatic production of albumin and α_1-acid glycoprotein can also alter the pharmacokinetics of highly protein-bound antimicrobials, producing increases in Vd and CL and, therefore, different dose requirements in this scenario (Barbot et al. 2003; Barre et al. 1987; Burkhardt et al. 2007; Joynt et al. 2001). The effect of hypoproteinemia on the excretion of renally cleared antimicrobials has to be considered when dosing hydrophilic antimicrobials.

13.6   Measurement of Vd and CL

13.6.1 Measurement of Vd

The estimation of Vd can be undertaken using tests that provide information about body composition. Therefore, for lipophilic drugs it is important to measure the amount of adipose tissue with consideration of the octanol/water coefficient (or published Vd data), whereas for hydrophilic drugs, estimation of the extracellular body water (EBW) is required.

There are several techniques for estimating the intravascular, intracellular and extra-cellular body water (EBW), and therefore the Vd of hydrophilic and lipophilic drugs:

Sodium bromide (NaBr) test: when NaBr is administered, the ion Br– distributes deeply into the extracellular fluid but is unable to penetrate the cells. The determination of the peak concentration allows calculating the EBW (Miller et al. 1989).

Total body bioelectrical impedance: allows the measurement of EBW and TBW depending on the frequency of the bioelectrical impedance waves. Low-frequency bioelectrical impedance waves cannot penetrate the cells, but are transmitted through the EBW and allow measurement of this parameter. On the other hand, at high frequencies, the bioelectrical current can penetrate all body tissues completely and flow through the extracellular and intracellular electrolyte solutions, giving then information about the TBW (Chumlea and Guo 1994).

Indocyanine green (ICG) test: ICG binds extensively to albumin in the bloodstream and due to the large volume of the complex with the protein is unable to distribute to extravascular water, being almost entirely cleared by the liver. The intravenous administration and monitoring of ICG pharmacokinetics in plasma gives information about intravascular volume and hepatic function (Jacob et al. 2007).

However, clinical use of these procedures is not available at the bedside and is mostly restricted to research purposes. The estimation of a drug's Vd by the clinicians is much more empirical, based on the nature and severity of sickness, fluid balance, individual patient characteristics (age, weight, height), clinical management and published data for the antimicrobial.

13.6.2 Measurement of CL

The estimation of CL in critically ill patients with MODS is dependent on the main organ responsible for drug metabolism and/or excretion to correlate the degree of organ dysfunction with the likely elimination rate. For renally excreted drugs, the performance of a 24-, 12- or 8-h urinary creatinine clearance has been demonstrated to be a suitable estimation of the glomerular filtration rate (GFR) (Pong et al. 2005; Wells and Lipman 1997). Other equations, such as the Cockroft-Gault or Modified Diet in Renal Disease (MDRD), are not appropriate as they are yet to be validated in critically ill patients (Cockroft and Gault 1976; Levey et al. 1999). A recent paper suggests that even a 2-h urinary CrCL can be used as a sufficient indicator of GFR (Herrera-Gutierrez et al. 2007). However, a urinary creatinine clearance collection is not useful when the patient has been prescribed RRT. The CL of hydrophilic drugs by RRT depends on many factors, mainly the modality and settings prescribed. Other factors that determine the extraction ratio are molecular weight (drugs with a molecular weight greater than the pores of the filter membrane cannot be removed by RRT), protein binding (only unbound molecules can be removed by RRT), drug affinity for adsorbing to the filter membrane, the "location" where replacement fluid is added to the circuit (either pre- or post-filter) and the ultrafiltration rate (Choi et al. 2009). Reference materials should be consulted for guidance on antimicrobial dose requirements during the form of RRT used at different institutions.

For hepatically cleared drugs, the estimation of the degree of liver dysfunction and its effects on drug metabolism and excretion is by the performance of static tests (serum activities of liver enzymes, albumin and coagulation factor hepatic synthesis and bilirubin levels) and/or dynamic tests (i.e., ICG, caffeine, bromosuphofthalein, galactose, $^{14}CO_2$ or lidocaine metabolite MEGX in serum tests) (Sakka 2007). Although easier, the use of static tests does not provide sufficient information on the influence of the degree of hepatic dysfunction on drug metabolism. Dynamic tests are related to the inner capacity of the liver to metabolize and eliminate different compounds, and provide a better insight on the functional status of the liver. Several dynamic tests exist that evaluate the hepatic clearance half-life, the elimination capacity and the metabolite formation as a surrogate to assess liver function (Sakka 2007). It is not within the scope of this chapter to refer to all of them, but the use of ICG and lidocaine metabolite MEGX tests would be more reliable and recommendable clinical tests, especially ICG due to its non-invasive and easy determination (Sakka 2007). However, as for the determination of CL, these tests are not available at real-time, and liver function is estimated empirically, based on static tests and the clinical presentation of the patient.

13.7   Optimizing Initial Dosing of Antimicrobials in MODS

Antimicrobials have complex dosing requirements because they have "silent" pharmacodynamics, which means that it is not possible to evaluate the clinical efficacy of treatment from moment to moment. Therefore, dosing titration based on clinical response is not possible, and appropriate dosing and inappropriate dosing appear clinically "the same" during initial dosing. It follows that it is crucial to ensure that individualized doses are prescribed to these patients according to their Vd and CL to ensure optimal treatment of the severe infections.

By pharmacokinetic principles, initial antimicrobial dosing must be driven by the predicted Vd. Due to a septic insult, Vd of hydrophilic drugs is frequently increased (even doubled) in critically ill patients, and dosing must be adjusted to compensate for this larger Vd (Roberts and Lipman 2006, 2009). The increased Vd results from aggressive fluid resuscitation, capillary leakage and fluid shifts into peripheral tissues (Plank and Hill 2000; van der Poll 2001). The larger extent of fluid distribution from the intravascular to the extravascular space creates an antimicrobial concentration gradient, causing increased antimicrobial movement from plasma into extravascular space and particularly peripheral tissues. Therefore, and perhaps paradoxically, patients with MODS will still require larger than standard initial dosing of hydrophilic antimicrobials to compensate for these increases in Vd and to ensure that timely therapeutic levels are achieved in the site of the infection. This has been recognized with the glycopeptide teicoplanin (Outman et al. 1990), but sparse data are available on other broadly used antimicrobials, such as β-lactams.

The case of lipophilic antimicrobials is quite different, as initial dosing must be guided by a chronic condition of the patient, i.e., amount of adipose tissue. In this scenario, total body weight should be considered for first day dosing, as patients with a higher proportion of adipose tissue will require larger than standard doses to achieve therapeutic concentrations (Allard et al. 1993). This is the same principle by which loading doses of other lipophilic drugs, such as amiodarone, are required

(Chow 1996; Richens 1979). Furthermore, in the case of obesity, there is evidence that supports that loading doses are required for even hydrophilic antimicrobials, as obesity is associated with an increase in the amount interstitial fluid, connective tissue and muscle mass (Bauer et al. 1983; Blouin et al. 1982). Nowadays, obesity is a very frequent condition in the ICU that must be considered for initial dosing, as larger than standard doses may be required. In this context, use of an equation that assists calculation of lean body weight should be used (Janmahasatian et al. 2005).

13.8 Optimizing Maintenance Dosing of Antimicrobials in MODS

By pharmacokinetic principles as well, maintenance dosing must be guided by predicted antimicrobial CL (Rowland and Tozer 1995). The previous section provides recommendations on how to estimate this CL depending on the organ system responsible for metabolism and/or elimination. In this section, we will individually consider the most relevant organ systems (mainly renal and hepatic systems) that may affect pharmacokinetics.

Figure 13.3 summarizes the scenarios likely to alter pharmacokinetics in MODS.

13.8.1 Renal Dysfunction

Hydrophilic antimicrobials are mainly cleared by the renal glomerular filtration and/or tubular secretion processes. Decreased drug clearance of these drugs is common in

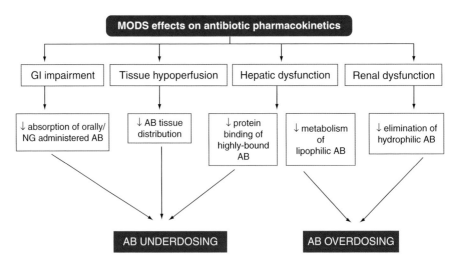

Fig. 13.3 Clinical scenarios frequently found in MODS that can produce variations in antimicrobial pharmacokinetics. *GI* gastrointestinal, *AB* antimicrobial, *NG* nasogastrically

renal failure, which necessitates dose reductions or extended dosing intervals to prevent drug accumulation and toxicity. This is especially important for drugs with narrow therapeutic ranges, such as glycopeptides and aminoglycosides (Gilbert et al. 2009). Use of therapeutic drug monitoring (TDM) should be used where possible as an effective strategy to maximize efficacy and prevent drug toxicity (Begg et al. 2001; MacGowan 1998). For antimicrobials where regular TDM "at the bedside" is not available, empirical dose reductions based on clinical evaluation of renal function are required.

For the purposes of dose reduction, it is useful to apply knowledge of antimicrobial pharmacodynamics to ensure attainment of pharmacodynamic targets. An example of this would be to reduce the dose rather than the frequency of administration for time-dependent antimicrobials as a strategy to preserve the $f_{T>MIC}$. On the contrary, for drugs like aminoglycosides with concentration-dependent activity, it is advisable to prolong the interval between doses rather than decreasing the dose and administer it with the usual frequency, which would also assist prevention of aminoglycoside-associated renal toxicity (Buijk et al. 2002; Roberts and Lipman 2009).

13.8.2 Renal Replacement Therapy (RRT)

The effects of RRT on hydrophilic antimicrobial CL are variable and heavily dependent on the modality and settings prescribed. Hemodialysis, hemofiltration, hemodiafiltration or peritoneal dialysis all have different mechanisms and can have different capacities for removing metabolic waste and drugs from the bloodstream. The implications of RRT on drug dosing have been recently reviewed (Choi et al. 2009), and due to space limitations are beyond the scope of this paper. However, Table 13.2 additionally provides some recommendations for dosing in RRT.

13.8.3 Hepatic Dysfunction

The liver is the primary organ system responsible for drug metabolism, and hepatic impairment can significantly impact on the CL of both lipophilic and hydrophilic drugs. Lipophilic drugs normally undergo phase I (mainly oxidation) and then phase II (mainly conjugation to hydrophilic molecules) metabolism in the liver to increase the hydrophilicity of the molecule to facilitate renal CL of the metabolites. Hepatic failure may compromise this capacity of the liver, leading to a decrease in the elimination and therefore accumulation and potential toxicity. Some examples of this phenomenon are nitroimidazole antimicrobials, extensively oxidized by the liver, where decreased CL has been observed in liver failure (Farrell et al. 1984), increasing the risk of toxicity (i.e., seizures, peripheral neuropathy). Similar dose reduction requirements apply for the triazole voriconazole, where mild to moderate hepatic failure (Child Pugh A and B) require 50% reductions in maintenance dosing. In this case, TDM is available in most of the institutions, and represents the gold standard to prevent accumulation and toxicity for triazole antifungals (Bruggemann et al. 2008).

Table 13.2 Principles for loading and maintenance dosing of antimicrobials in critically ill patients with MODS (Antibiotic Expert Group 2006; Donnelly et al. 2008; Roberts and Lipman 2009; MIMS Australia 2009)

Antimicrobial	Main organ systems responsible for CL	PD parameter associated with maximal activity	LD in patients with increased Vd	MD in acute kidney injury[a]	MD in hepatic failure[a]	MD dose in RRT[b]
β-lactams (i.e., penicillins, cephalosporins, carbapenems, monobactams)	Renal	$f_{T>MIC}$	Administer the standard MD for normal renal function as a LD on day 1	Reduce dose but maintain therapeutic interval where possible to maintain $f_{T>MIC}$	Normal dosing	Reduce dose but maintain therapeutic interval where possible to maintain $f_{T>MIC}$
Aminoglycosides	Renal	C_{max}/MIC	Administer a high dose (i.e., 7 mg/kg gentamicin) as a LD on day 1 to achieve a C_{max}/MIC ratio of 10	Monitor trough level (C_{min}) after 24 h aiming for levels <0.5 mg/L. Dosing q48h may be required for severe renal dysfunction	Normal dosing	Monitor trough level (C_{min}) after 24 h aiming for levels <0.5 mg/L and titrate dosing according to results
Glycopeptides	Renal	AUC_{0-24}/MIC	*Vancomycin:* 25–30 mg/kg LD *Teicoplanin:* 6 mg/kg q12h for 3 doses as LD	*Vancomycin:* Monitor trough level (C_{min}) on day 2 aiming for range 15–20 mg/L (20–25 mg/L if CI). Dosing must be titrated via TDM *Teicoplanin:* dose 3 mg/kg q12h from the 4th dose and titrate dosing on day 4 guided by TDM, aiming for C_{min} >10 mg/L	Normal dosing	*Vancomycin:* Monitor trough level (C_{min}) on day 3 aiming for range 15–20 mg/L (20–25 mg/L if CI). Dosing should be titrated to this range *Teicoplanin:* dose 3 mg/kg q12h from the 4th dose and titrate dosing on day 4 guided by TDM, aiming for C_{min} >10 mg/L

	Elimination	PK/PD index				
Fluoroquinolones	Renal and hepatic (ciprofloxacin, moxifloxacin), renal (levofloxacin)	AUC_{0-24}/MIC and C_{max}/MIC	Ciprofloxacin: 400 mg q8h on day 1; Levofloxacin: 500–750 mg q24h on day 1; Moxifloxacin: 400 mg q24h	Ciprofloxacin: 400 mg q12–24 h; Levofloxacin: 250 mg q24–48 h; Moxifloxacin: 400 mg q24h	Ciprofloxacin: 400 mg q12–24 h; Levofloxacin: 500–750 mg q24h; Moxifloxacin: 400 mg q24h	Ciprofloxacin: 400 mg q12–24 h; Levofloxacin: 500 mg q48h or 250 mg q24h; Moxifloxacin: 400 mg q24h
Lincosamides	Renal and hepatic	$f_{T>MIC}$	Administer 600 mg q8h as a LD on day 1	Lincomycin: 600 mg q12h; Clindamycin: 600 mg q8h	Lincomycin: reduce to 600 mg q12h; Clindamycin: 600 mg q12–24 h	No data for lincomycin, maintain normal dosing for clindamycin
Macrolides	Hepatic	$f_{T>MIC}$ (clarithromycin and erythromycin) and AUC_{0-24}/MIC (azithromycin)	Azithromycin: 500 mg q24h; Clarithromycin: 500 mg q12h	Azithromycin: 500 mg q24h; Clarithromycin: in severe renal failure, 250 mg q12h	Azithromycin: 500 mg q24h; Clarithromycin: 500 mg q12h	Azithromycin: 500 mg q24h; Clarithromycin: 500 mg q12h
Nitroimidazoles (metronidazole)	Hepatic	C_{max}/MIC	500 mg q8h	500 mg q8h	500 mg q12–24 h in severe hepatic failure	500 mg q8h
Daptomycin	Renal	C_{max}/MIC AUC_{0-24}/MIC	6 mg/kg LD on day 1	6 mg/kg q48h	Normal dosing	6 mg/kg q48h
Tigecycline	Hepatic	AUC_{0-24}/MIC	100 mg LD for 1 dose	After 12 h from LD, administer 50 mg q12h	After 12 h from LD, administer 25 mg q12h in severe hepatic failure	After 12 h from LD, administer 50 mg q12h
Linezolid	Hepatic	$f_{T>MIC}$	600 mg q12h	600 mg q12h	600 mg q12h – Monitor levels using TDM	600 mg q12h

(continued)

Table 13.2 (continued)

Antimicrobial	Main organ systems responsible for CL	PD parameter associated with maximal activity	LD in patients with increased Vd	MD in acute kidney injury[a]	MD in hepatic failure[a]	MD dose in RRT[b]
Triazole antifungals	Renal (fluconazole) Hepatic (voriconazole and posaconazole)	AUC_{0-24}/MIC and C_{max}/MIC	*Fluconazole*: 6 mg/kg q12h *Voriconazole*: 6 mg/kg 12 h *Posaconazole*: 200 mg q8h	*Fluconazole*: reduce dose by 50% *Voriconazole*: monitor trough level (C_{min}) on day 3 aiming for range 1–6 mg/L. Dosing must be titrated to fit in this range *Posaconazole*: not required	*Fluconazole*: not required *Voriconazole*: reduce dose to 50% in mild to moderate hepatic failure, Monitor trough level (C_{min}) on day 3 aiming for range 1–6 mg/L. Dosing must be titrated to fit in this range *Posaconazole*: not required	*Fluconazole*: not required (depends on settings) *Voriconazole*: change to oral, as the IV formulation vehicle may accumulate *Posaconazole*: unknown
Echinocandins	Hepatic (caspofungin), plasmatic esterases (anidulafungin)	AUC_{0-24}/MIC and C_{max}/MIC	70 mg q24h on day 1 (caspofungin), 200 mg (anidulafungin)	50 mg q24h (caspofungin), 100 mg (anidulafungin)	35 mg q24h (caspofungin), 100 mg (anidulafungin)	50 mg q24h (caspofungin), 100 mg (anidulafungin)
Amphotericin B	Hepatic and renal	Unknown	5 mg/kg/day	5 mg/kg/day	Unknown	Unknown

LD loading dose, *MD* maintenance dose, *RRT* renal replacement therapy, *Vd* volume of distribution, *q6h* 6-hourly, *q8h* 8-hourly, *q12h* 12-hourly, *q24h* once daily, *q48h* every second day, *CI* continuous infusion, *TDM* therapeutic drug monitoring

[a] Actual dose prescribed will be guided by the actual level of organ dysfunction

[b] Dose dependent on data available for dialysis settings

Another consequence of liver failure is a decreased biliary clearance of antimicrobials, such as the new tetracycline tigecycline, which is usually cleared unchanged by biliary excretion. A study comparing individuals with different degrees of hepatic failure found that systemic CL of the drug was reduced by 55% and $t_{1/2}$ was prolonged 43% in patients with severe hepatic impairment (Child Pugh C). In this context, a dose reduction of tigecycline is suggested to avoid toxicity (unpublished data, source: Tigacyl® product information).

Moreover, hypoproteinemia secondary to decreased production of albumin and α_1-acid glycoprotein in liver dysfunction, together with the transcapillary escape of these proteins due to capillary leakage (Fleck et al. 1985; Rothschild et al. 1969; Son et al. 1996), has the potential to contribute to altered pharmacokinetics of highly protein-bound antimicrobials (> 80% protein binding). In the case of hypoalbuminemia, significant increases in the Vd and CL of drugs, such as ceftriaxone (85–95% protein bound), ertapenem (85–95%) and teicoplanin (90–95%), have been observed, which may be clinically significant and lead to a failure to achieve pharmacodynamic targets (Barbot et al. 2003; Boselli et al. 2006; Brink et al. 2009; Burkhardt et al. 2005; Joynt et al. 2001). Decreased plasma concentrations of α_1-acid glycoprotein were reported to increase the Vd of the macrolide erythromycin (73–81% protein bound) substantially, whereas CL decreased by 60% because of metabolic impairment (Barre et al. 1987).

As a summary of this section, Table 13.2 provides some broad recommendations for optimizing initial and maintenance dosing in patients with MODS.

13.9   Conclusions

Optimal antimicrobial use in MODS is complex and dependent on drug-, disease- and patient-related factors. The contribution of an ICU pharmacist to optimization of antimicrobial use can be manifested in the provision of advice on dose adjustments that consider drug physicochemical and pharmacodynamic characteristics as well as disease-related alterations in antimicrobial pharmacokinetics. There are two important phases to be taken into account for improving antimicrobial dosing optimization in critically ill patients with MODS. During the initial phase of therapy, loading doses must be guided by the estimated Vd, which is likely to be increased for both lipophilic and hydrophilic antimicrobials in critically ill patients, although the function of the organ system(s) responsible for clearance might be impaired. From day 2 onward, maintenance dosing can be adjusted to the estimated level of impaired organ function. The dose requirements for each antimicrobial must be considered individually depending on the organ system that is failing, drug physicochemistry and clearance pathway. Due to the significant variability of organ function in critically ill patients with MODS, therapeutic drug monitoring should be regarded as a useful tool where available to individualize dosing on a daily basis to ensure appropriate exposure to the antimicrobial. Further research on dose adjustment in MODS is highly recommendable for improving patient quality of care and outcomes for ICU patients.

Acknowledgments We would like to acknowledge funding of the Burns, Trauma and Critical Care Research Centre by National Health and Medical Research Council of Australia (Project Grant 519702), Australia and New Zealand College of Anaesthetists (ANZCA 06/037 and 09/032), Queensland Health – Health Practitioner Research Scheme and the Royal Brisbane and Women's Hospital Research Foundation. Marta Ulldemolins is supported by CIBERES, AGAUR 09/SGR/1226 and FIS 07/90960. Dr. Roberts is funded by a fellowship from the National Health and Medical Research Council of Australia (Australian Based Health Professional Research Fellowship 569917).

Financial support
National Health and Medical Research Council of Australia (Project Grant 519702; Australian Based Health Professional Research Fellowship 569917), Australia and New Zealand College of Anaesthetists (ANZCA 06/037 and 09/032), CIBERES, AGAUR 09/SGR/1226 and FIS 07/90960.
Transparency Declarations
None to declare.

References

Allard S, Kinzig M, Boivin G, Sorgel F, LeBel M (1993) Intravenous ciprofloxacin disposition in obesity. Clin Pharmacol Ther 54:368–373

American College of Chest Physicians/Society of Critical Care Medicine (1992) American College of Chest Physicians/Society of Critical Care Medicine Consensus Conference: definitions for sepsis and organ failure and guidelines for the use of innovative therapies in sepsis. Crit Care Med 20:864–874

Antibiotic Expert Group (2006) Antibiotic therapeutic guidelines, vol 13. Therapeutic Guidelines Limited, Melbourne

Barbot A, Venisse N, Rayeh F, Bouquet S, Debaene B, Mimoz O (2003) Pharmacokinetics and pharmacodynamics of sequential intravenous and subcutaneous teicoplanin in critically ill patients without vasopressors. Intensive Care Med 29:1528–1534

Barre J, Mallat A, Rosenbaum J, Deforges L, Houin G, Dhumeaux D, Tillement JP (1987) Pharmacokinetics of erythromycin in patients with severe cirrhosis. Respective influence of decreased serum binding and impaired liver metabolic capacity. Br J Clin Pharmacol 23: 753–757

Bauer LA, Edwards WA, Dellinger EP, Simonowitz DA (1983) Influence of weight on aminoglycoside pharmacokinetics in normal weight and morbidly obese patients. Eur J Clin Pharmacol 24:643–647

Begg EJ, Barclay ML, Kirkpatrick CM (2001) The therapeutic monitoring of antimicrobial agents. Br J Clin Pharmacol 52(Suppl 1):35S–43S

Blouin RA, Bauer LA, Miller DD, Record KE, Griffen WO Jr (1982) Vancomycin pharmacokinetics in normal and morbidly obese subjects. Antimicrob Agents Chemother 21:575–580

Boselli E, Breilh D, Saux MC, Gordien JB, Allaouchiche B (2006) Pharmacokinetics and lung concentrations of ertapenem in patients with ventilator-associated pneumonia. Intensive Care Med 32:2059–2062

Brink AJ, Richards GA, Schillack V, Kiem S, Schentag J (2009) Pharmacokinetics of once-daily dosing of ertapenem in critically ill patients with severe sepsis. Int J Antimicrob Agents 33:432–436

Bruggemann RJ, Donnelly JP, Aarnoutse RE, Warris A, Blijlevens NM, Mouton JW, Verweij PE, Burger DM (2008) Therapeutic drug monitoring of voriconazole. Ther Drug Monit 30: 403–411

Buijk SE, Mouton JW, Gyssens IC, Verbrugh HA, Bruining HA (2002) Experience with a once-daily dosing program of aminoglycosides in critically ill patients. Intensive Care Med 28:936–942

Burkhardt O, Majcher-Peszynska J, Borner K, Mundkowski R, Drewelow B, Derendorf H, Welte T (2005) Penetration of ertapenem into different pulmonary compartments of patients undergoing lung surgery. J Clin Pharmacol 45:659–665

Burkhardt O, Kumar V, Katterwe D, Majcher-Peszynska J, Drewelow B, Derendorf H, Welte T (2007) Ertapenem in critically ill patients with early-onset ventilator-associated pneumonia: pharmacokinetics with special consideration of free-drug concentration. J Antimicrob Chemother 59:277–284

Choi G, Gomersall CD, Tian Q, Joynt GM, Freebairn R, Lipman J (2009) Principles of antibacterial dosing in continuous renal replacement therapy. Crit Care Med 37:2268–2282

Chow MS (1996) Intravenous amiodarone: pharmacology, pharmacokinetics, and clinical use. Ann Pharmacother 30:637–643

Chumlea WC, Guo SS (1994) Bioelectrical impedance and body composition: present status and future directions. Nutr Rev 52:123–131

Cockroft D, Gault M (1976) Prediction of creatinine clearance from serum creatinine. Nephron 16:31–41

Craig WA (1998) Pharmacokinetic/pharmacodynamic parameters: rationale for antibacterial dosing of mice and men. Clin Infect Dis 26:1–10

Donnelly AJ, Baughman VL, Gonzales JP, Golembiewski J, Tomsik EA (2008) Anesthesiology and critical care drug handbook. Lexi-Comp, Hudson

Farrell G, Baird-Lambert J, Cvejic M, Buchanan N (1984) Disposition and metabolism of metronidazole in patients with liver failure. Hepatology 4:722–726

Fleck A, Raines G, Hawker F, Trotter J, Wallace PI, Ledingham IM, Calman KC (1985) Increased vascular permeability: a major cause of hypoalbuminaemia in disease and injury. Lancet 1: 781–784

Garnacho-Montero J, Garcia-Garmendia JL, Barrero-Almodovar A, Jimenez-Jimenez FJ, Perez-Paredes C, Ortiz-Leyba C (2003) Impact of adequate empirical antibiotic therapy on the outcome of patients admitted to the intensive care unit with sepsis. Crit Care Med 31:2742–2751

Gilbert B, Robbins P, Livornese LL Jr (2009) Use of antibacterial agents in renal failure. Infect Dis Clin North Am 23:899–924

Greenfield RA, Gerber AU, Craig WA (1983) Pharmacokinetics of cefoperazone in patients with normal and impaired hepatic and renal function. Rev Infect Dis 5(Suppl 1):S127–S136

Herrera-Gutierrez ME, Seller-Perez G, Banderas-Bravo E, Munoz-Bono J, Lebron-Gallardo M, Fernandez-Ortega JF (2007) Replacement of 24-h creatinine clearance by 2-h creatinine clearance in intensive care unit patients: a single-center study. Intensive Care Med 33: 1900–1906

Heyland DK, Tougas G, King D, Cook DJ (1996) Impaired gastric emptying in mechanically ventilated, critically ill patients. Intensive Care Med 22:1339–1344

Jacob M, Conzen P, Finsterer U, Krafft A, Becker BF, Rehm M (2007) Technical and physiological background of plasma volume measurement with indocyanine green: a clarification of misunderstandings. J Appl Physiol 102:1235–1242

Janmahasatian S, Duffull SB, Ash S, Ward LC, Byrne NM, Green B (2005) Quantification of lean bodyweight. Clin Pharmacokinet 44:1051–1065

Jones AE, Puskarich MA (2009) Sepsis-induced tissue hypoperfusion. Crit Care Clin 25:769–779

Joukhadar C, Frossard M, Mayer BX, Brunner M, Klein N, Siostrzonek P, Eichler HG, Muller M (2001) Impaired target site penetration of beta-lactams may account for therapeutic failure in patients with septic shock. Crit Care Med 29:385–391

Joynt GM, Lipman J, Gomersall CD, Young RJ, Wong EL, Gin T (2001) The pharmacokinetics of once-daily dosing of ceftriaxone in critically ill patients. J Antimicrob Chemother 47:421–429

Kollef MH, Sherman G, Ward S, Fraser VJ (1999) Inadequate antimicrobial treatment of infections: a risk factor for hospital mortality among critically ill patients. Chest 115:462–474

Kumar A, Roberts D, Wood KE, Light B, Parrillo JE, Sharma S, Suppes R, Feinstein D, Zanotti S, Taiberg L et al (2006) Duration of hypotension before initiation of effective antimicrobial therapy is the critical determinant of survival in human septic shock. Crit Care Med 34: 1589–1596

Levey AS, Bosch JP, Lewis JB, Greene T, Rogers N, Roth D (1999) A more accurate method to estimate glomerular filtration rate from serum creatinine: a new prediction equation. Modification of Diet in Renal Disease Study Group. Ann Intern Med 130:461–470

MacGowan AP (1998) Pharmacodynamics, pharmacokinetics, and therapeutic drug monitoring of glycopeptides. Ther Drug Monit 20:473–477

MacLaren R, Bond CA, Martin SJ, Fike D (2008) Clinical and economic outcomes of involving pharmacists in the direct care of critically ill patients with infections. Crit Care Med 36:3184–3189

Marshall JC (2001) Inflammation, coagulopathy, and the pathogenesis of multiple organ dysfunction syndrome. Crit Care Med 29:S99–S106

Miller ME, Cosgriff JM, Forbes GB (1989) Bromide space determination using anion-exchange chromatography for measurement of bromide. Am J Clin Nutr 50:168–171

MIMS Australia (http://www.mims.com.au/), MIMS Australia Pty Ltd. Accessed on Dec 2009

Outman WR, Nightingale CH, Sweeney KR, Quintiliani R (1990) Teicoplanin pharmacokinetics in healthy volunteers after administration of intravenous loading and maintenance doses. Antimicrob Agents Chemother 34:2114–2117

Pannu N, Nadim MK (2008) An overview of drug-induced acute kidney injury. Crit Care Med 36:S216–S223

Paul S, Escareno CE, Clancy K, Jaklitsch MT, Bueno R, Lautz DB (2009) Gastrointestinal complications after lung transplantation. J Heart Lung Transplant 28:475–479

Pharmaceutical Research and Manufactures of America http://www.phrma.org/newmedicines/. Accessed on Dec 2009

Plank LD, Hill GL (2000) Similarity of changes in body composition in intensive care patients following severe sepsis or major blunt injury. Ann N Y Acad Sci 904:592–602

Pong S, Seto W, Abdolell M, Trope A, Wong K, Herridge J, Harvey E, Kavanagh BP (2005) 12-hour versus 24-hour creatinine clearance in critically ill pediatric patients. Pediatr Res 58:83–88

Rello J, Gallego M, Mariscal D, Sonora R, Valles J (1997) The value of routine microbial investigation in ventilator-associated pneumonia. Am J Respir Crit Care Med 156:196–200

Richens A (1979) Clinical pharmacokinetics of phenytoin. Clin Pharmacokinet 4:153–169

Roberts JA, Lipman J (2006) Antibacterial dosing in intensive care: pharmacokinetics, degree of disease and pharmacodynamics of sepsis. Clin Pharmacokinet 45:755–773

Roberts JA, Lipman J (2009) Pharmacokinetic issues for antibiotics in the critically ill patient. Crit Care Med 37:840–851

Roberts JA, Kruger P, Paterson DL, Lipman J (2008) Antibiotic resistance–what's dosing got to do with it? Crit Care Med 36:2433–2440

Roberts JA, Kirkpatrick CM, Roberts MS, Robertson TA, Dalley AJ, Lipman J (2009a) Meropenem dosing in critically ill patients with sepsis and without renal dysfunction: intermittent bolus versus continuous administration? Monte Carlo dosing simulations and subcutaneous tissue distribution. J Antimicrob Chemother 64:142–150

Roberts JA, Roberts MS, Robertson TA, Dalley AJ, Lipman J (2009b) Piperacillin penetration into tissue of critically ill patients with sepsis – bolus versus continuous administration? Crit Care Med 37:926–933

Rothschild MA, Oratz M, Zimmon D, Schreiber SS, Weiner I, Van Caneghem A (1969) Albumin synthesis in cirrhotic subjects with ascites studied with carbonate-14C. J Clin Invest 48:344–350

Rowland M, Tozer TN (1995) Clinical pharmacokinetics. Concepts and applications. Lippincott Williams & Wilkins, Philadelphia

Ryan DM (1993) Pharmacokinetics of antibiotics in natural and experimental superficial compartments in animals and humans. J Antimicrob Chemother 31(Suppl D):1–16

Sakka SG (2007) Assessing liver function. Curr Opin Crit Care 13:207–214

Singh G, Harkema JM, Mayberry AJ, Chaudry IH (1994) Severe depression of gut absorptive capacity in patients following trauma or sepsis. J Trauma 36:803–808

Son DS, Hariya S, Shimoda M, Kokue E (1996) Contribution of alpha 1-acid glycoprotein to plasma protein binding of some basic antimicrobials in pigs. J Vet Pharmacol Ther 19: 176–183

Spellberg B, Guidos R, Gilbert D, Bradley J, Boucher HW, Scheld WM, Bartlett JG, Edwards J Jr (2008) The epidemic of antibiotic-resistant infections: a call to action for the medical community from the Infectious Diseases Society of America. Clin Infect Dis 46:155–164

Thijs LG, Schneider AJ, Groeneveld AB (1990) The haemodynamics of septic shock. Intensive Care Med 16(Suppl 3):S182–S186

van der Poll T (2001) Immunotherapy of sepsis. Lancet Infect Dis 1:165–174

Wan L, Bagshaw SM, Langenberg C, Saotome T, May C, Bellomo R (2008) Pathophysiology of septic acute kidney injury: what do we really know? Crit Care Med 36:S198–S203

Wells M, Lipman J (1997) Measurements of glomerular filtration in the intensive care unit are only a rough guide to renal function. S Afr J Surg 35:20–23

Westphal JF, Brogard JM (1993) Clinical pharmacokinetics of newer antibacterial agents in liver disease. Clin Pharmacokinet 24:46–58

Improving Outcomes in Sepsis and Septic Shock: Getting it Right the First Time

14

Duane Funk, Shravan Kethireddy, and Anand Kumar

14.1 Introduction

Infections among critically ill patients have convincingly been shown to directly increase mortality, prolong hospital length of stays, and increase healthcare costs (Chastre and Fagon 2002; Rello et al. 2002). In the past the general approach to antimicrobial therapy of infection involved an escalation strategy wherein patients were started on the narrowest reasonable antimicrobial regimen expected to cover a majority of common pathogens. In addition to mild and moderately ill patients, this strategy was also applied to the critically ill at high risk of death. Only if clinical failure occurred was therapy broadened or otherwise adjusted. While this approach is effective in the management of relatively minor infections in ambulatory patients, its application to seriously ill patients at significant risk of death was problematic.

The current approach to optimizing outcomes of serious infections among ICU patients, developed and refined in recent decades, derives from studies identifying specific remediable risk factors for poor outcomes in those same patients. Adequacy of initial antimicrobial therapy has emerged as a significant, modifiable risk factor determining patient outcomes and has become a cornerstone of the treatment

D. Funk • S. Kethireddy
Section of Critical Care Medicine, University of Manitoba,
Winnipeg, MB, Canada

A. Kumar (✉)
Section of Critical Care Medicine, Section of Infectious Diseases,
University of Manitoba, Winnipeg, MB, Canada

Section of Critical Care Medicine, JJ399d, Health Sciences Centre,
Winnipeg, MB, Canada

Robert Wood Johnson Medical School, University of Medicine and Dentistry,
Piscataway, NJ, USA
e-mail: akumar61@yahoo.com

J. Rello (eds.), *Sepsis Management*,
DOI 10.1007/978-3-642-03519-7_14, © Springer-Verlag Berlin Heidelberg 2012

paradigm of life-threatening infections. Whether treating healthcare-associated pneumonia, bacteremia, or septic shock, the principles of appropriate empiric antimicrobial therapy remain the same; the regimen should exhibit in vitro activity against the isolated pathogen and take into consideration current clinical practice guidelines regarding the dosing, route, and pattern of administration (McGregor et al. 2007; Moellering 2009).

Nonetheless, some studies evaluating differences in outcomes have failed to report a survival advantage with initiation of appropriate therapy (Ammerlaan et al. 2009; Cheng and Buising 2009). Despite the intuitive benefits of "getting it right" early, studies reporting a lack of mortality advantage compel us to better understand what, in fact, constitutes appropriate antimicrobial therapy. In this context, McGregor and colleagues identified five major aspects to consider when evaluating whether a therapeutic regimen is appropriate (McGregor et al. 2007).

The choice of an antimicrobial regimen involves more than just ensuring in-vitro sensitivity on standard testing. For example, some antimicrobials not active in vitro (especially those that are heavily concentrated intracellularly) may have significant in-vivo activity appropriate for clinical management (e.g., macrolides for *L. pneumophila* pneumonia). Secondly, the correct route of administration and duration of therapy are vital to ensure that the antibiotic penetrates the site of infection for a long enough period of time. Dosing the antibiotic based on minimum inhibitory concentrations (MIC) of the infecting pathogen as well as utilizing combination therapy over monotherapy when indicated (e.g., for therapy of serious enterococcal infections) are both important components of an adequate regime. Finally the method by which mortality benefits are assessed will undoubtedly have an impact on determining whether appropriate antimicrobial therapy is truly effective. It is with this framework that we will summarize data on appropriate antimicrobial therapy in various categories of ICU-related infections.

This chapter will focus on the evidence behind the concept of timely administration of appropriate antimicrobial chemotherapy. We look at several different infectious diseases as a model for the overall concept of early appropriate therapy. Specifically we will look at healthcare-acquired pneumonia (HCAP), community-acquired pneumonia (CAP), intra-abdominal infections, candidemia/bacteremia, and septic shock. We will then discuss the overall methodological limitations of some of the studies on early appropriate therapy and explore key concepts as to what constitutes appropriate therapy.

14.2 Healthcare-Acquired Pneumonia

The approach to antibiotic treatment of healthcare- and hospital-acquired pneumonia outlined in the ATS/IDSA and AMMI guidelines provides important, practical components of the de-escalation approach (Niederman et al. 2005; Rotstein et al. 2008). A key decision when considering initial empiric therapy in this situation is the potential for infection by multidrug-resistant pathogens (Micek et al. 2007). Anticipating the presence of resistant organisms can prevent crucial delays in treating infections with appropriate antimicrobials. Alvarez-Lerma et al. showed that attributable mortality from hospital-acquired pneumonia was significantly higher among patients who required modification of their initial treatment regimen (24.7% vs. 16.2% $p=0.034$); greater than 25% of cases required modification due to isolation of a resistant pathogen (Alvarez-Lerma and the ICU-acquired Pneumonia Study Group 1996).

Recently Depuydt and colleagues showed that isolation of multidrug-resistant organisms does not increase the risk of death among ICU patients in settings where rates of early and appropriate antimicrobial therapy are high (Depuydt et al. 2008).

Dosing of antibiotics in HAP/VAP patients is another important aspect to consider when selecting an initial regimen. For example, optimal vancomycin dosing in MRSA pneumonia has been suggested to improve clinical and bacteriological outcomes if the 24-h area under the curve of serum vancomycin divided by the minimum inhibitory concentration of the organism (AUC/MIC ratio) is >400 µg/mL (Moise et al. 2004). This highlights the importance of not only starting a drug in a timely fashion, but also dosing it accordingly. While clinicians should be aware of national/international guidelines for appropriate antimicrobial therapy of HCAP, knowledge of local antibiotic susceptibility profiles (particularly for local hospitals and ICUs) is critical (Kaufman et al. 1998; Bantar et al. 2007). Several studies have demonstrated an increased frequency of appropriateness of antimicrobial therapy with the judicious use of infectious disease consultation and antibiogram data (Byl et al. 1999; Raineri et al. 2008).

14.3 Community-Acquired Pneumonia

Treatment of severe community-acquired pneumonia illustrates several other key aspects of the correct approach to initiation of appropriate empiric antimicrobials. Patients with severe community-acquired pneumonia requiring intensive care should receive an empiric combination, as per current national guidelines, in order to ensure that at least one antimicrobial is active against the pathogen (Mandell et al. 2007).

In their clinical trial comparing levofloxacin against combination therapy with cefotaxime and ofloxacin, Leroy and colleagues found a trend towards inferior outcomes among patients requiring mechanical ventilation and receiving monotherapy (Leroy et al. 2005). Based on this as well as other observational and retrospective data, patients with community-acquired pneumonia associated with septic shock or requiring mechanical ventilation should be treated with intravenous empiric combination therapy for at least 48 h (Mandell et al. 2007). Patients not as severely ill can be treated adequately with monotherapy (Mandell et al. 2007).

Timeliness of antibiotic administration has also been studied in a large cohort of Medicare patients with community-acquired pneumonia. This retrospective analysis found that patients experienced improved 30-day mortality when antimicrobials were administered within 4 h, leading to recommendations that patients with severe community-acquired pneumonia receive antimicrobials in the emergency room prior to inpatient hospitalization (Houck et al. 2004). Others have found similar results with 8-h cutoffs(Meehan et al. 1997; Gacouin et al. 2002).

14.4   Intra-Abdominal Infections

Intra-abdominal infections (IAIs) are one of the most common infection-related causes of hospital admission and are a significant source of morbidity. Community-acquired IAIs are associated with low mortality, but nosocomial infections carry significant mortality and are a burden on hospital resources. Unlike community-acquired pneumonia, in most cases antimicrobial treatment of IAIs serves only as an adjunct to cure, with source control (either with operative or percutaneous interventions) playing a major role.

The treatment of IAIs is complicated by the fact that many of these infections are polymicrobial and many of the organisms encountered in IAIs have broad resistance patterns. There have been few studies that address the question of appropriateness of antimicrobial therapy in IAIs with respect to mortality. The few studies that do specifically examine IAI consistently suggest worse clinical outcomes and increased length of hospital and ICU stay with inappropriate therapy (Sitges-Serra et al. 2002; Sturkenboom et al. 2005; Bare et al. 2006; Tellado et al. 2007a).

In a retrospective multicenter study involving patients with community-acquired IAIs requiring surgery, inappropriate antimicrobial chemotherapy reduced the clinical success rate and increased hospital length of stay (LOS) (Krobot et al. 2004). A similar study from Spain involving 425 patients with community-acquired IAIs found similar results with respect to clinical failure and increased LOS (Tellado et al. 2007b). In this retrospective study, patients receiving inappropriate therapy were less likely to have clinical success (79% vs. 26%), were more likely to require further therapy (40% vs. 7%) and were more likely to require re-admission to hospital within 30 days of discharge (18% vs. 3%). All three measured parameters were significantly different statistically from the group that received appropriate therapy. This study was not able to demonstrate an increase in mortality with inappropriate therapy, most likely a reflection of the low baseline risk of death (4%) between both groups. This study did, however, demonstrate a significant increase in hospital costs associated with inappropriate therapy.

Falagas et al. studied patients with IAIs and skin/soft tissue infections in an attempt to determine what factors affected outcome (Falagas et al. 1996). In this retrospective, case-matched study, 90 patients with IAIs were assessed for risk factors of clinical failure (as defined by the need for repeat surgical intervention or the need to receive prolonged courses of antibiotics). Multivariate analysis revealed that the strongest predictor of clinical failure was the administration of inappropriate empiric antimicrobial therapy, resulting in an almost 15-fold increase in the rate of clinical failure. While this study suffers from methodological flaws and enlists a rather broad definition of failure, it adds further credence to the need for appropriate therapy in IAIs. While no patients died in this study, APACHE II scores were quite low (mean 5, interquartile range 3–8, predicted mortality 4.4–8.7%).

Kollef et al. looked at hospital mortality of critically ill patients who received inappropriate antimicrobial therapy with a high risk of death (15.6%) (Kollef et al. 1999). This study found that inappropriate therapy resulted in a significantly increased risk of death (52.1% vs. 12.2%, RR 4.26; 95% CI 3.22–5.15; $p < 0.001$) in all patients. The study also analyzed patients by source of infection and found that, in the subset with IAI (90 patients), the risk of death was greater in the group that received inappropriate antimicrobial therapy. Using a logistical regression model, inappropriate antimicrobial therapy was the strongest predictor of hospital mortality (OR 4.27, 95% CI 3.35–5.44, $p < 0.001$).

Similarly, Kumar and colleagues have recently published data on the impact of inappropriate initial empiric therapy in cases of septic shock (Kumar et al. 2009). Among the 1,041 patients with septic shock caused by intra-abdominal infections, survival to hospital discharge was 48.5% in those receiving appropriate therapy and 11.5% among those receiving inappropriate therapy (OR 7.66).

All of the trials looking at appropriate antimicrobial therapy in patients with IAIs are limited by small sample size, retrospective nature, inadequate power, differing definitions of inappropriate therapy, and different outcome variables. However, based on the current evidence it would appear that inadequate treatment of IAIs results in longer hospital stays and increased costs. Mortality does not seem to be increased when the baseline mortality is low, but might be increased in the patient population at higher risk of death (i.e., those that require intensive care unit admission).

14.5   Bacteremia/Candidemia

Studies examining the impact of initiation of inappropriate antimicrobial therapy in bacteremia date back at least to the work of McCabe and colleagues in 1962 (Mccabe and Jackson 1962). Since then, a large number of studies have examined the outcome of bacteremia caused by a wide variety of pathogens in relationship to the initiation of inappropriate empiric antibiotic therapy (McGregor et al. 2007). The majority of these studies clearly suggest inferior clinical outcomes and an increase in mortality (using logistic regression analysis) if inappropriate empiric therapy is initiated.

In one of the early, comprehensive examinations of the subject, Kreger and colleagues, in 1980, demonstrated a doubling of the risk of septic shock (23%–49%) and death (19–37%) among 612 patients with gram-negative bacteremia empirically treated with an inappropriate regimen (Kreger et al. 1980). Further, they showed that the risk of death among those with gram-negative septic shock treated with inappropriate antimicrobials was increased approximately 50% (from 41% to 59%).

Kollef et al. reported on approximately 500 patients with positive blood cultures admitted to the ICU in a single center (Ibrahim et al. 2000). Initiation of inappropriate therapy was associated with a risk ratio for death of 2.2 relative to those receiving appropriate empiric therapy. Receipt of previous antibiotics during the hospitalization and isolation of *Candida spp.* in blood were two major correlates of receiving inappropriate initial therapy. Two of the largest studies (>2,000 patients each) examining this issue were those of Leibovici and colleagues, who demonstrated that inappropriate initial empiric therapy was associated with a 60–100% increase in mortality risk in two separate studies (Leibovici et al. 1997, 1998). In one study, the adverse impact of inappropriate therapy held when assessed together with other variables associated with outcome in logistic regression (Leibovici et al. 1998).

Several studies have extended the observations of the impact of initiation of inappropriate antimicrobial therapy to candidemia and invasive candida infection. Laupland and colleagues have demonstrated that initiation of inappropriate therapy for invasive candida infection was associated with a significant increase in mortality (26% vs. 46%) (Parkins et al. 2007). Several other authors have shown that initiation of appropriate antifungal therapy within 12–24 h of blood cultures, eventually found positive for *Candida spp.*, results in improved survival compared to later initiation of appropriate therapy (i.e., many patients had inappropriate initial therapy) (Morrell et al. 2005; Garey et al. 2006).

14.6 Sepsis and Septic Shock

Over the past several years the treatment of septic shock from the emergency department to the ICU has undergone a paradigm shift. In the past, the speed of resuscitation of patients with severe sepsis and septic shock in the emergency room was not viewed as a priority to the same degree as trauma or myocardial infarction with shock. With the publication of Rivers' study on early goal-directed therapy in the emergency department showing that mortality could be reduced (46.5–30.5%) with rapid, aggressive resuscitation, the concept of the "golden hour" was extended to sepsis (Rivers et al. 2001).

The intervention in this study was a bundle of procedures and therapies aimed at providing adequate organ blood flow with the use of fluids, vasopressors, red blood cell transfusions, and inotropic therapy. Antimicrobial therapy was not specifically prioritized as part of the resuscitation. Nonetheless, antimicrobial therapy was given to 86.3% of patients in the goal-directed group within the first 6 h, and 96.7% of patients received appropriate antibiotics. Of note, 92.4% of patients in the control group received antibiotics within 6 h, and in 94.3% the antibiotics were adequate. Since this was a bundled approach to severe sepsis and septic shock, it was unclear what affect each individual therapy had on the overall mortality. Although usually interpreted to support early aggressive goal-directed fluid and blood product-oriented resuscitation, other interpretations of the results are possible.

Although antimicrobial therapy was not randomized and should not have been different between groups, it is difficult to understand how the experimental group, which was assigned greater fluid resuscitation and a higher level of monitoring (oximetric central venous catheter, etc.), and most likely would have received greater attention than the "standard care" group, would not benefit with more rapid non-randomized therapeutics given the unblinded study design. The reporting method describing the time to antimicrobials could easily obscure major group-associated variations in the distribution of antimicrobial times given that the usual median time to antimicrobials in emergency room environments is approximately 4 h (i.e., a shortening of time to antimicrobial therapy in the experimental group could easily be missed given the reporting methodology). Given the potential impact of even modest reductions in time to antimicrobial therapy in septic shock and the distinct possibility that variation time

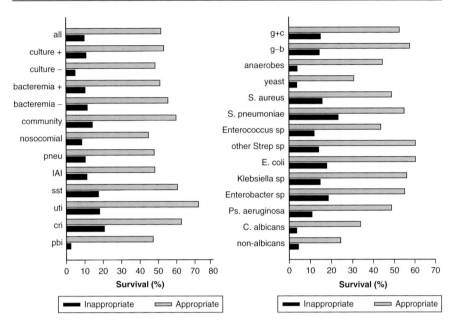

Fig. 14.1 Antimicrobial appropriateness and survival in septic shock subgroups. *Culture +* culture positive infections, *culture −* culture negative infections, *bacteremia +* bacteremic infections, *bacteremia −* non-bacteremic infections, *community* community acquired infections, *nosocomial* nosocomial infections, *pneu* all infections of the respiratory tract including pneumonia and empyema, *IAI* all intra-abdominal infections including peritonitis, cholangitis, cholecystitis, intra-abdominal abscess, ischemic bowel, etc., but excluding infections of the abdominal wall, *UTI* all infections of the urinary tract including pyelonephritis (with or without obstruction) and perinephric abscesses but exclusive of infections of the reproductive tract, *sst* skin and soft tissue infections including fascial or skeletal muscle excluding surgical wound infections, *cri* catheter-related infections including central venous, dialysis, pulmonary artery and arterial catheters, *pbi* primary blood stream infections, *g + c* infections caused by gram-stain positive cocci, *g−b* infections caused by gram negative bacilli, *yeast* Candida and other yeast infections excluding blastomycosis and filamentous fungi such as Aspergillus, *sp* species (Adapted from Kumar et al. (2009))

to antimicrobials went unrecognized, it seems likely that at least some of the improvement in outcome in this study is related to this factor.

To examine the specific impact of early appropriate antimicrobial therapy on survival in septic shock, Kumar et al. retrospectively looked at the duration of hypotension before initiation of effective antimicrobial therapy (Kumar et al. 2006). They found that each hour delay in instituting therapy resulted in a 7.6% decrease in survival. Interestingly, patients in this study only received initially appropriate therapy 80% of the time. In a subsequent study, Kumar et al. found that the administration of inappropriate antibiotics resulted in a significant decrease in survival (52% vs. 10.3%, OR 9.45 95% CI 7.7–11.5, $p < 0.0001$) in patients with septic shock (2009). The decrease in survival varied from 2.3-fold for pneumococcal pneumonia to 17.6-fold with primary bacteremia (Fig. 14.1). After adjustment for various comorbidities (including the number of presenting organ failures), therapeutic variables (use of mechanical ventilation, drotrecogin-alfa activated and low-dose steroids), and severity of illness (APACHE II score), inappropriate therapy was the strongest correlate of death (adjusted OR 8.99, 95% CI 6.0–12.23).

Inappropriate therapy was similarly associated with an odds ratio of death of approximately 8 compared to those receiving initially appropriate therapy among ICU patients with sepsis and septic shock in Spain (Garnacho-Montero et al. 2003). Similar survival data have been shown for patients with *Candida albicans* blood stream infection and septic shock who received appropriate antifungal therapy within 15 h of the first positive blood culture result (Patel et al. 2009).

Six hundred fifty-five patients with either community-acquired or nosocomial infection requiring admission to the ICU were assessed in another retrospective study (Kollef et al. 1999). Inappropriate therapy was more common in those admitted with nosocomial infection (particularly those initially admitted with infection from the community before acquiring a nosocomial infection). Higher APACHE II scores (i.e., sicker patients) and those having received recent antimicrobial therapy had a significantly higher probability of being administered inappropriate empiric antimicrobial therapy. Mortality was most closely related to the initial receipt of inappropriate antimicrobial therapy. Initiation of inappropriate empiric antimicrobial therapy was more closely associated with mortality than APACHE II score, the number of presenting organ system dysfunctions, and the use of pressors, findings later replicated in septic shock in the study of Kumar et al. (Kumar et al. 2009). The same group has recently shown that combination therapy provided a higher degree of antimicrobial appropriateness and better survival in 760 patients with bacteremic gram-negative sepsis (Micek et al. 2010).

Similarly, Harbarth and colleagues assessed the impact of inappropriate empiric antimicrobial therapy in a retrospective analysis of data from a randomized, double-blind trial of an immunomodulatory agent for sepsis (Harbarth et al. 2003). Fifty-two percent of the subjects were bacteremic. Of the 23% of the 904 patients enrolled who received inappropriate initial therapy, mortality was significantly higher (39% vs. 24%, $p < 0.001$). Even after adjustment for comorbid conditions, severity of illness, site of infection, and the propensity score, inappropriate antimicrobial therapy was independently associated with increased mortality (odds ratio = 1.8; 95% confidence interval: 1.2–2.6) (Harbarth et al. 2003).

In another Spanish study of patients with septic shock, inappropriate antimicrobial therapy was again associated with a fourfold increase in mortality. The authors of this study tried to determine the attributable mortality to ineffective therapy and found that attributable mortality increased with the severity of the illness at the time of ICU admission. Attributable mortality was 10.7% with an APACHE II score of <15 and 41.8% with an APACHE II score of ≥25 when inappropriate antibiotics were given (Valles et al. 2003).

Further evidence that appropriate empiric antimicrobial administration is key to survival in sepsis and septic shock is a study from the University of Pennsylvania that has an early goal-directed therapy protocol for patients including early antibiotic administration (Gaieski et al. 2010). In this retrospective study, effects of different time cutoffs for administration of appropriate antimicrobial therapy were analyzed. Much like the Kumar paper, this study found a relationship between time to antibiotic administration and survival. When only those patients who received appropriate therapy were considered, there was a significant difference in survival between patients who received their therapy in less than an hour after triage compared with those that received treatment greater than 1 h after triage. However, with the institution of inappropriate therapy, there was no significant difference between time of antibiotic and survival, probably because antimicrobial administration was delayed and survival very low in patients receiving inappropriate initial empiric therapy. This study suggests that the use of initially appropriate therapy is only beneficial if that appropriate therapy is provided within an early window of opportunity.

Interestingly, in most of the studies looking at time and appropriateness of antibiotic therapy, anywhere from 20% to 40% of patients receive inadequate treatment. It is therefore critically important to institute broad-spectrum antimicrobial therapy based on presumed source of sepsis, antibiogram at the particular institution (or even within the ICU), and risk factors for resistant organisms if effective therapy is to be implemented.

The current weight of evidence clearly supports the early institution of appropriate antimicrobial therapy in all patients with life-threatening infection, particularly sepsis and septic shock. However, an examination of the studies looking at these questions suggests that patients at the highest risk of death (i.e., those with septic shock) seem to derive a greater mortality benefit, whereas those at a lower risk of death seem to have a more limited mortality benefit. There is evidence of a benefit to these less acutely ill patients with respect to decreases in length of stay and hospital costs with an appropriate empiric antimicrobial regime.

14.7 Risk Factors for Inappropriate Antimicrobials

One of the most problematic aspects in effective early initiation of appropriate antimicrobials is the failure of clinicians to appreciate the risk of infection with antibiotic-resistant organisms. An appropriate antimicrobial regimen should take into account the likely anatomic site of infection, patient-associated risk factors including immune status, and local organism resistance patterns. Risk factors for infection with resistant organisms include previous or prolonged hospital stay, previous antimicrobial usage, immunosuppression, and high frequency of antibiotic resistance in the community or specific hospital (Kollef 2000). Several investigators have studied the risk factors associated with inappropriate antimicrobial administration. In their observations of a large multicenter cohort, Harbarth et al. found that patients with multiresistant organisms had a nearly fivefold increased risk of inappropriate therapy (OR 4.7; 95% CI: 3.0–7.4) (Harbarth et al. 2003). Similarly, Lodise et al. found among patients with *Pseudomonas* bacteremia that antibiotic resistance was associated with a nearly fivefold increased risk of inappropriate therapy (AOR 4.6; 95% CI: 1.9–11.2, $p = 0.001$) and subsequent increase

Table 14.1 Indication for extended empiric antibiotic therapy of severe sepsis/septic shock

↑ Gram-negative coverage	1. Nosocomial infection
	2. Neutropenic or immunosuppressed
	3. Immunocompromised due to chronic organ failure (liver, renal, lung, heart, etc.)
↑ Gram-positive coverage (vancomycin, daptomycin, etc.)	1. High level endemic MRSA (community or nosocomial)
	2. Neutropenic patient
	3. Intravascular catheter infection
	4. Nosocomial pneumonia
Fungal/yeast coverage (triazole, echinocandin, amphotericin B)	1. Neutropenic fever or other immunosuppressed patient unresponsive to standard antibiotic therapy
	2. Prolonged broad-spectrum antibiotic therapy
	3. Positive relevant fungal cultures
	4. Consider empiric therapy if high-risk patient with severe shock

MRSA methicillin resistant *Staphylococcus aureus*

in 30-day mortality (Lodise et al. 2007). The prospective study by Ibrahim and colleagues reported that bloodstream infections by several different antibiotic-resistant pathogens were associated not only with the greatest rates of inadequate therapy, but also with increased hospital mortality when compared to adequate therapy. Similar associations have been identified by other investigators on a variety of pathogens (Hyle et al. 2005; Peralta et al. 2007; Tumbarello et al. 2008). This data should impress upon clinicians that anticipation of pathogen resistance and appropriate antibiotic targeting, while an obstacle, is crucial.

Strategies to reduce the risk of inappropriate antimicrobial therapy include using local antibiograms and antibiotic practice guidelines as well as obtaining an infectious disease consultation. Clinical decision support through the use of individual hospital-tailored antibiograms can guide empiric antibiotic choices. It is important, however, to understand that not all antibiograms are created equal. Comparability and accuracy are markedly affected by the type of calculation algorithms used, and so hospital laboratories should refer to antibiogram development guidelines published by the Clinical and Laboratory Standards Institute (CLSI) (Hindler and Stelling 2007). In addition, a substantial body of literature suggests that pathogen distribution and resistance patterns may vary according to hospital ward with suboptimal coverage when hospital-wide antibiograms are utilized (Whipple et al. 1991; Valles et al. 2003). Unit-specific antibiograms may be necessary to afford optimal data for initiation of appropriate antimicrobial therapy.

Several investigators have shown that consultation with an infectious disease specialist can improve outcomes. Fowler et al. showed that patients with *Staphylococcus aureus* bacteremia experienced improved cure rates (79.5% vs. 64.4%, $p=0.01$) and lower rates of relapsed infection (6.3% vs. 18.2%, $p<0.01$) when physicians followed the advice of an infectious disease specialist (Fowler et al. 1998). Similarly, among 428 episodes of bacteremia evaluated, Byl et al. found a marked increase in appropriate empiric antibiotic administration with infectious disease consultation (78% vs. 54%,

$p < 0.001$) as well as a concomitant decrease in mortality with appropriate therapy (adjusted OR 0.47; 95% CI: 0.25–0.87; $p = 0.017$) (Byl et al. 1999).

Finally, antibiotic practice guidelines published by various expert panels, i.e., the American Thoracic Society (ATS) and Infectious Disease Society of America (IDSA), can further assist clinicians not only in determining appropriate antibiotic choices, but also in administering antibiotics at the appropriate dosages with respect to targeted anatomic sites, patient immune status, and minimum levels of drug concentrations needed to effectively treat the infection. Table 14.1 illustrates modifications of empiric regimens targeted towards drug-resistant organisms in specific high-risk cases with severe sepsis.

14.8   Research Limitations

As with all therapeutic interventions, there are potential adverse consequences associated with the institution of early broad-spectrum antimicrobial therapy. Some studies have failed to show an improvement in patient outcome with early appropriate therapy (McGregor et al. 2007; Kim et al. 2009). In the absence of a tangible benefit, "appropriate" empiric therapy, which usually involves broader spectrum, more expensive antibiotics, may lead to increased hospital costs and possibly greater adverse effects from drug toxicity. The issue of antibiotic stewardship also becomes important as treatment with broad-spectrum antibiotics without de-escalation of the initial empiric regime may increase selection pressure and lead to an increase in antibiotic-resistant pathogens. Unfortunately, there is limited consensus among infectious disease specialists and intensive care physicians as to what constitutes ideal appropriate empiric therapy, the duration of this therapy, what pattern of de-escalation should occur, and treatment duration in patients with negative cultures. This section will discuss the limitations of the current research on this subject.

Past research in this area (as outlined in the previous sections) has been limited by significant methodological flaws. First, most of these studies were small and retrospective in nature. Randomized trials of early versus delayed therapy would, for obvious ethical reasons, never be conducted. Retrospective studies, for all their weaknesses, remain the best clinical research alternative. Second, the definition of appropriate therapy does differ between studies. The timeline of therapy undoubtedly plays a significant role in treatment success. Baseline mortality of patients also has to be taken into account when determining outcomes. Finally, the benefit of early aggressive therapy has to be assessed for potential adverse effects, including overall costs, and potential for creating resistance patterns.

14.9   Definition of Appropriate Therapy

When describing appropriate therapy, many factors must be taken into account. Most of the current studies on appropriate therapy have defined this as the selection of an antibiotic that has in vitro activity against the organism that was isolated from the index culture. Other studies have defined appropriate as consistent with current practice guidelines for the particular site of infection (i.e., ventilator-acquired pneumonia). When defining appropriate therapy, the use of culture results should be the gold standard, as the antibiograms of organisms at different institutions shows great variability. However, this definition, while microbiologically sound, ignores the unique pharmacokinetics and pharmacodynamics of antibiotics, particularly in the critically ill.

Even if the antibiotic selected is appropriate, the route of administration of the drug may play a role in the ability of the drug to have activity against the organism. This problem is magnified in the critically ill patient who may have alterations in gut motility due to the postoperative state, ileus, or use of narcotics that might alter bowel motility. In these patients, the use of an oral antibiotic, even if it had in vitro activity against the causative pathogen, may not reach the site of infection at all, or it may do so at an inadequate concentration, rendering it less effective, and with the potential of increasing resistance.

The dose of the antibiotic also needs to be taken into account in the critically ill as these patients often have altered volumes of distribution based on fluid overload and the use of renal replacement therapy. For example, aminoglycosides are primarily distributed in extracellular water, but patients with septic shock may undergo >10 L of saline resuscitation/volume expansion in the first 24 h of resuscitation (a 50% increase in extracellular volume in a 100-kg patient). In such patients, standard dosing will result in suboptimal blood concentrations for some antibiotics, particularly aminoglycosides with less than ideal clinical response (Franson et al. 1988; Whipple et al. 1991). Further, patients might have altered clearance of antibiotics based on intrinsic or acquired hepatic or renal disease. Again, an antibiotic with in vitro activity might be ineffective in the situation where it is given in an inadequate dose based on the patient's volume of distribution or in a dose that does not take into account the patient's ability to metabolize and clear these drugs.

As an example, aminoglycosides and β-lactams are metabolized remarkably rapidly in patients with extensive burn injury owing to their distribution in extracelluar fluid (which is lost rapidly through the area of the burn). Augmented renal clearance in hyperdynamic states associated with sepsis can also be an issue (Roberts and Lipman 2006; Udy et al. 2009). This problem is easily solved in those situations where there is time and drug levels can be monitored. In that circumstance, therapy can be titrated for the individual patient, but unfortunately most antibiotics do not have levels that are easily measured in hospital laboratories, and if the first hours of therapy are critical, time may not allow necessary titration.

Another pharmacokinetic factor that plays a role in the definition of appropriate therapy is the difference between in vitro and in vivo susceptibility, which can be an issue in patients with intra-abdominal abscesses or other clinical scenarios where the antibiotic cannot reach the infected site at an appropriate concentration (e.g., meningitis, necrotizing soft tissue infections, infections of ischemic limbs, and pancreatic infections). Some pathogens, particularly *Legionella sp.*, are primarily intracellular pathogens. Antibiotics that can be effective in vitro but have limited intracellular penetration (β-lactams, aminoglycosides) have been shown to be ineffective clinically, while agents with limited activity in vitro but that are intracellularly concentrated (macrolides, fluoroquinolones) can be highly effective clinically.

The ability of most antibiotics to kill bacteria is dependent on either a concentration- or time-dependent effect. For example, the efficacy of aminoglycoside and fluoroquinolone antimicrobial effects is dependent on their peak concentrations or the area under the curve. For drugs such as penicillins, the time that the drug concentration is above the minimum inhibitory concentration (MIC) for the bacteria determines the effectiveness of killing. Again, when defining appropriate therapy, these factors must be taken into account as a drug that is dependent on concentration-based killing that does not reach high peak levels will be ineffective. Similarly, a drug that relies on time-dependent killing and does not have an optimal time above MIC will have sub-maximal clinical activity even if in vitro sensitivity is demonstrated (e.g., cefotaxime for serious *S. aureus* infections). Close consultation with the microbiology laboratory, the infectious disease service, and pharmacy is the only way to ensure the adequate dosing and delivery of antibiotics to critically ill patients (Byl et al. 1999; Raineri et al. 2008).

The majority of studies on antimicrobial therapy have demonstrated that the time to institution of effective antimicrobial therapy is an independent determinant of a good outcome in patients. In those who are critically ill the delayed administration of antibiotics has been shown to increase mortality (Kumar et al. 2006). This mortality effect does not seem to be present when the patient population has a low baseline mortality (Cheng and Buising 2009). When analyzing the literature on appropriate therapy, very few studies mention the time to institution of appropriate therapy. Future studies in this area must also take this into account when describing appropriate versus inappropriate therapy. Delays in therapy of even 1–2 h can cause an increase in mortality that abrogates the benefit of appropriate therapy against the organism.

The assessment of appropriateness of antimicrobial therapy and the results of studies addressing this issue must also specifically take into account the baseline risk of death of patients. Patients with a low risk of death might not see the same benefit of early appropriate therapy as those who are more acutely ill. Patients who are less ill might also derive a benefit, but the sample sizes would have to be significantly larger to detect a difference. On the other hand, those patients at exceptionally high mortality risk due to underlying comorbidities or due to the severity of the infectious process (or due to very late antimicrobial initiation) may not be salvageable despite optimal antimicrobial therapy (Fig. 14.2). In a recent analysis of combination antimicrobial therapy in severe infections, we have shown that the benefit of combination therapy is restricted to high-risk patients, particularly those with septic shock (Kumar et al. 2010). It is likely that the adverse impact of inappropriate therapy is similarly restricted.

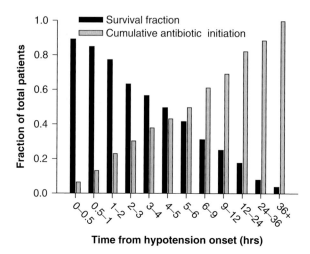

Fig. 14.2 Cumulative effective antimicrobial initiation following onset of septic shock-associated hypotension and associated survival. *X axis* represents time (hours) following first documentation of septic shock-associated hypotension. *Orange bars* represent the fraction of patients surviving to hospital discharge and the *white bars* represent the cumulative fraction of patients having received effective antimicrobials at any given time point (Adapted from Kumar et al. (2006))

14.10 Conclusion

Numerous factors are responsible for the relative efficacy of early and appropriate antimicrobial therapy. The definition of appropriate, pharmacokinetic, and pharmacodynamic issues, time course of administration, and the effect of baseline mortality all factor into the end result of the utility of this therapy. From a practical standpoint, the clinician who is presented with a patient with a life-threatening infection must make a rapid decision as to the source and potential microbial etiology of the infection. Then, the rapid administration of appropriate antimicrobials must be viewed as an equally important task as restoring hemodynamics. The logistical hurdles in this are not insignificant and realistically are only surmounted when a systems-based approach is taken. This involves developing an antibiogram based on past institutional culture results, the development of a protocol (in consultation with infectious disease experts) for treatment of these infections, and ensuring that pharmacy, transport, and nursing services are adequate to dispense, deliver, and administer the drugs to patients, with a similar minimum "door to needle" time as is done with thrombolytic therapy for acute myocardial infarction.

References

Alvarez-Lerma F, ICU-acquired Pneumonia Study Group (1996) Modification of empiric antibiotic treatment in patients with pneumonia acquired in the intensive care unit. Intensive Care Med 22:387–394

Ammerlaan H, Seifert H et al (2009) Adequacy of antimicrobial treatment and outcome of *Staphylococcus aureus* bacteremia in 9 Western European countries. Clin Infect Dis 49: 997–1005

Bantar C, Alcazar G et al (2007) Are laboratory based antibiograms reliable to guide the selection of empirical antimicrobial treatment in patients with hospital acquired infections? J Antimicrob Chemother 59:140–143

Bare M, Castells X et al (2006) Importance of appropriateness of empiric antibiotic therapy on clinical outcomes in intraabdominal infections. Int J Technol Assess Health Care 22:242–248

Byl B, Clevenbergh P et al (1999) Impact of infectious diseases specialists and microbiological data on the appropriateness of antimicrobial therapy for bacteremia. Clin Infect Dis 29:60–66

Chastre J, Fagon JY (2002) Ventilatory-associated pneumonia. Am J Respir Crit Care Med 265:867–903

Cheng AC, Buising KL (2009) Delayed administration of antibiotics and mortality in patients with community acquired pneumonia. Ann Emerg Med 53(5):618–624

Depuydt PO, Vandijck DM et al (2008) Determinants and impact of multidrug antibiotic resistance in pathogens causing ventilator-associated-pneumonia. Crit Care Med 12(6)

Falagas ME, Barefoot L et al (1996) Risk factors leading to clinical failure in the treatment of intra-abdominal or skin/soft tissue infections. Eur J Clin Microbiol Infect Dis 15(12):913–921

Fowler VG, Sanders LL et al (1998) Outcome of staphylococcus aureus bacteremia according to compliance with recommendations of infectious diseases specialists: experience with 244 patients. Clin Infect Dis 27:478–486

Franson TR, Quebbeman EJ et al (1988) Prospective comparison of traditional and pharmacokinetic aminoglycoside dosing methods. Crit Care Med 16(9):840–843

Gacouin A, Le Tulzo Y et al (2002) Severe pneumonia due to Legionella pneumophila: prognostic factors, impact of delayed appropriate antimicrobial therapy. Intensive Care Med 28(6):686–691

Gaieski DF, Mikkelsen ME et al (2010) Impact of time to antibiotics on survival in patients with severe sepsis or septic shock in whom early goal-directed therapy was initiated in the emergency department. Crit Care Med 38(4):1045–1053

Garey KW, Rege M et al (2006) Time to initiation of fluconazole therapy impacts mortality in patients with candidemia: a multi-institutional study. Clin Infect Dis 43:25–31

Garnacho-Montero J, Garcia-Garmendia JL et al (2003) Impact of adequate empirical antibiotic therapy on the outcome of patients admitted to the intensive care unit with sepsis. Crit Care Med 31(12):2742–2751

Harbarth S, Garbino J et al (2003) Inappropriate initial antimicrobial therapy and its effect on survival in a clinical trial of immunomodulating therapy for severe sepsis. Am J Med 115:529–535

Hindler JF, Stelling J (2007) Analysis and presentation of cumulative antibiograms: a new consensus guideline from the Clinical and Laboratory Standards Institute. Clin Infect Dis 44(6): 867–873

Houck PM, Bratzler DW et al (2004) Timing of antibiotic administration and outcomes for medicare patients hospitalized with community-acquired pneumonia. Arch Intern Med 164: 637–644

Hyle EP, Lipworth AD, Zaoutis TE, Nachamkin I, Bilker WB, Lautenbach E. Impact of inadequate initial antimicrobial therapy on mortality in infections due to extended-spectrum beta-lactamase-producing enterobacteriaceae: variability by site of infection. Arch Intern Med. 2005 Jun 27;165(12):1375–80

Ibrahim EH, Sherman G et al (2000) The influence of inadequate antimicrobial treatment of bloodstream infections on patient outcomes in the ICU setting. Chest 118(1):146–155

Kaufman D, Haas CE et al (1998) Antibiotic Susceptibility in the surgical Intensive care unit compared with the hospital wide antibiogram. Arch Surg 133:1041–1045

Kim SH, Park WB et al (2009) You only find what you look for: the importance of high creatinine clearance in the critically ill. Anaesth Intensive Care 37(1):11–13

Kollef MH (2000) Inadequate antimicrobial treatment: an important determinant of outcome for hospitalized patients. Clin Infect Dis 31(Suppl 4):S131–S138

Kollef MH, Sherman G et al (1999) Inadequate antimicrobial treatment of infections: a risk factor for hospital mortality among critically ill patients. Chest 115(2):462–474

Kreger BE, Craven DE et al (1980) Gram negative bacteremia IV. Reevaluation of clinical features and treatment in 612 patients. Am J Med 68:344–355

Krobot K, Yin D et al (2004) Effect of inappropriate initial empiric antibiotic therapy on outcome of patients with community-acquired intrabdominal infections requiring surgery. Eur J Clin Microbiol Infect Dis 23:682–687

Kumar A, Roberts D et al (2006) Duration of hypotension before initiation of effective antimicrobial therapy is the critical determinant of survival in human septic shock. Crit Care Med 34: 1589–1596

Kumar A, Ellis P et al (2009) Initiation of inappropriate antimicrobial therapy results in a fivefold reduction of survival in human septic shock. Chest 136:1237–1248

Kumar A, Safdar N et al (2010) The survival benefit of combination antibiotic therapy for serious infections associated with sepsis and septic shock is contingent on the risk of death: a meta-analytic/meta-regression study. Crit Care Med 38(8):1651–1664

Leibovici L, Paul M et al (1997) Monotherapy versus beta-lactam aminoglycoside combination treatment for gram negative bacteremia: a prospective, observational study. Antimicrob Agents Chemother 41:1127–1133; (erratum appears in AAC 1997 Nov;41(11):2595)

Leibovici L, Shraga I et al (1998) The benefit of appropriate empirical antibiotic treatment in patients with bloodstream infection. J Intern Med 244:379–386

Leroy O, Saux P et al (2005) Comparison of levofloxacin and cefotaxime combined with ofloxacin for ICU patients with community-acquired pneumonia: a retrospective study and meta-analysis. Chest 128:172–183

Lodise TP, Patel N et al (2007) Predictors of 30-day mortality among patients with pseudomonas aeruginosa bloodstream infections: impact of delayed appropriate antibiotic selection. Antimicrob Agents Chemother 51(10):3510–3515

Mandell LA, Wunderink RG et al (2007) Infectious Disease Society of America/American Thoracic Society guidelines on management of community acquired pneumonia in adults. Clin Infect Dis 44:S27–S72

Mccabe WR, Jackson GG (1962) Gram negative bacteremia II. Clinical, laboratory, and therapeutic observations. Arch Intern Med 110:856–864

McGregor JC, Rich SE et al (2007) A systematic review of the methods used to assess the association between appropriate antibiotic therapy and mortality in bacteremic patients. Clin Infect Dis 45:329–337

Meehan TP, Fine MJ et al (1997) Quality of care, process, and outcomes in elderly patients with pneumonia. JAMA 278(23):2080–2084

Micek ST, Kollef KE et al (2007) Health care-associated pneumonia and community -acquired pneumonia: a single center experience. Antimicrob Agents Chemother 51(10):3568–3573

Micek ST, Welch EC et al (2010) Empiric combination antibiotic therapy is associated with improved outcome against sepsis due to Gram-negative bacteria: a retrospective analysis. Antimicrob Agents Chemother 54(5):1742–1748

Moellering RC (2009) What is inadequate antibacterial therapy. Clin Infect Dis 49:1006–1008

Moise PA, Forrest A et al (2004) Pharmacodynamics of vancomycin and other antimicrobials in patients with *Staphylococcus aureus* lower respiratory tract infections. Clin Pharmacokinet 43:925–942

Morrell M, Fraser VJ et al (2005) Delaying the empiric treatment of Candida bloodstream infection until positive blood culture results are obtained: a potential risk factor for hospital mortality. Antimicrob Agents Chemother 49:3640–3645

Niederman MS, Craven DE et al (2005) Guidelines for the management of adults with hospital acquired, ventilator-associated, and healthcare-associated pneumonia. Am J Respir Crit Care Med 171:388–416

Parkins MD, Sabuda DM et al (2007) Adequacy of empiric antifungal therapy and effect on outcome among patients with invasive Candida species infections. J Antimicrob Chemother 60:613–618

Patel GP, Simon D et al (2009) The effect of time to antifungal therapy on mortality in Candidemia associated septic shock. Am J Ther 16(6):508–511

Peralta G, Sanchez MB, Garrido JC, De Benito I, Cano ME, Martinez-Martinez L, Roiz MP. Impact of antibiotic resistance and of adequate empirical antibiotic treatment in the prognosis of patients with Escherichia coli bacteraemia. J Antimicrob Chemother. 2007 Oct;60(4):855–63

Raineri E, Pan A et al (2008) Role of the infectious diseases specialist consultant on the appropriateness of antimicrobial therapy prescription in an intensive care unit. Am J Infect Control 36:283–290

Rello J, Ollendorf DA et al (2002) Epidemiology and outcomes of ventilator-associated pneumonia in a large US database. Chest 122:2121

Rivers E, Nguyen B et al (2001) Early goal-directed therapy in the treatment of severe sepsis and septic shock. N Engl J Med 345(19):1368–1377

Roberts JA, Lipman J (2006) Antibacterial dosing in intensive care: pharmacokinetics, degree of disease and pharmacodynamics of sepsis. Clin Pharmacokinet 45(8):755–773

Rotstein C, Evans G et al (2008) AMMI Canada guidelines-clinical practice guidelines for hospital acquired pneumonia and ventilator-associated pneumonia in adults. Can J Infect Dis Med Microbiol 19:19–53

Sitges-Serra A, Lopez MJ et al (2002) Postoperative enterococcal infection after treatment of complicated intra-abdominal sepsis. Br J Surg 89:361–367

Sturkenboom MCJM, Goettsch WG et al (2005) Inappropriate initial treatment of secondary intraabdominal infections leads to increased risk of clinical failure and costs. Br J Clin Pharmacol 60:438–443

Tellado JM, Sen SS et al (2007a) Consequences of inappropriate initial empiric parenteral antibiotic therapy among patients with community acquired intraabdominal infections in Spain. Scand J Infect Dis 39:947–955

Tellado JM, Sen SS et al (2007b) Consequences of inappropriate initial empiric parenteral antibiotic therapy among patients with community-acquired intra-abdominal infections in Spain. Scand J Infect Dis 39(11–12):947–955

Tumbarello M, Sali M, Trecarichi EM, Leone F, Rossi M, Fiori B, De Pascale G, D'Inzeo T, Sanguinetti M, Fadda G, Cauda R, Spanu T. Bloodstream infections caused by extended-spectrum-beta-lactamase- producing Escherichia coli: risk factors for inadequate initial antimicrobial therapy. Antimicrob Agents Chemother. 2008 Sep;52(9):3244–52

Udy A, Roberts JA et al (2009) You only find what you look for: the importance of high creatinine clearance in the critically ill. Anaesth Intensive Care 37(1):11–13

Valles J, Rello J et al (2003) Community-acquired bloodstream infection in critically ill adult patients: impact of shock and inappropriate antibiotic therapy on survival. Chest 123(5):1615–1624

Whipple JK, Ausman RK et al (1991) Effect of individualized pharmacokinetic dosing on patient outcome. Crit Care Med 19(12):1480–1485

Index

J. Rello (eds.), *Sepsis Management*,
DOI 10.1007/978-3-642-03519-7, © Springer-Verlag Berlin Heidelberg 2012

Printing: Ten Brink, Meppel, The Netherlands
Binding: Stürtz, Würzburg, Germany